The Vascular Surgery In-Training Examination Review (VSITE)

Allen Murga
Theodore H. Teruya
Ahmed M. Abou-Zamzam Jr
Christian Bianchi
Editors

The Vascular Surgery In-Training Examination Review (VSITE)

Springer

Editors

Allen Murga
Department of Vascular Surgery
Loma Linda University
Loma Linda, CA, USA

Ahmed M. Abou-Zamzam Jr
Chief of Vascular Surgery of
Loma Linda
Loma Linda University
Loma Linda, CA, USA

Theodore H. Teruya
Department of Surgery
Loma Linda University
Loma Linda, CA, USA

Christian Bianchi
Department of Vascular Surgery
Loma Linda University
Loma Linda, CA, USA

ISBN 978-3-031-24120-8 ISBN 978-3-031-24121-5 (eBook)
https://doi.org/10.1007/978-3-031-24121-5

This Springer imprint is published by the registered company Springer Nature Switzerland AG
The registered company address is: Gewerbestrasse 11, 6330 Cham, Switzerland

Dedicated to my wonderful wife who has supported me through this journey, as well as my kids and my mom for their enduring support.

Preface

The Vascular Surgery In-Training Exam (VSITE) is taken every year by integrated vascular surgery residents and vascular surgery fellows. Much of the stress associated with this exam stems from the enormous amount of material that needs to be covered. As well, as the importance that it plays in their careers.

As the ABSITE for general surgery, the VSITE aims to evaluate the trainee's knowledge in different areas within vascular surgery. In addition, training programs use this test as a tool of measurement for how well the residents and fellows are progressing and provide feedback and promotion through the program.

The field of vascular surgery has evolved over the last couple of years and continues to rapidly change to date. Because of this, study guides are needed to help with keeping things concise and high yield for trainees to prepare for this rigorous exam.

The VSITE review book is a high-yield bullet point format that allows trainees to navigate through all the different subjects within vascular surgery. This book by no means is intended to substitute as the sole material for studying vascular surgery.

My goal is that this book will serve as a guide for students, residents, fellow and vascular surgeons as they navigate and prepare for the VSITE, written and oral boards.

Loma Linda, CA — Allen Murga
Loma Linda, CA — Theodore H. Teruya
Loma Linda, CA — Ahmed M. Abou-Zamzam Jr
Loma Linda, CA — Christian Bianchi

Contents

Contributors

Ahmed M. Abou-Zamzam Jr Division of Vascular Surgery, Loma Linda University Health, Loma Linda, CA, USA

Olamide Alabi Department of Surgery, Emory University School of Medicine, Atlanta, GA, USA

Cassra N. Arbabi Department of Vascular Surgery, Cedars-Sinai Medical Center, Beverly Hills, CA, USA

Christian Bianchi Vascular Surgery of Loma Linda, Loma Linda University, Loma Linda, CA, USA

Department of Vascular Surgery, Loma Linda University Medical Center, Loma Linda Veteran Affairs Medical Center, Riverside University Health System, Loma Linda, CA, USA

Vascular Surgery, Loma Linda University, Loma Linda, CA, USA

Hans Keenan Boggs Department of Surgery, Loma Linda University Medical Center, Loma Linda, CA, USA

Kristine Bonnick Department of Surgery, Loma Linda University, Loma Linda, CA, USA

Shayna Brathwaite Department of Vascular Surgery, Emory University, Atlanta, GA, USA

Megan Brenner University of California Riverside School of Medicine, Moreno Valley, CA, USA

B. S. Chloe Dominguez Division of Vascular Surgery, Loma Linda University Health, Loma Linda, CA, USA

Carlos Chavez de Paz Department of Surgery, Cary Medical Center, Caribou, ME, USA

Emaad Farooqui University of Southern California/Keck School of Medicine, Los Angeles, CA, USA

Joshua A. Gabel Department of Surgery, Loma Linda University, Loma Linda, CA, USA

Nephtali R. Gomez Department of General Surgery, Endocrine Surgery and Surgical Oncology, Loma Linda University, Loma Linda, CA, USA

Cameron Hand Department of Family Medicine, Pomona Valley Hospital Medical Center, Pomona, CA, USA

Sukgu M. Han University of Southern California/Keck School of Medicine, Los Angeles, CA, USA

Division of Vascular Surgery and Endovascular Therapy, Comprehensive Aortic Center at Keck Hospital of University of Southern California, Los Angeles, CA, USA

Sandeep Jhajj Department of Surgery, Loma Linda University, Loma Linda, CA, USA

Rahul Kar Department of Vascular Surgery, Loma Linda University, Loma Linda, CA, USA

Christopher B. Khoury Department of Surgery, Loma Linda University, Loma Linda, CA, USA

Sharon Kiang Department of Vascular Surgery, Loma Linda University Medical Center, Loma Linda, CA, USA

Division of Vascular Surgery, Institutional Review Board (IRB) Committee, Vascular Non-Invasive Laboratory, Va Loma Linda Healthcare System, Loma Linda, CA, USA

Department of Surgery, Division of Vascular Surgery, Center of Excellence for Surgical Research, Loma Linda Surgery, Loma Linda University|School of Medicine, Loma Linda, CA, USA

Paul Pyoungkang Kim Department of General Surgery, Loma Linda University School of Medicine, Loma Linda University Medical Center, Loma Linda, CA, USA

Stephanie Hyejin Kim Department of General Surgery, Loma Linda University School of Medicine, Loma Linda University Medical Center, Loma Linda, CA, USA

Lucyna Krzywon Department of Surgery, Loma Linda University, Loma Linda, CA, USA

Isabella J. Kuo Surgery, University of California, Irvine, Orange, CA, USA

University of California Irvine, Orange, CA, USA

Beatriz Valdovinos Leong Department of Surgery, Loma Linda University, Loma Linda, CA, USA

University of California Irvine, Orange, CA, USA

Shelley Maithel Surgery, University of California, Irvine, Orange, CA, USA

Kristyn Mannoia Department of Surgery, Loma Linda University, Loma Linda, CA, USA

Miguel Francisco Manzur Vascular Surgery, LAC+USC/Keck Medical Center of USC, Los Angeles, CA, USA

Brittany Mead Division of Vascular Surgery, Department of Surgery, Cook County Health, Chicago, IL, USA

Rush University Medical Center, Chicago, IL, USA

Tyler Miskin Vascular and Interventional Radiology, Department of Radiology, Loma Linda University Medical Center, Loma Linda, CA, USA

Allen Murga Department of Vascular Surgery, Loma Linda University, Loma Linda, CA, USA

Thomas F. O'Donnell Jr. Tufts University School of Medicine, The Cardiovascular Center at Tufts Medical Center, Boston, MA, USA

Christian Ochoa Vascular Surgery, Keck Medical Center of USC, Los Angeles, CA, USA

Seyed Saeed Pairawan Division of Vascular Surgery, Loma Linda University Health, Loma Linda, CA, USA

Sheela T. Patel Department of Surgery, Loma Linda University, Loma Linda, CA, USA

Alyssa Pyun Division of Vascular Surgery, Department of Surgery, University of Southern California, Los Angeles, CA, USA

Anna Romagnoli University of Maryland Shock Trauma Center, Baltimore, MD, USA

Alexander M. Schurman Department of Surgery, University of California-Riverside/Riverside University Health System, CA, USA

Neha Sheng Division of Vascular Surgery, Department of Surgery, Cook County Health, Chicago, IL, USA

Agustin Sibona General Surgery, Loma Linda University Health, Loma Linda, CA, USA

Andrew Son Department of Surgery, Division of Vascular Surgery, Loma Linda University School of Medicine, Coleman Pavilion, Loma Linda, CA, USA

Morvarid Tavassoli Department of General Surgery, Riverside University Health System, Moreno Valley, CA, USA

Theodore H. Teruya Department of Surgery, Loma Linda University, Loma Linda, CA, USA

Roger Tomihama Vascular and Interventional Radiology, Department of Radiology, Loma Linda University Medical Center, Loma Linda, CA, USA

Shauna Trinh Department of General Surgery, Riverside University Health System, Moreno Valley, CA, USA

Kenneth R. Ziegler Division of Vascular Surgery, Department of Surgery, University of Southern California, Los Angeles, CA, USA

1 Embryology of the Vascular System

Kristyn Mannoia and Lucyna Krzywon

Embryology of the Vascular System

Timeline of embryologic development [1, 2].

- 4th week: development of the cardiovascular system
  - Dorsal aortas fuse to create thoracic and abdominal aorta.
  - Venous systems develop.
  - Day 22: First heartbeat.
  - Day 24: Heart starts circulating blood.
  - Day 26–30: Aortic arches 2–6 form from mesenchyme.
- 5–6th week: lymphatic system develops
- 8–9th week: liver, bone marrow, spleen, and thymus begin blood cell production.

Formation of blood vessels: early angiogenesis

- Splanchnic mesodermal cells differentiate into angioblasts, aggregate in the chorion, yolk sac, embryo, and splanchnic mesoderm.

K. Mannoia (✉) · L. Krzywon
Department of Surgery, Loma Linda University, Loma Linda, CA, USA
e-mail: Kmannoia@llu.edu; lkrzyqwon@llu.edu

A. Murga et al. (eds.), *The Vascular Surgery In-Training Examination Review (VSITE)*,
https://doi.org/10.1007/978-3-031-24121-5_1

- Vasculogenesis: Angioblasts flatten into endothelium to form vessel cords which combine to form vessels.

  Mediating factors:

- Vascular endothelial growth factor (VEGF):
  - Stabilizes and organizes capillary networks.
  - Promotes growth of additional blood vessels.
- Hypoxia:
  - Upregulates genes and increases angiogenesis in a localized region.
  - Mechanism by which exercise improves claudication symptoms in PAD.
- Hematopoietic stem cells:
  - Blood source for embryo until day 60, then liver, bone marrow, spleen, and thymus begin production.

  Aortic arch (Fig. 1.1) [1, 2].

- Normal arch development: present in only ~65% of the population.
  - The dorsal aortas fuse and become the thoracic/abdominal aorta at C7 vertebrae.
  - 1st, 2nd and 5th Aortic arches disappear and have no lasting adult structures
  - 3rd Aortic arches become the common carotid arteries and proximal internal carotid arteries
  - 4th Aortic arches are asymmetric

    Left 4th arch becomes incorporated into the adult aortic arch between the left common carotid artery and left subclavian artery.

    Right 4th arch becomes the proximal right subclavian artery.

    The right and left 7th intersegmental arteries become the right and left subclavian arteries.

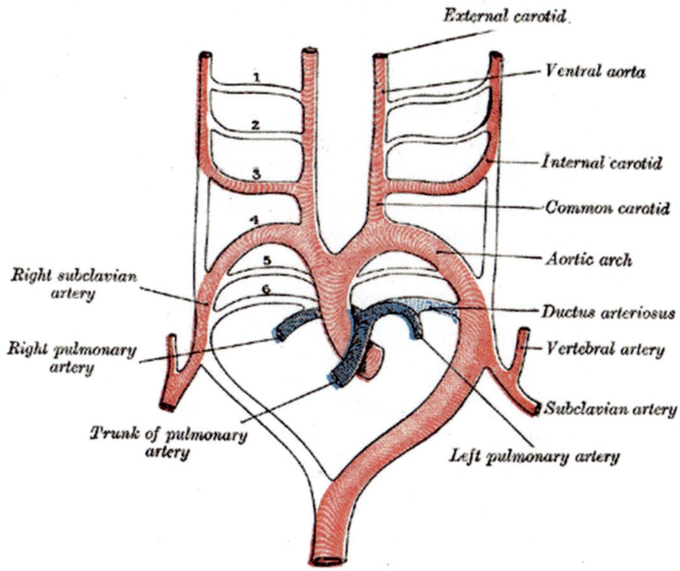

Fig. 1.1 Embryologic development of the aorta. Henry Vandyke Carter - Henry Gray (1918) Anatomy of the Human Body Bartleby.com: Gray's Anatomy, Plate 473, Public Domain, https://commons.wikimedia.org/w/index.php?curid=567240

- 6th Aortic arches become pulmonary arteries and ductus arteriosus from the distal left 6th aortic arch
  - The ductus arteriosus will become the ligamentum arteriosum.
- Abnormal aortic arch variants [1, 2].
  - Bovine arch (22%): left common carotid artery of brachiocephalic trunk.
    - Most common arch abnormality.
  - Patent ductus arteriosus (PDA):
    - Shunts blood from developing fetal lungs to systemic circulation.
    - Most common vascular abnormality.
    - Usually constricts at birth in response to high blood O_2 concentration, forms ligamentum arteriosum.

Pulmonary hypertension results if persistent PDA due to shunting between high pressure thoracic aorta and low pressure pulmonary arteries.

- Coarctation of the aorta:

  Most commonly occurs distal to ligamentum arteriosum.

  Pre-ductal if occurs proximal to ligamentum arteriosum (check with pulse ox on finger and toe).

  Unclear etiology, possibly same as closure of ductus arteriosus.

  Inferior notching on XR of ribs 3–8 due to collateralization via intercostals.

- Double aortic arch:

  Failure of the right dorsal aorta to involute.

  Results in vascular ring with right dorsal aortic arch posterior to esophagus and left aortic arch anterior to trachea.

  Symptoms from compression of both trachea and esophagus.

- Right aortic arch:

  Persistence of right with involution of the left dorsal aorta distal to the left 7th intersegmental artery.

  Ligamentum arteriosum comes from distal right 6th arch.

  Arch may pass right to left posterior to the trachea and esophagus forming a vascular ring with the ligamentum arteriosum anterior.

  May pass anterior to the trachea and esophagus, will have mirrored branching.

  - Increased rate of heart malformations with infantile cyanosis.
  - Tetralogy of Fallot.

- Replaced right subclavian artery:

  Abnormal involution of the right 4th aortic arch, with right subclavian origin distal to the left subclavian artery, usually courses retroesophageal.

  5% of patients have compression of the esophagus: dysphagia Lusoria

Kommerell diverticulum: aneurysm of the abnormal artery. Can compress other structures, rupture, or be the source of emboli.

Descending aorta (thoracic and abdominal) [2, 3].

- Dorsal aortas fuse at 4th week to create the thoracic and abdominal aorta.
- Thoracic:
  - Dorsal branches off aorta form intercostal arteries.
  - Ventral branches form superior thoracic, internal thoracic, and superior epigastric arteries.
- Abdominal:
  - Dorsal branches form common iliac arteries,
  - Ventral branches form allantoic and vitelline vessels.

    Allantoic vessels become umbilical arteries, later internal iliacs.

    Vitelline vessels form celiac, superior and inferior mesenteric arteries.
- Lateral segmental arteries: supply primitive urogenital ridge that forms gonads and kidneys.
  - With horseshoe or ectopic kidney, look for additional anomalous arterial supply.
  - Separate lateral segmental branches form adrenal and gonadal arteries.

Limb development [4].

- Limb buds come from the embryonic trunk.
  - Blood vessels come from segmental aortic branches and cardinal veins.
- Upper Limb.
  - Normal development is primarily from the 7th cervical intersegmental artery which combines with the limb bud axillary artery.
  - Can have high takeoff of radial artery above antecubital fossa.

- Lower limb.
  - Common iliac arteries are formed by the fusion of umbilical arteries with 5th lumbar intersegmental arteries.
  - The external iliac arteries form from the 2nd branches of the 5th lumbar intersegmental arteries and create the iliofemoral arteries.
  - The sciatic artery joins the iliofemoral system at the popliteal fossa, usually regresses before birth.

    May persist if iliofemoral artery fails to develop.
    - Runs with sciatic nerve, through sciatic notch and is superficial in the gluteal region, therefore susceptible to trauma.
    - Persistent sciatic may become aneurysmal, cause compressive symptoms.
    - Absent femoral but present popliteal pulse.
  - Popliteal artery is formed by combining the deep popliteal artery from the sciatic system and the superficial popliteal artery from the iliofemoral system.

    Popliteal entrapment: abnormal relationship between popliteal vessels and muscles causes claudication, possible aneurysms.

Venous system *(*Fig. 1.2*)* [2, 3].

- At week 4 embryonic veins develop from enlarging capillary networks into 3 paired venous systems.
  - Vitelline veins drain the yolk sac and developing GI system.

    The right vitelline vein becomes the ductus venosus and IVC.

    Vitelline anastomoses remodel to form the splenic and inferior mesenteric veins.
  - Umbilical veins return oxygenated blood to the heart from the placenta.

    Right umbilical vein regresses.

    Left umbilical vein anastomoses with the ductus venosus to directly enter the IVC.

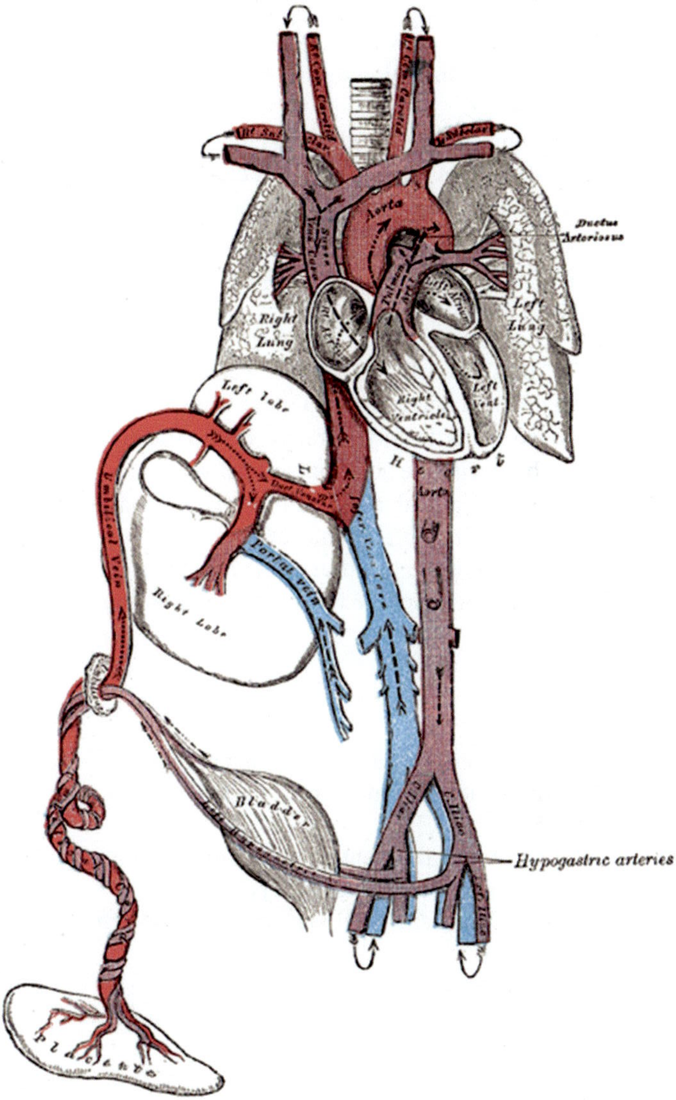

Fig. 1.2 Venous system variants. By Henry Vandyke Carter - Henry Gray (1918) Anatomy of the Human Body Bartleby.com: Gray's Anatomy, Plate 502, Public Domain, https://commons.wikimedia.org/w/index.php?curid=560282

At birth the left umbilical vein regresses to become the ligamentum teres within the falciform ligament and the ductus venosus regresses to become the ligamentum venosum.

  - Cardinal veins return blood to the embryo heart.

    Enlargement of the right anterior cardinal and right common cardinal veins forms the right atrium.

    Left common cardinal vein becomes the coronary sinus.

    Posterior cardinal veins contribute to the IVC and azygous systems.

- Superior vena cava [2, 4].
  - Cranial portions of the paired anterior cardinal veins become internal and external jugular veins.
  - Subclavian veins form separately in the upper limb buds and combine with the anterior cardinal veins.
  - The left and right anterior cardinal veins anastamose at week 7 to form the left brachiocephalic vein.
  - SVC forms from the junction of the left and right brachiocephalic veins to enter the heart at the right atrium.

SVC anomalies

- Double SVC.
  - Caudal left anterior cardinal vein fails to regress.
  - Brachiocephalic veins may or may not be present.
- Left-sided SVC.
  - Caudal section of the right anterior cardinal vein regresses and the left anterior cardinal vein persists.
  - Brachiocephalic vein will connect right and left anterior cardinal veins.
- Inferior vena cava [1, 2].
  - Formed from right vitelline vein in the liver, posterior cardinal veins, subcardinal veins.

    Posterior cardinal veins become the distal IVC, common iliac veins, and azygous vein.

    Right subcardinal vein enlarges to become the renal portion of the IVC; branches become the right renal and gonadal veins.

    - Left subcardinal vein becomes the left renal vein and left gonadal vein.
  - Supracardinal veins develop last and become the primary vessels to drain the body wall.
    - Right thoracic supracardinal vein and posterior cardinal vein become azygous vein.
    - Left thoracic supracardinal vein becomes hemiazygos vein.
- IVC Anomalies [1, 5].
  - IVC duplication from failure of the left supracardinal vein to regress with persistence of right supracardinal vein.
  - Left-sided IVC from failure of the left supracardinal vein to regress and regression of the right supracardinal vein.
    - Right adrenal and gonadal veins empty into the right renal vein instead of the IVC.
    - Left adrenal and gonadal veins empty directly into the IVC.
- Renal vein anomalies.
  - Retro-aortic left renal vein if posterior left subcardinal vein fails to regress.
  - Left circumaortic renal veins if both anterior and posterior renal veins persist.

Lymphatic system [1, 2].

- Believed to develop as buds from venous system.
- Week 5–6, 6 lymph sacs develop in a cranial to caudad sequence.
  - Cisterna chyli is last and located by the 3rd and 4th lumbar levels.
    - Meet extensions from the jugular lymph to form the thoracic lymph vessels that drain bilaterally into the internal jugular and subclavian junction.
    - Both tracts eventually fuse and become right-to-left directed.
  - Lymphatic vessels are not found in the CNS, meninges, eyes, internal ear canals, epidermis, or spleen.

Questions

1. A 64-year-old male presents with several months of calf cramping with exercise more than 50 ft. After thorough history and physical, you determine he suffers from claudication and advise a supervised exercise regimen. You explain this is the best way to build collaterals and improve his symptoms. What is the primary stimulus for angiogenesis in this patient's calves?
   (a) Hematopoietic stem cells.
   (b) Hypoxia.
   (c) Angioblasts.
   (d) VEGF.
   (e) Calf muscle pump.
2. A 36-year-old female presents with dysphagia and is found to have a Kommerell diverticulum. Which structure failed to regress during embryologic development?
   (a) Left dorsal aorta.
   (b) 7th intersegmental artery
   (c) Ductus arteriosus.
   (d) Right 6th aortic arch.
   (e) Right 4th aortic arch.
3. A 58-year-old man presents to the ED with painful blue spots on his right toes. A thorough history and physical exam reveals palpable femoral artery on the left, non-palpable on the right and bilateral popliteal, dorsalis pedis and posterior tibial pulses are palpable. What is the most likely diagnosis?
   (a) Aneurysmal persistent sciatic artery with emboli to the toes.
   (b) Abdominal aortic aneurysm with emboli to the toes.
   (c) Peripheral arterial disease in the right femoropopliteal segment.
   (d) Atrial fibrillation.
   (e) Paradoxical emboli from DVT.

Answer: 1. (b) 2. (e) 3. (a).

References

1. Davies M, Guest PJ. Developmental abnormalities of the great vessels of the thorax and their embryological basis. Br J Radiol. 2003;76(907):491–502. https://doi.org/10.1259/bjr/14043447.
2. Endean E. Embryology and developmental anatomy. In: Sidawy AN, Perler BA, editors. Rutherford's vascular surgery and endovascular therapy. Elsevier; 2019. p. 13–29.
3. Greenfield LJ, Mulholland MW. Vascular disease. In: Greenfield LJ, Mulholland MW, editors. Surgery: scientific principles and practice. Lippincott Williams & Wilkins; 2001.
4. Rodriguez-Niedenfuhr M, et al. Development of the arterial pattern in the upper limb of staged human embryos: normal development and anatomic variations. J Anat. 2001;199(4):407–17. https://doi.org/10.1046/j.1469-7580.2001.19940407.x.
5. Giordano JM, Trout HH. Anomalies of the inferior vena cava. J Vasc Surg. 1986;3(6):924–8. https://doi.org/10.1016/0741-5214(86)90162-x.

2 Hematology and Coagulation

Kristyn Mannoia and Lucyna Krzywon

Hematology and Coagulation

General:

- Banked blood is low in 2,3 DPG which increases Hgb affinity for O_2.
- Vitamin K required for factors II, VII, IX, X and protein C and S synthesis in liver.
- Protein C breaks down factors V and VIII. Protein S is cofactor.
- Factor VIII is the only factor not made in liver (made by reticuloendothelial system).
- PT is best test for liver synthetic function.
- Aspirin irreversibly binds to cyclooxygenase, lasts life of the platelet is approximately 7 days.
- Clopidogrel irreversibly inhibits ADP receptor, inhibits platelet aggregation.

K. Mannoia (✉) · L. Krzywon
Department of Surgery, Loma Linda University, Loma Linda, CA, USA
e-mail: Kmannoia@llu.edu; lkrzyqwon@llu.edu

A. Murga et al. (eds.), *The Vascular Surgery In-Training Examination Review (VSITE)*,
https://doi.org/10.1007/978-3-031-24121-5_2

Platelets [1]:

- Form initial hemostatic plug after vascular injury.
- 2 platelet activation routes release platelet granules
  - No direct tissue damage — > Extrinsic pathway with tissue factor (TF) activation via factor VII.
  - Direct tissue damage — > Intrinsic pathway with exposed subendothelial collagen binding vWF, which directly binds GpIb receptor on platelet.
- Aggregation mediated by receptors.
  - B1: mediates platelet interaction with cells, collagen, fibronectin, laminin.
  - B2: LeuCAM on leukocytes and other inflammatory cells.
  - B3: cytoadhesion via GpIIb/IIIa binding fibrinogen, von Willebrand factor (vWF), fibronectin/vitronectin, and thrombospondin.
  - GpIIb/IIIa sites become accessible once platelets are activated.
- Platelet plug formation allows coagulation protein assembly.
  - Leukocyte adhesion to platelets recruits tissue factor.
  - Tissue factor activates extrinsic pathway.

Extrinsic pathway (Fig. 2.1):

- Factors: VII.
- TF complexes with factor VIIa — > activates factors IX, X into IXa and Xa.
- Factor Xa and Va activate factor II (prothrombin) into factor IIa (thrombin).
- Thrombin creation enhanced via prothrombin complex = Xa, Va, Ca2+, IIa.
- Thrombin cleaves factor XIII into XIIIa, and fibrinogen into fibrin to create cross-linked fibrin plug as well as further activate platelets and factors V, VIII.

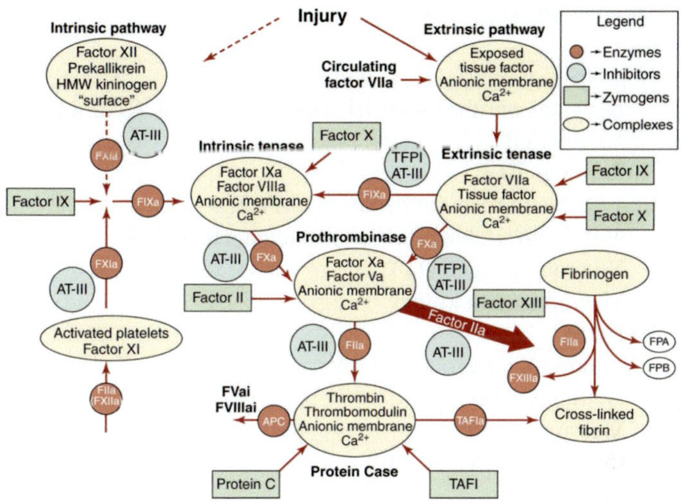

Fig. 2.1 Overview of hemostasis. (Reproduced with permission from Sidawy, Anton N., and Bruce A. Perler. 2019. Rutherford's vascular surgery and endovascular therapy)

Intrinsic pathway (Fig. 2.1):

- Factors: XII, XII, IX, VIII.
- Activation of XI into XIa via activation of factor XII, prekallikrein, HMWK, and thrombin.
- Factor XIa activates factor XIa and IXa,
- Factor VIIIa dissociates from vWF to form Xase complex with factor IXa, X, Ca2+ to create activated factor Xa for further thrombin amplification.

Common pathway:

- Factors: X, V, II, XIII.

Medications [1]:

- Heparin.
  - Activates antithrombin III which inactivates factors IX, X, XI, and XII.
  - Prolongs PTT.
- Low-molecular weight heparin (LMWH).
  - 90% bioavailable after sub-cutaneous injection
  - No monitoring of PTT.
  - Metabolized in kidney.
- Warfarin.
  - Vitamin K antagonist inhibits production of Vit K-dependent clotting factors.
  - Measure with PT.
  - Reverse with Vit K, FFP.
- Argatroban.
  - Direct thrombin inhibitor. When bridging to coumadin, has combined effect on INR so only stop argatroban when INR >5.
  - Metabolized in liver.
- Bivalirudin.
  - Direct thrombin inhibitor.
  - Metabolized in kidney.
- Tissue plasminogen activator.
  - Fibrinolytic enzyme produced in endothelial cells.
  - Secretion caused by epinephrine, thrombin, histamine, acetylcholine.
  - Primary agent used for lytic therapy.

    Bleeding is the most common risk. Intracranial, GI, retroperitoneal, and access site.

    Monitor fibrinogen during lysis therapy. Stop if <100 mg/dL. Cryoprecipitate if bleeding.

    Risk factors for bleeding: tumors, uncontrolled hypertension, stroke in last 3 months, recent trauma, spine operation, lysis longer than 48 h.
  - Antidote is e-aminocaproic acid.

Natural anticoagulant mechanisms [2].

- Goal is to restrict thrombin activity to localized area of vascular injury.
- Antithrombin III is the central anticoagulant molecule.
  - Glycoprotein, 70 kDa.
  - Binds thrombin to inhibit removal of FPA and FPB from fibrinogen.
  - Inhibits activation of factors V, VIII and platelet aggregation.
  - Directly inhibits factors IXa, Xa, XIa.
- Protein C inactivates factors Va, VIIIa, — > decreases Xase and prothrombinase complex activity.
  - Vitamin K-dependent.
  - Protein S is a cofactor of activated protein C, regulated by complement C4b-binding protein and decreased in SLE.
- Heparin cofactor II regulates thrombin activity in extravascular tissues.
- Tissue factor pathway inhibitor.
  - Binds TF-VIIa complex to inhibit activation of factor X and prothrombinase complex.

Fibrinolysis

- Clot lysis to prevent thrombus formation outside of area of injury.
- Plasmin: main fibrinolytic enzyme, to provide localized proteolysis.
  - Substrates include: fibrin, fibrinogen.
  - Activated by tissue plasminogen activator (tPA), urokinase, intrinsic factors (factor XII, prekallikrein, HMWK),
  - APC inactivates the tPA inhibitor.
- Fibrin digestion yields fragment E + 2 molecules of fragment D (D-dimer).
- Elevated d-dimer following DVT treatment predicts ongoing risk of VTE.

Hypercoagulable states.

- Heparin-associated thrombocytopenia (HIT) [1].
  - Occurs in up to 30% of patients who receive heparin.
  - Severe cases associated with thrombosis.
  - IgG antibody binds to heparin-platelet factor 4 complex resulting in platelet aggregation.
  - 3–14 days after initiating heparin therapy
  - Diagnose: 50% platelet decrease, platelet count decrease <100 k/mL.
  - Gold standard: ELISA for anti-heparin-PF4 complex, previously serotonin release assay. Excellent negative predictive value.
  - Treatment: stop all heparin administration, start direct thrombin inhibitors: argatroban (liver), fondaparinux, lepirudin, danaparoid, bivalirudin (kidney).
  - Start warfarin when thrombocytopenia has resolved otherwise venous gangrene due to rapid reduction in Vit K-dependent clotting factors.
- Antithrombin III deficiency [1].
  - Serine protease inhibitor of thrombin, kallikrein, VIIa, IXa, Xa, XIa, XIIa.
  - Autosomal dominant inheritance, 2% of the population, heterozygous inheritance has an increase in risk of VTE, AT levels 70% of normal.
  - Acquired by liver disease, malignancy, sepsis, DIC, malnutrition.
  - Type I: quantitative, type II: qualitative.
  - Treatment is administration of antithrombin III concentrate or fresh frozen plasma followed by anticoagulation with heparin or oral anticoagulation with direct thrombin inhibitors (argatroban, bivalirudin).
  - Lifelong anticoagulation after first VTE episode.
- Protein C and S deficiency (clinically identical) [1, 2].
  - Autosomal dominant inheritance for deficiencies (type 1: quantitative, type 2: qualitative).

  - Homozygous deficiency: purpura fulminans- > death in infancy due to unrestricted clotting and fibrinolysis.
  - Heterozygous deficiency: 60% of normal protein c levels.
  - Acquired deficiency due to liver failure, DIC, nephrotic syndrome.
  - Diagnose: plasma levels of protein C (antigen and antibody) and protein S antigen.
  - Treatment: anticoagulation initially with heparin, then life-long oral anticoagulation after the first thrombotic event.
  - Watch for transient hypercoagulable states when initiating oral anticoagulation due to the inhibition of vitamin K-dependent factors with short half-lives (VII, protein C) compared to factors II, IX, X with longer half-lives -> microcirculation thrombosis and warfarin-induced skin necrosis.
- Factor V Leiden mutation [1].
  - 20–60% of idiopathic VTE. Most common hereditary cause of VTE
  - Factor V that is resistant to APC inactivation due to point mutation (replacement of arginine with glutamine).
  - Homozygous mutation has increased relative risk, heterozygous mutation has increased relative risk of VTE.
  - Diagnose: clot-based functional assay and genetic analysis to differentiate between homo and heterozygous states.
  - Treatment: anticoagulation for homozygous, heterozygous same as general population.
  - After first VTE, increased risk of second event.
- Lupus anticoagulant/antiphospholipid syndrome [1, 2].
  - Caused by phospholipid antibodies against cardiolipin and lupus anticoagulant.
  - Prolonged PTT that does not correct with FFP.
  - Falsely + RPR test for syphilis.
  - Symptoms: thrombosis, pregnancy loss.
  - Treatment: Lifetime anticoagulation.
- Hyperhomocysteinemia [1, 2].
  - Increased risk of VTE.

  - Associated with MTHFR mutation.
  - Other causes: smoking, increased age, coffee consumption, low folate, B6, B12, DM, lupus, cancer, metformin, anticonvulsants, levodopa.
  - Treat with folate supplementation to decrease homocysteine levels to normal.
- Prothrombin G20210A [1, 2].
  - Prothrombin (factor II) is vitamin K-dependent.
  - Activated into thrombin.
  - Genetic polymorphism from guanine to adenine on 20,210 nucleotide of prothrombin gene causes elevated prothrombin levels.
  - 2nd most common cause of hypercoagulability in Caucasians
  - Treatment: recurrent VTE episodes or carriers of factor V Leiden and G20210A polymorphism, lifelong anticoagulation.
- Warfarin-induced thrombosis.
  - Formation of fibrin clots in microvasculature due to early inhibition of anticoagulants protein C and S with later inhibition of procoagulant clotting factors.
  - Petechiae and punctate areas of skin necrosis, most commonly breasts, buttocks, thighs, and penis.
  - Treatment: immediate cessation of warfarin. Give IV Vit K, FFP, and alternative anticoagulant once INR is subtherapeutic.
- Cigarette smoking.
  - Causes endothelial cell damage and altered function.
  - Increases platelet adhesion and permeability of endothelial surfaces to fibrinogen.
  - Decreases nitric oxide availability and impairs vascular tone.
- Pregnancy.
  - More likely to develop VTE 2/2 anatomic compression and hormone-related clotting factor induction.
  - Low-risk thrombophilia—observe: heterozygous FVL, prothrombin G20201A heterozygous, protein C or S deficiency.

  - High-risk thrombophilia—prophylactic LMWH throughout pregnancy and postpartum: FVL homozygous, antithrombin deficiency, prothrombin G20201A homozygous.

Abnormal platelet aggregation [1, 2].

- Possibly associated with diabetes mellitus as it is known to have hyperactive platelets and hyperlipidemia.
- Hyperactive platelets associated with graft thrombosis in peripheral arterial reconstructions.
- Not recommended to follow bleeding time.
- Both arterial and venous episodes.
- Consider platelet aggregation assays.
- Therapy: aspirin and clopidogrel can be considered.
- Can be due to heparin or H2 Inhibitors.
- Glanzmann's thrombocytopenia: GpIIb/IIIa receptor deficiency.
  - Platelets cannot bind to each other, usually linked by fibrin.
  - Give platelets.
- Bernard-Soulier-GpIb receptor deficiency.
  - Platelets cannot bind to collagen, usually linked by vWF.
  - Give platelets.
- Uremia (BUN>60–80).
  - Platelet function inhibited by decreased vWF release.
  - Tx: hemodialysis, DDAVP (rapid reversal), cryoprecipitate if moderate-to-severe bleeding.

Disseminated intravascular coagulation

- Acute thrombosis caused by sepsis, pancreatitis, trauma, obstetric complications, transplant rejection, malignancies, and liver failure.
- Tumor factor release into vasculature causing unregulated activation of the coagulation cascade, leading to massive thrombin and fibrin production which then causes consumption of clotting factors and depletion of fibrinogen.
- Fibrinolysis then occurs leading to hemorrhage.

- Diagnosis: clinical.
  - Labs: down-trending platelets, decreased fibrinogen, increased PT, Increased fibrin split products, + D-dimer.
- Treatment: support and reverse underlying condition.

Bleeding disorders [1, 2].

- Hemophilia A.
  - Factor VIII deficiency, X-linked recessive.
  - Most common symptom = hemarthrosis, other symptoms: joint bleeding, epistaxis, hematuria, intracerebral hemorrhage.
  - Prolonged PTT, normal PT.
  - Check PTT q8hrs post-op.
  - Need VIII levels at 100% pre-op and within 80–100% until POD 10–14.
  - Tx: recombinant factor VIII, cryoprecipitate.
- Hemophilia B,
  - Aka Christmas disease.
  - Factor IX deficiency, X-linked recessive.
  - Prolonged PTT, normal PT.
  - Tx: recombinant factor IX or FFP.
- von Willebrand disease.
  - Most common congenital bleeding disorder.
  - Most common symptom: epistaxis or bleeding after dental procedures.
  - 3 types:

    Type 1: most common, usually mild symptoms, reduced quantity of vWF, autosomal dominant.

    Type 2: defect in vWF molecule making it less effective (qualitative), autosomal dominant.

    Type 3: complete vWF deficiency.
  - Treat with recombinant factor VIII, vWF, cryoprecipitate.
  - DDAVP ineffective for type 3.

Questions

1. A 62-year-old female presents to the emergency room with acute onset of leg swelling. Her medical history includes CKD 4 and liver cirrhosis. She reports that she has a history of heparin-induced thrombocytopenia on a prior admission for DVT. What would be the anticoagulant of choice for this patient?
   (a) Heparin.
   (b) Argatroban.
   (c) Bivalirudin.
   (d) Fondaparinux.
   (e) Lovenox.
2. A 47-year-old female presents to the emergency room with petechiae over her breasts and thighs. She was recently started on warfarin for acute DVT. Her INR is 2.7. Which of the following is NOT a part of her initial treatment plan?
   (a) Stop warfarin.
   (b) Start heparin drip.
   (c) Administer IV Vit K.
   (d) Transfuse FFP.
   (e) Resect the areas of petechiae.
3. Mechanism of action of clopidogrel?
   (a) Inhibits H2 receptors.
   (b) Inactivates APC.
   (c) Inhibits activation of fibrinogen.
   (d) Inhibits ADP receptor.
   (e) Inactivates cyclooxygenase.

Answers: 1. (d), 2. (b), 3. (d).

References

1. Mulholland MW, Greenfields LJ. Surgery: scientific principles and practice. Lippincott, Williams & Wilkins; 2016.
2. Sidawy AN, Perler BA. Rutherford's vascular surgery and endovascular therapy. Elsevier; 2019.

3 Fluids, Electrolytes, and Nutrition

Paul Pyoungkang Kim, Stephanie Hyejin Kim, and Nephtali R. Gomez

Fluids

1. *Fluid Compartments* [1]
    (a) Total body weight (TBW) = is $\frac{2}{3}$ water: $\frac{2}{3}$ is intracellular, $\frac{1}{3}$ is extracellular ($\frac{2}{3}$ interstitial, $\frac{1}{3}$ plasma)
    (b) Proteins (primarily albumin) = osmotic pressure between the plasma and interstitial compartments
    (c) Sodium and glucose = osmotic pressure between intracellular and extracellular compartments
    (d) Disturbances in fluid balance include: change in volume, change in concentration, and/or change in composition

P. P. Kim · S. H. Kim
Department of General Surgery, Loma Linda University School of Medicine, Loma Linda University Medical Center, Loma Linda, CA, USA
e-mail: Pkim1@llu.edu; stkim2@llu.edu

N. R. Gomez (✉)
Department of General Surgery, Endocrine Surgery and Surgical Oncology, Loma Linda University, Loma Linda, CA, USA
e-mail: NRgomez@llu.edu

A. Murga et al. (eds.), *The Vascular Surgery In-Training Examination Review (VSITE)*,
https://doi.org/10.1007/978-3-031-24121-5_3

(e) In surgical patients, significant gains and losses of bodily fluids occur in the extracellular compartment (i.e. the "third space"), easily measured by weighing the patient

(f) Calculated serum osmolality $= 2[\mathrm{Na}] + \frac{[Glucose]}{18} + \frac{[BUN]}{2.8}$, Normal: 280–295 mOsm/kg

2. *Volume Disturbances*

(a) The most common cause of volume depletion in surgical patients is loss of *GI fluids* (Tables 3.1 and 3.2)

(b) *Volume Depletion* [2]

- Diagnosis: Basic metabolic panel (BMP) is typically sufficient (↓K, ↓Cl, $\uparrow HCO_3$)BUN/Cr ratio > 20, fractional excretion of Na (FENa) (urine Na/Cr)/(plasma Na/Cr) <1% = Pre-renal, urine osmolality >500 mOsm

Table 3.1 Common causes of volume disturbances

Volume depletion	Volume overload
• GI losses (nasogastric suctioning, emesis, diarrhea, fistulas) • Dehydration • Trauma • Burns • GI bleeding • Diuretic-use • Excessive sweating • Dialysis • Renal failure • Adrenal insufficiency • Osmotic diuresis due to diabetes mellitus • Central diabetes insipidus • SIADH • Third-space losses (e.g. intraperitoneal, retroperitoneal, intestinal lumen)	• Heart failure • Renal failure • Nephrotic syndrome • Cirrhosis • Pregnancy • Premenstrual edema

Data taken from: de Moya M, Stearns DA, Yeh D. c1996–2021. Chicago, IL. American College of Surgeons Blended Surgical Education and Training for Life: Fluids and Electrolytes and Brunicardi CF, Anderson DK, Billiar TR, Dunn DL, Kao LS, Hunter JG, Matthews JB, et al. *Schwartz's Principles of Surgery, 9th edition*. "Chapter 3: Fluid and Electrolyte Management of the Surgical Patient"

Table 3.2 Signs and symptoms of volume disturbances

	Volume depletion	Volume overload
General	Weight loss, lethargy, confusion, skin turgor	Weight gain, peripheral edema
Cardiovascular	Tachycardia, hypotension with narrowed pulse pressure, orthostasis, delayed capillary refill, collapsed neck veins	Systolic hypertension and systolic murmur due to increased cardiac output, distended neck veins
Respiratory	Tachypnea	Pulmonary edema
Gastrointestinal	Ileus, nausea, emesis	Intestinal edema
Oral	Dry mucous membranes	
Renal	Oliguria, thirst	
Musculoskeletal	Weakness	

Data taken from: de Moya M, Stearns DA, Yeh D. c1996–2021. Chicago, IL. American College of Surgeons Blended Surgical Education and Training for Life: Fluids and Electrolytes and Brunicardi CF, Anderson DK, Billiar TR, Dunn DL, Kao LS, Hunter JG, Matthews JB, et al. *Schwartz's Principles of Surgery, 9th edition*. "Chapter 3: Fluid and Electrolyte Management of the Surgical Patient"

- Treatment:
  - Intraoperatively and 24-h post-op: lactated ringer.
  - >24-h post-op: D5 0.45% normal saline with 20 mEq K+
  - Maintenance fluid can be calculated: 4 cc/kg/h for first 10 kg, 2 cc/kg/h for second 10 kg, 1 cc/kg/h for each kg after that.
  - Monitor urine output (UOP) for effective volume repletion therapy. Minimum expected UOP should be >0.5 mL/kg/h.

(c) *Volume Overload* [3]

- Diagnosis: Primarily clinical (peripheral edema, pulmonary edema, shortness of breath)
  - 24-h urinalysis for proteinuria may help distinguish between acute renal failure vs. non-renal causes

- Treatment:
  - Treat the underlying cause.
    May require diuretics, dialysis, paracentesis, dietary salt restriction, management of heart failure or renal disease
  - Monitor daily weights to track therapy progression.

Electrolytes and Acid Balance (Table 3.3)

1. *Sodium* (normal requirement: 1.5 mEq/kg/day) [4].
   (a) *Hyponatremia.*
   - Common causes:
     - High volume status: dilutional (most common), increased ADH secretion, pharmacologic (e.g. diuretics, ACE inhibitors, antipsychotics, tricyclic antidepressants).
     - Normal volume status: hyperglycemia, SIADH, diuretics.
     - Low volume status: decreased sodium intake, GI losses, primary renal disease, diuretics.
   - Treatment:
     - Asymptomatic: free water restriction.
     - Symptomatic or neurologic symptoms present: free water restriction, followed by diuresis and IV hypertonic saline.
     - Increase the serum sodium by 4–6 $\frac{\text{mEq}}{\text{L}}$ over a period of 4–24 h, but do not exceed 8 $\frac{\text{mEq}}{\text{L}}$ in a 24-h period; rapid correction can cause central pontine myelinolysis.

   (b) *Hypernatremia.*
   - Common causes:
     - High volume status: iatrogenic sodium intake, mineralocorticoid excess, Cushing's disease, congenital adrenal hyperplasia, hyperaldosteronism (rarely).

Table 3.3 Signs and symptoms of electrolyte abnormalities

Hyponatremia	Headache, confusion, increased intracranial pressure, seizures, coma, nausea, vomiting, watery diarrhea, weakness, muscle cramping, fatigue, hypertension, bradycardia, lacrimation, salivation, oliguria
Hypernatremia	Restlessness, ataxia, delirium, seizures, coma, weakness, hypotension, tachycardia, oliguria, dry and sticky mucous membranes, decreased secretions (saliva, tears)
Hypokalemia	Ileus, constipation, fatigue, diminished reflexes, weakness, paralysis, cardiac arrest
Hyperkalemia	Nausea, vomiting, colic, diarrhea, weakness, paralysis, cardiac arrhythmias, cardiac arrest
Hypocalcemia	Hyperactive reflexes, peripheral and perioral paresthesia, twitching with facial tapping (Chvostek's sign), cardiac arrhythmias, carpopedal spasm (Trousseau's sign), seizures
Hypercalcemia	Abdominal pain, nausea, vomiting, bone pain, weakness, confusion, hypertension, cardiac arrhythmias, polyuria, polydipsia
Hypomagnesemia	Hyperactive reflexes, tetany, cardiac arrhythmias
Hypermagnesemia	Diminished reflexes, weakness, lethargy, nausea, vomiting, respiratory depression, hypotension, cardiac arrest
Hypophosphatemia	Clinical symptoms usually absent; severe hypophosphatemia may include cardiac and muscle dysfunction
Hyperphosphatemia	Clinical symptoms are usually absent

Data taken from: de Moya M, Stearns DA, Yeh D. c1996–2021. Chicago, IL. American College of Surgeons Blended Surgical Education and Training for Life: Fluids and Electrolytes and Brunicardi CF, Anderson DK, Billiar TR, Dunn DL, Kao LS, Hunter JG, Matthews JB, et al. *Schwartz's Principles of Surgery, 9th edition*. "Chapter 3: Fluid and Electrolyte Management of the Surgical Patient"

- Normal volume status: water loss (e.g. skin, GI), diabetes insipidus, diuretics, renal disease.
- Low volume status: water loss (e.g. skin, GI), dehydration, diabetes insipidus, aquaretics, renal disease, adrenal failure.

- Treatment:
  - Replacement of water deficit with hypotonic fluid (e.g. D5W, 5% dextrose in 0.9% normal saline).
    $\text{Water deficit} = \text{TBW} \times \frac{\text{Serum Na} +}{140} - 1$, with TBW estimated to be 50% of lean body weight.
  - Acute hypernatremia: replace entire water deficit in a 24-h period; measure serum sodium every 1–2 h until it is 145 mEq.
  - Chronic hypernatremia: replace a portion of the water deficit in a 24-h period until serum sodium is lowered by 10 $\frac{\text{mEq}}{\text{L}}$.
  - Monitor rate of infusion, as rapid correction can cause *cerebral edema*

2. Potassium (normal requirement: 1 mEq/kg/day).
   (a) *Hypokalemia* [5].
   - Common causes:
     - Dietary deficiency, GI losses (diarrhea, fistulas, nasogastric suctioning, emesis), renal losses, potassium-deficient IV therapies, hyperaldosteronism, pharmacologic therapies (e.g. diuretics), increased potassium excretion, metabolic alkalosis, excess insulin
   - Treatment:
     - Correct hypomagnesemia if present, as low magnesium can inhibit potassium repletion
     - For every 10 mEq of potassium given you can expect an increase of 0.1 $\frac{\text{mEq}}{\text{L}}$ increase in serum potassium
     - Do not give potassium faster than 10 mEq/h intravenously
     - Example: for symptomatic or severe hypokalemia (<2.5 $\frac{\text{mEq}}{\text{L}}$): IV repletion with 60 mEq KCl in 1 L of 0.9% NaCl over 6 h.

    - Closely monitor with serial serum potassium measurements and continuous EKG monitoring; proceed with caution if oliguria or renal dysfunction is present

(b) *Hyperkalemia* [6].

- Common causes:
    - Increased potassium intake (e.g. dietary, supplements), renal insufficiency, adrenal insufficiency, potassium-sparing diuretics, acidosis, hyperglycemia, cellular injury (e.g. GI hemorrhage, crush injury, hemolysis)
- Treatment:
    - Discontinue potassium supplementations
    - If ECG changes (peaked T waves) present → Calcium chloride or calcium gluconate 1 g IV given over 2 h (caution with digitalis toxicity)
    - SQ injection 10 units of regular insulin with 50 mL D50W or in 500 mL of D10W over a period of 60 min (causes intracellular shift of potassium)
    - Beta-agonists (e.g. Albuterol: nebulization of 10–20 mg in 5 mL normal saline)
    - Sodium polystyrene sulfonate (Kayexalate): binds potassium in the colon in exchange for sodium

      Oral administration: 50 g in 30 mL of sorbitol solution.

      Rectal administration (faster onset of action than oral): 50 g in a retention enema.
    - Dialysis if refractory

3. *Calcium, Magnesium, Phosphate*.

(a) Hypocalcemia.

- Common causes:
    - Hypoparathyroidism, pancreatitis, necrotizing fasciitis, renal failure, GI fistulas, tumor lysis syndrome, toxic shock syndrome, thyroid/parathyroid surgery, malignancy, blood transfusions

- Treatment:
  - Address concurrent hypomagnesemia and/or hypokalemia if present
  - Asymptomatic: oral administration of 1–2 g of elemental calcium per day given as calcium gluconate or calcium carbonate
  - Symptomatic: 10 mL of IV 10% calcium gluconate over 10 min; administer repeat boluses or a continued infusion with 20–30 mL of 10% calcium gluconate in 1 L of D5W over a 12–24 h period as needed

(b) *Hypercalcemia* [7].

- Common causes:
  - Primary hyperparathyroidism, malignancy (e.g. breast cancer)
- Treatment:
  - IV volume repletion (1–2 L of 0.9% NaCl over 1 h to achieve a urine output of 200 $\frac{mL}{h}$), followed by diuresis (e.g. 10–20 mg IV furosemide) if needed
  - Lactated ringer and thiazide diuretics contraindicated

(c) *Hypomagnesemia*.

- Common causes:
  - Pharmacologic therapies (e.g. diuretics), inadequate intake (e.g. chronic TPN), alcohol dependence, increased renal excretion, GI losses (e.g. diarrhea, malabsorption, acute pancreatitis, ostomy or fistula output)
- Treatment:
  - Mild symptoms or asymptomatic: oral magnesium gluconate 500 mg 2–3 times/day
  - Symptomatic or severely deficient: IV repletion (e.g. 1–2 g magnesium sulfate diluted in 50–100 mL D5W over 5–60 min, followed by a continuous IV infusion of 0.5–1 $\frac{g}{h}$)

    - Address concurrent hypokalemia and/or hypocalcemia if present
    - Calcium gluconate may be used should magnesium toxicity arise during repletion

(d) *Hypermagnesemia*
- Common causes:
    - Severe renal insufficiency, excess intake, iatrogenic etiology during repletion or correction of hypomagnesemia
- Treatment:
    - Eliminate exogenous sources of magnesium
    - Address volume deficits and acidosis if present
    - Administer calcium chloride for acute symptoms
    - Hemodialysis if refractory to above therapies

(e) *Hypophosphatemia.*
- Common causes:
    - Inadequate intake, malabsorption, intracellular shift of phosphorus (e.g. respiratory alkalosis from hyperventilation, excess insulin, refeeding syndrome, hungry bone syndrome), excess excretion
- Treatment:
    - Oral (1 g sodium phosphate or potassium phosphate three times/day) or parenteral nutrition (IV potassium phosphate 0.17 $\frac{\text{mL}}{\text{kg}}$ of body weight over 6 h; use sodium phosphate if renal impairment is present) depending on the level of depletion and tolerance to enteral feeds

(f) *Hyperphosphatemia.*
- Common causes:
    - Excess intake, decreased excretion due to renal failure, hypothyroidism, hyperthyroidism, cellular injury

- Treatment:
  - Sucralfate, aluminum-containing antacids, calcium acetate tablets if hypocalcemia is also present

4. *Acid-Base Regulation and Acid-Base Disorders.*
   (a) Unlike the rapid respiratory response to metabolic derangements in acid-base homeostasis, metabolic renal compensations in response to ventilatory disruptions in acid-base homeostasis may not occur until 6–8 h and may persist for several days.
   - Anion gap = Na − (HCO_3 + Cl) (Tables 3.4, 3.5, and 3.6)

5. *Maintenance Fluid and Electrolyte Therapy.*
   (a) When selecting the appropriate type of fluid therapy (e.g. crystalloid versus colloid), consider:
   - The patient's volume status, weight, caloric needs, and co-morbidities
   - The presence of electrolyte or compositional abnormality

   (b) Common applications.
   - Lactate ringer and normal saline are commonly used to replenish GI losses and restore extracellular volume losses
   - Dextrose provides calories, diminishing the demand for muscle catabolism; however, dextrose is not used in resuscitation therapy due to osmotic diuresis (Table 3.7)

Table 3.4 Arterial blood gas in respiratory and metabolic acid-base disturbances

	Acute (without compensation)			Chronic (with compensation)		
	pH (7.35–7.45)	PCO_2 (35–45 mmHg)	Plasma HCO3- (22–28 mmol/L)	pH (7.35–7.45)	PCO_2 (35–45 mmHg)	Plasma HCO3- (22–28 mmol/L)
Respiratory acidosis	↓↓	↑↑ Hyperventilation	–	↓	↑↑	↑
Respiratory alkalosis	↑↑	↓↓ Hypoventilation	–	↑	↓↓	↓
Metabolic acidosis	↓↓	–	↓↓	↓	↓ Hypoventilation	↓
Metabolic alkalosis	↑↑	–	↑↑	↑	↑ Hyperventilation	↑

Table 3.5 Common causes of respiratory and metabolic acid-base disturbances

Respiratory acidosis	*Hypoventilation*: Narcotics, CNS injury, pulmonary etiology (mucus plug, atelectasis, pneumonia, secretions, pleural effusion), pain, impaired diaphragmatic excursion, ascites, abdominal compartment syndrome, abdominal distension
Respiratory alkalosis	*Hyperventilation*: Pain, anxiety, CNS injury or disorders, drugs (e.g. salicylates), infection, hypoxemia, thyrotoxicosis
Metabolic acidosis	*Increased anion gap*: Lactic acidosis, exogenous acid, salicylates, methanol, ethylene glycol, endogenous acid production, ketoacidosis, renal insufficiency, uremia, paraldehyde, isoniazid *Normal anion gap*: GI losses (e.g. ileostomies, fistulas), exogenous acid, loss of bicarbonate, renal tubular acidosis, carbonic anhydrase inhibitor
Metabolic alkalosis	*Impaired excretion of bicarbonate*: Mineralocorticoid excess, massive potassium depletion, GI losses, diuretics, acetate in parenteral nutrition, citrate, antacids, bicarbonate, milk-alkali syndrome *Increased generation of bicarbonate*: Decreased GFR, increased bicarbonate absorption

Table 3.6 Treatment for respiratory and metabolic acid-base disturbances

Respiratory acidosis	Relieve airway obstruction if present, restore adequate ventilation (e.g. intubation, BiLevel), restore level of consciousness
Respiratory alkalosis	Ventilation control (i.e. control or improve pain and/or anxiety); may need pericentesis
Metabolic acidosis	Address underlying cause, supplement with sodium bicarbonate until $pH > 7.20$
Metabolic alkalosis	Address underlying cause, administer 0.9% normal saline for chloride-responsive alkalosis with correction of potassium deficit, as metabolic acidosis can be worsened by hypokalemia

Tables 3.4–3.6 Data taken from: Doherty GM. *Current Diagnosis and Treatment: Surgery, 15th edition.* "Chapter 9: Fluid, Electrolyte, and Acid-Base Disorders." McGraw Hill. 2015.

Table 3.7 Composition of common electrolyte solutions (mEq/L)

	Na+	Cl-	K+	HCO3-	Ca2+	Mg2+	mOsm
Extracellular fluid	142	103	4	27	5	3	280–310
Lactated ringer	130	109	4	28	2.7	–	273
0.9% NaCl	154	154	–	–	–	–	308
D5 0.45% NaCl	77	77	–	–	–	–	407
D5W	–	–	–	–	–	–	253
3% NaCl	513	513	–	–	–	–	1026

Data taken from: de Moya M, Stearns DA, Yeh D. c1996–2021. Chicago, IL. American College of Surgeons Blended Surgical Education and Training for Life: Fluids and Electrolytes

Nutrition

1. *Effect of Surgery, Illness, and Injury on Nutritional Requirements.*
   (a) Effect of Surgery on Nutritional Status.
   - Iatrogenic and Pre-operative Measures: Pre-operative fasting and surgery provoke an inflammatory response that mediates tissue healing and proper tissue perfusion [8], but predisposes to infection [9].
   - Post-operative Course and Healing: Malnutrition and decreased energy stores are associated with worse clinical outcomes in children undergoing surgery [10] while post-operative oral nutrition supplementation improved a wide variety of outcome measures [11].

   (b) *Effect of Illness and Injury on Nutritional Status.*
   - Acute Effects: Acute illness episodes (e.g. sickle cell disease) appear to decrease appetite as indicated by body fat measures and inadequate intake of macronutrients [12], while increased appetite is associated with better quality of life (QoL) in post-operative gastric cancer patients [13].

- Chronic Disease: Though modern medicine has increased longevity, this change predisposes a growing number of people to diseases of old age that may affect appetite and ability to swallow that leads to altered food intake and impaired nutritional status [14].

2. *Nutritional Assessment and Indications.*
   (a) *Age and Implications of Aging Processes.*
   - Aging is accompanied by normal changes that may limit intake of soft foods that lead to decreased overall intake. Overlying malabsorptive changes may lead to micronutrient deficiencies in the face of decreased overall basal metabolic rate (BMR) requirements that may lead to overconsumption of raw calories (leading to obesity and its accompanying problems) [14].
   - Age alone demonstrates a significant and independent effect on assessments on nutritional status, with increasing age associated with poor clinical outcomes [15].

   (b) *Anthropometric Assessments of Nutrition.*
   - Proper nutrition can have significant effect on easily preventing common diseases. There are available several anthropometric measures to quickly assess nutritional status [16].
   - Assessment Methods Available at the Bedside (Table 3.8):

   (c) Biochemical Assessments (Table 3.9).
   (d) Clinical Assessments/Physical Exam (Table 3.10).
   (e) Summary.
   - At the bedside, nutritional status can be assessed using the "ABCs"
     - A = anthropometric measures (e.g. BMI, muscle cross-sectional areas, etc.)

Table 3.8 Bedside assessments for estimation of nutritional status

Measure	Formula/method	Indication
[a]Body mass index (BMI)	BMI = weight (kg)/height^2 (m)	BM > 40 = grade 3/severe obesity BMI 35–39.9 = grade 2 obesity BMI 30–34.9 = grade 1 obesity BMI 25–29.9 = overweight
Waist circumference [16]		>40in/102 cm (male) = high risk >35in/88 cm (female) = high risk
[b]Arm circumference(s)	MAMC = MAC − (3.14 × TSF)	>90th percentile = obesity
[c]Measurement of body fat	TSF measured using calipers and compared to table	>95th percentile = obesity Body fat % > 25% (male) = obesity Body fat % >33% (female) = obesity
Broka's index [16]	Ideal body weight (kg) = height (cm) − 100	
Psoas muscle index (PMI) [17]	Psoas cross-sectional area taken at L3	<15.2 cm^2 (male) = LBM <39.0 cm^2 (female) = LBM

MAC = Mid-arm circumference, midpoint of non-dominant arm
MAMC = Mid-arm muscle circumference
TSF = Triceps skinfold measurement, taken at midpoint of non-dominant arm between acromion and olecranon bone by pulling subcutaneous tissue away from underlying triceps and measuring with calipers to compare to reference table
Broka's index can only be valid for adults [18]
Psoas cross-sectional area can be used as an indicator for lean body mass (LBM) and low LBM on admission in critically ill patients has been associated with higher mortality rates, less ventilator-free days, less ICU-free days, and less likely to discharge to home [17]
[a] Data from CDC https://www.cdc.gov/obesity/adult/defining.html
[b] Data from https://nutritionalassessment.mumc.nl/en/anthropometry
[c] Data from https://nutritionalassessment.mumc.nl/en/skinfold-measurements

Table 3.9 Biochemical markers for nutritional status

Indicator	Normal value	Half-life
Albumin	3.5–5.0 g/dL	20 days
Transferrin	170–370 mg/dL	8–10 days
Transthyretin/prealbumin	16–30 mg/dL	2–4 days
Retinol binding protein	3.0–7.5 mg/dL	10 h

Source: Hood [19]

Table 3.10 Physical exam findings suggestive for nutritional deficits

System	Finding(s)	Common deficiency indicated
General	Fatigue ability	Anemia
Hair	Thin, sparse, dry, brittle, dyspigmented, flag signs Follicular hyperkeratosis	Kwashiorkor Scurvy (vit C deficiency)
Face	Periorificial lesions Moon face, nasolabial dyssebacia	Hypozincemia Pellagra (vit B3 deficiency)
Eyes	Pale conjunctiva Corneal xerosis, keratomalacia, Bitot's spot	Anemia Vit A deficiency
Lips	Angular stomatitis, cheilosis	Iron or vit B deficiencies
Tongue	Pale Scarlet Atrophic glossitis	Anemia Vit B12 deficiency Iron or vit B deficiencies
Skin	Diffuse petechiae Phrynoderma	Scurvy (vit C deficiency) Vit A deficiency
Neuro	Peripheral neuropathy	Vit B6 deficiency

Source: Galimberti [20], Upadhyay [16]

- B = biochemical measures (e.g. serum albumin, transferrin, micronutrients, etc.)
- C = clinical assessment (e.g. general appearance of face and features)

3. *Nutritional Requirements.*
   (a) Recommendations for General Nutrition (Table 3.11).
      - Fat supplies 9 calories/g, protein(s) and oral carbohydrates supply 4 calories/g, and dextrose supplies 3.4 calories/g [22].

   (b) Other considerations for total parenteral nutrition (TPN) formulation [23].
      - TPN formulations must also contain all essential vitamins and minerals
      - Children and patients with fevers have elevated daily energy requirements (up to 120 kcal/kg for children and 12% increased caloric need for every 1*C of fever)
      - Certain medical conditions require modified formulations, such as:
        - Reduced protein and high essential amino acids in renal insufficiency.
        - Reduced fluid intake in cardiac or renal failure.
        - Elevated lipid content in respiratory failure (to minimize CO_2 production).

4. *Choice of Route for Nutritional Support.*
   (a) Enteral Nutrition (ETF, enteral tube feeding).
      - Indications [24]
        - If oral intake is not tolerated post-operatively, ETF should be considered within POD 1–2 in the severely malnourished, POD 3–5 in the moderately malnourished, and within POD 7 in the normally nourished.
        - Early post-pyloric ETF is generally safe and effective in post-operative patients even in the setting of apparent ileus
        - Bolus feeding may cause bloating and diarrhea, but is generally preferred over continuous infusion which may promote bacterial overgrowth

Table 3.11 Recommended daily nutritional intake guidelines

Component	Recommended daily intake
Water	30–40 mL/kg body weight
Energy	30–35 kcal/kg body weight (standard medical patient) 30–45 kcal/kg body weight (post-operative patient) 45 kcal/kg body weight (hypercatabolic states)
Protein	1.0 g/kg body weight (standard medical patient), 2.0 g/kg body weight (post-operative patient), 3.0 g/kg body weight (hypercatabolic patient).
Essential fatty acids (omega-3 s)	1.6 g/day (males) or 1.1 g/day (females)

Source: NIH [21]

- Contraindications
  - Do not use ETF for patients with traumatic injury to the bowel, obstructions, and open routes for leakage (high output enterocutaneous fistula) [25].
- Potential Complications [26]
  - Diarrhea leading to potential need for conversion to TPN.

    If diarrhea is present, consider less calorically or osmotically dense formula.

    Causes for diarrhea include: antibiotic-associated bacterial imbalance (namely C. difficile), gut neurohormonal changes due to bypassing of cephalic phase of feeding, infected diets, hypoalbuminemia [27].
  - Refeeding syndrome in the severely malnourished.
  - Potential microbial contamination and infection of feeds.

    Avoiding gastric acid suppression and allowing feed breaks to restore gastric pH can help mitigate bacterial overgrowth.

(b) Parenteral Nutrition (PN).
- Indications [28]
  - Enteral is preferred but if not possible, parenteral is the alternative.

    Barriers to ETF include: short bowel syndrome, intestinal obstruction, prolonged ileus, malabsorptive processes, hypercatabolic states, lymphatic leaks not responding to diet modifications.
  - Supplemental PN recommended for at-risk patients within 7–10 days of admission if not able to meet 60% of energy and protein requirements.
- Contraindications [29]
  - Where oral intake or ETF is possible.
  - Patients in good nutrition that only require a predicted short term TPN (<2 weeks)
  - Irreversibly decerebrate patients or patients with severe cardiovascular instability.
  - Lack of specific therapeutic goal where TPN is to only prolong life in the setting of inevitable death.
- Potential Complications [29]
  - Metabolic complications such as hyper/hypoglycemia, metabolic acidosis, and micronutrient deficiencies.
  - Catheter complications such as pneumo/hemothorax, cardiac tamponade, hemorrhage, air embolism, and catheter thrombosis.
  - Prolonged TPN associated with hepatobiliary complications (liver enzyme elevations, steatosis, steatohepatitis, cholestasis, fibrosis, cirrhosis) and intestinal complications (changes in gut morphology, intestinal blood flow, cell proliferation/apoptosis, enzymatic functions, immune defenses and barrier integrity, motility, and bacterial ecology) [30]

Selected Review Questions

1. A patient with renal insufficiency develops hyperkalemia and is started on a treatment course with sodium polystyrene sulfonate (Kayexalate). What is the mechanism of action of this drug?
   (a) increase urinary excretion of potassium,
   (b) increase GI excretion of potassium via sodium exchange,
   (c) increase cellular uptake of potassium,
   (d) decreased GI absorption of potassium.
2. A patient presents with tachycardia and dry mucous membranes. Which of the additional findings would be most consistent with volume depletion?
   (a) hematocrit of 30%,
   (b) urine output of >0.5 mL/kg/h,
   (c) serum sodium of >145 mEq/L,
   (d) serum sodium of <145 mEq/L.
3. According to ESPEN guidelines, which of the following is an indicator for severe nutritional risk in a patient?
   (a) Weight loss >10–15% within last 6 months.
   (b) BMI <19.
   (c) Caloric intake <2000 calories.
   (d) Serum albumin <4.5 g/dL.
4. Which of the following is NOT a potential cause for diarrhea in a patient on ETF?
   (a) antibiotic-associated bacterial imbalance,
   (b) gut neurohormonal changes,
   (c) infected diets,
   (d) hypo-osmotic formulation.
5. Which of the following gives the best indication of acute (<24 h) changes in nutritional status?
   (a) Albumin.
   (b) Prealbumin.
   (c) Transferrin.
   (d) Transthyretin.
   (e) Retinol binding protein.

Answers: 1 (b), 2 (c), 3 (a), 4 (d), 5 (e)

References

1. Shires GT. Chapter 3. Fluid and electrolyte management of the surgical patient. In: Brunicardi FC, Andersen DK, Billiar TR, Dunn DL, Hunter JG, Matthews JB, et al., editors. Schwartz's principles of surgery [internet]. 9th ed. New York, NY: The McGraw-Hill Companies; 2010. [cited 2019 Oct 31]. accessmedicine.mhmedical.com/content.aspx?aid=5011700.
2. Lewis JL. Volume depletion - endocrine and metabolic disorders [internet]. Merck Manuals Professional Edition. 2018 [cited 2019 Oct 31]. https://www.merckmanuals.com/professional/endocrine-and-metabolic-disorders/fluid-metabolism/volume-depletion.
3. Zhan HT, Purcell ST, Bush RL. Preoperative optimization of the vascular surgery patient. Vasc Health Risk Manag. 2015;11:379–85.
4. Rassam SS, Counsell DJ. Perioperative electrolyte and fluid balance. Contin Educ Anaesth Crit Care Pain. 2005;5(5):157–60.
5. Kardalas E, Paschou SA, Anagnostis P, Muscogiuri G, Siasos G, Vryonidou A. Hypokalemia: a clinical update. Endocr Connect. 2018;7(4):R135–46.
6. Hollander-Rodriguez JC, Calvert JF. Hyperkalemia. AFP. 2006;73(2):283–90.
7. Mirrakhimov AE. Hypercalcemia of malignancy: an update on pathogenesis and management. N Am J Med Sci. 2015;7(11):483–93.
8. Gillis C, Wischmeyer PE. Pre-operative nutrition and the elective surgical patient: why, how and what? Anaesthesia. 2019;74(S1):27–35.
9. Visser M, Niessen HWM, Kok WEM, Cocchieri R, Wisselink W, van Leeuwen PAM, et al. Nutrition before and during surgery and the inflammatory response of the heart: a randomized controlled trial [Internet]. J Nutr Metab. 2015;2015:123158. https://doi.org/10.1155/2015/123158.
10. Radman M, Mack R, Barnoya J, Castañeda A, Rosales M, Azakie A, et al. The effect of preoperative nutritional status on postoperative outcomes in children undergoing surgery for congenital heart defects in San Francisco (UCSF) and Guatemala City (UNICAR). J Thorac Cardiovasc Surg. 2014;147(1):442–50.
11. Jull A. Postoperative oral nutritional supplementation improved nutritional status and quality of life in malnourished patients. Evid Based Nurs. 2001;4:22.
12. Malinauskas BM, Gropper SS, Kawchak DA, Zemel BS, Ohene-Frempong K, Stallings VA. Impact of acute illness on nutritional status of infants and young children with sickle cell disease. J Am Diet Assoc. 2000;100(3):330–4.

13. Kundes MF, Kement M, Yegen F, Alkan M, Kaya S, Kaptanoglu L. Effects of clinical factors on quality of life following curative gastrectomy for gastric cancer. Niger J Clin Pract. 2019;22(5):661.
14. Leslie W, Hankey C. Aging, nutritional status and health. Healthcare (Basel). 2015;3(3):648–58.
15. Forster S, Gariballa S. Age as a determinant of nutritional status: a cross sectional study. Nutr J. 2005;4(1):28.
16. Upadhyay R, Tripathi K. How can we assess the nutritional status of an individual? J Nutr Food Sci. 2017;7(6):1–2.
17. Looijaard WGPM, Molinger J, Weijs PJM. Measuring and monitoring lean body mass in critical illness. Curr Opin Crit Care. 2018;24(4):241.
18. Rao KV, Balakrishna N. Feasibility of Broka's index for the nutritional status of adults. Indian J Med Res. 1995;102:173–8.
19. Hood AW. Nutritional status assessment in adults laboratory medicine [internet]. Medscape 2015 [cited 2019 Oct 31]. https://emedicine.medscape.com/article/2141861-labs.
20. Galimberti F, Mesinkovska NA. Skin findings associated with nutritional deficiencies. [cited 2019 Oct 31]; https://www.mdedge.com/ccjm/article/114635/dermatology/skin-findings-associated-nutritional-deficiencies.
21. Office of Dietary Supplements - Omega-3 Fatty Acids [Internet]. National Institutes of Health. 2019 [cited 2019 Oct 31]. https://ods.od.nih.gov/factsheets/Omega3FattyAcids-HealthProfessional/.
22. Fiser S. Ch. 4: Fluids and electrolytes. In: The ABSITE review. 4th ed. Philadelphia: Lippincott Williams & Wilkins; 2014.
23. Thomas DR. Total parenteral nutrition (TPN) - nutritional disorders [Internet]. Merck manuals professional edition. [cited 2019 Oct 31]. https://www.merckmanuals.com/professional/nutritional-disorders/nutritional-support/total-parenteral-nutrition-tpn.
24. Stroud M, Duncan H, Nightingale J. Guidelines for enteral feeding in adult hospital patients. Gut. 2003;52(suppl 7):vii1–vii12.
25. Seron-Arbeloa C, Zamora-Elson M, Labarta-Monzon L, Mallor-Bonet T. Enteral nutrition in critical care. J Clin Med Res. 2013;5(1):1–11.
26. Pearce CB, Duncan HD. Enteral feeding. Nasogastric, nasojejunal, percutaneous endoscopic gastrostomy, or jejunostomy: its indications and limitations. Postgrad Med J. 2002;78(918):198–204.
27. Bowling TE. Diarrhoea in the enterally fed patient. Frontline Gastroenterol. 2010;1(3):140–3.
28. Wilkinson RE, Dickerson RN. "New" indications for parenteral nutrition. Hosp Pharm. 2016;51(10):795–7.
29. Maudar K. Total parenteral nutrition. Med J Armed Forces India. 1995;51(2):122–6.
30. Guglielmi FW, Boggio-Bertinet D, Federico A, Forte GB, Guglielmi A, Loguercio C, et al. Total parenteral nutrition-related gastroenterological complications. Dig Liver Dis. 2006;38(9):623–42.

Medications in Vascular Surgery

4

Joshua A. Gabel and Allen Murga

Medications in Vascular Surgery

Anti-thrombotic therapy:

Anti-coagulants

- Heparin.
  - Unfractionated Heparin (UFH).

    Mechanism of action: Binds to antithrombin (AT) and thrombin leading to increased inactivation of factor Xa and decreased conversion of fibrinogen to fibrin.

    Administration: Subcutaneous or intravenous.

    Half-life/clearance: 1–2 h/depolymerization and desulfation.

    Dosing (therapeutic): 80 units/kg; followed by 15–18 units/kg/h.

    Monitoring: Activated partial thromboplastin time (aPTT) and activated clotting time (ACT).

    Risk of heparin induced thrombocytopenia (HIT, 2.6% risk with exposure >4 days).

J. A. Gabel · A. Murga (✉)
Department of Surgery, Loma Linda University, Loma Linda, CA, USA
e-mail: amurga@llu.edu

A. Murga et al. (eds.), *The Vascular Surgery In-Training Examination Review (VSITE)*,
https://doi.org/10.1007/978-3-031-24121-5_4

    Contraindications:
    Protamine reversal.
    - Forms stable salt with heparin.
    - 1 mg to neutralize 90 units of UFH
    - Side effects: Hypotension, anaphylaxis.
  - Low-molecular weight heparin (LMWH).
    Mechanism of action: Binds AT leading to increased inactivation of factor Xa.
    Administration: Subcutaneous.
    Half-life/clearance: 4.5–7 h/hepatic.
    Dosing (therapeutic): 1 mg/kg twice daily.
    Monitoring: Anti-factor Xa activity (uncommon).
    Risk of HIT (0.2% risk).
    Contraindications:
    Indicated for use in treatment of VTE in setting of malignancy, renal disease, and Cr clearance <30 mL/min, pregnancy or pregnancy risk.
- Warfarin.
  - Mechanism of action: Binds vitamin-K epoxide reductase enzyme complex, thereby reducing the total amount of active forms of factors (II, VII, IX, X) and anticoagulant proteins C and S.
  - Administration: Oral.
  - Half-life/clearance: 20–60 h/hepatic excretion via cytochrome P-450.
  - Dosing: 5 mg daily, followed by INR-based dose adjustment on third day [1].
  - Monitoring: Prothrombin time (PT) and international normalized ratio (INR).
  - Contraindications: Elderly patients might have increased sensitivity and increased anticoagulation with smaller dose, hepatic dysfunction, pregnancy, blood dyscrasias.
  - Risk: Warfarin-induced skin necrosis occurs due to acquired protein C deficiency, leading to paradoxical activation of the coagulation cascade, occurs 3–6 days after drug is started.

Treatment: Stop medication, fresh frozen plasma or activated protein C and wound care with surgical debridement if needed.

- Direct Thrombin Inhibitors.
  - Argatroban.

    Mechanism of action: Direct thrombin inhibitor, reversible.

    Administration: Intravenous.

    Half-life/clearance: 39–51 min/hepatic via hydroxylation and aromatization of the 3-methyltetrahydroquinoline ring.

    - Excreted primarily via biliary secretions.

    Monitoring: aPTT or ACT.

    Synthetic arginine derivative.

    Indicated for anticoagulation in presence of HIT.
  - Bivalirudin (Angiomax).

    Mechanism of action: Direct inhibitor of thrombin, reversible.

    Administration: Intravenous.

    Half-life/clearance: 25 min with normal renal function, dialysis dependent patients up to 3.5 h/renal excretion and proteolytic cleavage.

    Monitoring: aPTT or ACT.

    Indicated for anticoagulation in presence of HIT, acute coronary syndromes.
  - Dabigatran (Pradaxa®).

    Mechanism of action: Competitive, direct thrombin inhibitor.

    Administration: Oral.

    Half-life/clearance: 12–17 h/renal.

    Monitoring: Dabigatran drug level (uncommon).

    Requires lead-in therapy with UFH or LMWH.

    Reversal with Idarucizumab (first line) or prothrombin complex concentrate (second line).

    Increased GI symptoms and GI bleed compared to other anti-coagulants.

- Direct Oral Anti-Coagulants (DOACs) also known as novel oral anti-coagulants (NOACs).
  - Fondaparinux.

    Mechanism of action: Reversible AT mediated inhibition of factor Xa.

    Administration: Subcutaneous.

    Half-life/clearance: 17–21 h/renal.

    Monitoring: Anti-factor Xa (uncommon).

    Reversal with Andexanet Alfa (first line) or prothrombin complex concentrate (second line).
  - Rivaroxaban (Xarelto®).

    Mechanism of action: Direct competitive inhibition of factor Xa.

    Administration: Oral.

    Half-life/clearance: 5–9 h/one-third hepatic, two-thirds renal.

    Monitoring: Anti-factor Xa (uncommon).

    Reversal with Andexanet Alfa (first line) or prothrombin complex concentrate (second line).
  - Apixaban (Eliquis®).

    Mechanism of action: Direct reversible inhibition of factor Xa.

    Administration: Oral.

    Half-life/clearance: 8–15 h/three-fourths hepatic, one-fourth renal.

    Monitoring: Anti-factor Xa (uncommon).

    Reversal with prothrombin complex concentrate.
  - Edoxaban (Savaysa®).

    Mechanism of action: Direct reversible inhibition of factor Xa.

    Administration: Oral.

    Half-life/clearance: 10–14 h/both hepatic and renal.

    Monitoring: Anti-factor Xa (uncommon).

    Requires lead-in therapy with UFH or LMWH.

Anti-platelet Therapy

- Aspirin.
  - Mechanism of action: Irreversible non-selective inhibition of cyclooxygenase 1 and 2.
  - Administration: Oral.
  - Half-life/clearance: 3 h/Renal.
  - Dosing: 75–150 mg once daily, with 81 mg being the most common dose.
  - Effect will last 5–7 days.
- Thienopyridines.
  - Clopidogrel (Plavix®).

    Mechanism of action: Irreversible inhibition of P2Y12 component of the ADP receptor.

    Administration: Oral.

    Half-life/clearance: 6 h/Hepatic.

    Dosing: 300 mg (loading dose), 75 mg once daily [2, 3].

    Reduced effectiveness with PPI [4].
  - Ticlopidine (Ticlid®).

    Mechanism of action: Irreversible inhibition of P2Y12 component of the ADP receptor.

    Administration: Oral.

    Half-life/clearance: 13 h/Hepatic.

    Monitoring: Signs of bleeding.

    Potent alternative anti-platelet medication in setting of Clopidogrel resistance.
  - Prasugrel (Effient®).

    Mechanism of action: Irreversible inhibition of P2Y12 component of the ADP receptor.

    Administration: Oral.

    Half-life/clearance: 7 h/Hepatic.

    Monitoring: Signs of bleeding.

    Potent alternative anti-platelet medication in setting of Clopidogrel resistance.
  - Ticagrelor (Brilinta®).

    Mechanism of action: Reversible inhibition of P2Y12 receptor.

    Administration: Oral.

  Half-life/clearance: 7 h/Hepatic.
  Monitoring: Signs of bleeding.
  Faster anti-platelet effects than Clopidogrel (1 h vs. 8 h) [5].
- Tirofiban (Aggrastat®)/Eptifbatide (Integrilin®).
  Mechanism of action: Reversible inhibition of glycoprotein IIb/IIIa receptor.
  Administration: Intravenous.
  Half-life/clearance: 2–2.5 h/Renal.
  Monitoring: aPTT or ACT.
  Limited historical use in peripheral vascular interventions [6].

Thrombolytics

- Alteplase (tPA).
  - Mechanism of action: Binds fibrin and converts plasminogen to plasmin.
  - Administration: Intravenous.
  - Half-life/clearance: 5 min/Plasma.
  - Monitoring: Signs of bleeding.
- Streptokinase.
  - Mechanism of action: Binds and activates plasminogen.
  - Administration: Intravenous.
  - Half-life/clearance: 80 min/Plasma.
  - Monitoring: Signs of bleeding.
  - Limited use due to immunogenic potential.

Treatment of Claudication

- Cilostazol (Pletal®).
  - Mechanism of action: cyclic AMP phosphodiesterase III inhibitor.
  - Administration: Oral.
  - Half-life/clearance: 12 h/Hepatic via cytochrome P-450 enzymes.
  - Dosing: 100 mg twice daily.

  - Monitoring: Periodic serum WBC and platelet counts.
  - Contraindicated in heart failure.
  - Improved maximal walking and pain-free walking distances compared to placebo [7].
- Pentoxifylline.
  - Mechanism of action: Increases red blood cell deformity and decreases viscosity.
  - Administration: Oral.
  - Half-life/clearance: 0.5 h/Renal.
  - Monitoring: Periodic renal function assessment.
  - Less commonly used due to variable outcomes and decreased effectiveness compared to Cilostazol [8].

Lipid-Lowering Therapy

- Statin [9]: Rosuvastatin, Atorvastatin, Simvastatin, Pravastatin.
  - Mechanism of action: Inhibit HMG-CoA reductase.
  - Administration: Oral.
  - Indicated for primary and secondary prevention of cardiac events in patients with peripheral arterial disease and diabetes.
  - Lowers LDL by 20–60%, increases HDL by 5–15%, and lowers triglycerides by 10–30%.
  - Side effects: Myalgias, Myositis, Transaminitis.
- Cholesterol absorption inhibitor: Ezetimibe.
  - Mechanism of action: Intestinal brush border inhibition of sterol transporter.
  - Administration: Oral.
  - Lowers LDLs, increases HDL, and decreases Triglycerides.
  - Side effects: Myalgias, headache.
  - Useful in patients with maximal statin therapy and need further reduction of LDLs.
  - For patients who do not tolerate high statin doses.
- PCSK9 inhibitors [10]: Evolocumab, Alirocumab.
  - Mechanism of action: Inhibits PCSK9 liver enzyme decreasing degradation of hepatic LDL receptors.

  - Administration: Subcutaneous.
  - Lowers LDL by 50%, increases HDL and lowers triglycerides.
  - Adjunct to lowering LDL in patients on statin therapy.
  - Side effects: Injection site reaction reported in up to 10% of patients.
- Fibrates [11]: Gemfibrozil, Bezafibrate, Fenofibrate, Fenofibric acid.
  - Mechanism of Action: Activation of nuclear transcription receptor PPAR- α, increasing fatty acid transport.
  - Administration: Oral.
  - Limited efficacy in patients with triglycerides greater than 200 mg/dL.
  - Side effects: transaminitis, GI disturbance, myopathy.
- Bile acid Sequestrants: Cholestyramine.
  - Mechanism of action: Binds bile acid in intestine preventing enterohepatic reuptake.
  - Administration: Oral.
  - Mainly works on lower LDLs.
  - Side effects: GI disturbance, transaminitis.
- Nicotinic acid [12]: Niacin.
  - Mechanism of action: Unclear.
  - Administration: Oral.
  - Lower LDL increases HDL and decreases triglycerides.
  - No additional benefit in patients on statin therapy.
  - Side effects: Flushing, transaminitis, hyperglycemia, hyperuricemia.
- Omega-3 fatty acids [13].
  - Mechanism of action: Beta-oxidation of fatty acids, inhibition of triglyceride synthesis, increased extrahepatic lipolysis.
  - Administration: Oral.
  - Main effect is to lower triglycerides.
  - Small decrease in cardiac and vascular death when combined with statin therapy.
  - Side effects: Nausea.

Smoking Cessation Therapy

- Varenicline (Chantix).
  - Mechanism of action: Neuronal nicotinic acetylcholine receptor partial agonist.
  - Administration: Oral.
  - Side effects: Nausea and sleep disorders (common).
  - No increased risk of suicide (Black box warning removed in 2016) [14].
  - Increased smoking cessation and maintenance of cessation compared to nicotine patch or placebo [15].
- Bupropion (Zyban®).
  - Mechanism of action: Weak inhibitor of dopamine and noradrenaline reuptake.
  - Administration: Oral.
  - Side effects: GI disturbance, lowers seizure threshold.
  - Contraindicated in patients with history of seizure disorder.

Adjuncts in Prevention of Contrast-Induced Nephrop athy

- Sodium bicarbonate.
  - Mechanism of action: Alkalization of renal tubular fluid.
  - Administration: Intravenous.
  - Dosing: 3 mL/kg per hour for 1 h before and 1 mL/kg per hour for 6 h after contrast exposure [16].
  - Variable historical efficacy; most recent data suggests no benefit over intravenous sodium chloride among patients at high risk of renal complications undergoing angiography [17].
- N-acetylcysteine.
  - Mechanism of action: Direct scavenging of superoxide radicals, increases glutathione synthesis.
  - Administration: Intravenous.
  - Variable historical efficacy; most recent data suggests no benefit over intravenous sodium chloride among patients at high risk of renal complications undergoing angiography [17].

Questions

1. A 50-year-old male with new onset right lower extremity DVT is started on Coumadin. On the third day of starting the medication he presents to the ED with right buttock pain and bullae. The next best step in management?
   (a) Obtain intravenous access and start antibiotics.
   (b) Cessation of warfarin with administration of fresh frozen plasma.
   (c) Obtain CT abdomen and pelvis.
   (d) Angiography with thrombolysis.
   (e) Administration of systemic thrombolytic agent.
2. The mechanism of action of aspirin is?
   (a) Reversible selective inhibition of prostaglandin synthesis.
   (b) Irreversible selective inhibition of production of thromboxane A1.
   (c) Irreversible non-selective inhibition of cyclooxygenase 1 and 2.
   (d) Reversible non-selective inhibition of P2Y12 receptor.
   (e) Irreversible competitive inhibition of ADP receptor.
3. The mechanism of action of Clopidogrel is?
   (a) Reversible inhibition of cyclooxygenase enzymes.
   (b) Irreversible inhibition of P2Y12 ADP receptors on platelets.
   (c) Reversible inhibition of P2Y12 ADP receptors on platelets.
   (d) Selective reversible inhibition of glycoprotein GPIIb/IIIa complex.
   (e) Irreversible inhibition of P2Y1 ADP receptors on platelets.

Answers:

1. (b)
2. (c)
3. (b)

References

1. Adfa Garcia P, Ruiz W, Loza MC. Warfarin initiation nomograms for venous thromboembolism. Cochrane Database Syst Rev. 2016;29:CD007699.
2. CAPRIE Steering Committee. A randomised, blinded, trial of clopidogrel versus aspirin in patients at risk of ischaemic events (CAPRIE). Lancet. 1996;348:1329–39.
3. Gerhard-Herman MD, Gornik HL, Barrett C, et al. 2016 AHA/ACC guideline on the management of patients with lower extremity peripheral artery disease: a report of the American College of Cardiology/American Heart Association task force on clinical practice guidelines. Circulation. 2017;135(12):e726–79.
4. Li XQ, Andersson TB, Ahalström M, et al. Comparison of inhibitory effects of the proton pump-inhibiting drugs omeprazole, esomeprazole, lansoprazole, pantoprazole and rabeprazole on human cytochrome P450 activities. Drug Metab Dispos. 2004;32(8):821–7.
5. Storey RF, Angiolillo DJ, Patil SB, et al. Inhibitory effects of ticagrelor compared with clopidogrel on platelet function in patients with acute coronary syndromes: the PLATO (PLATelet inhibition and patient outcomes) PLATELET substudy. J Am Coll Cardiol. 2010;56:1456–62.
6. Allie DE, Hebert CJ, Lirtzman MD, et al. A safety and feasibility report of combined direct thrombin and GP IIb/IIIa inhibition with bivalirudin and tirofiban in peripheral vascular disease intervention: treating critical limb ischemia like acute coronary syndrome. J Invas Cardiol. 2005;17:427–32.
7. Allie DE, Hebert CJ, Lirtzman MD, et al. A safety and feasibility report of combined direct thrombin and GP IIb/IIIa inhibition with bivalirudin and tirofiban in peripheral vascular disease intervention: treating critical limb ischemia like acute coronary syndrome. J Invasive Cardiol. 2005;17:427–32.
8. Salhiyyah K, Senanayake E, Abdel-Hadi M, Booth A, Michaels JA. Pentoxifylline for intermittent claudication. Cochrane Database Syst Rev. 2012;1:CD005262.
9. Jones PH, Davidson MH, Stein EA, et al. Comparison of the efficacy and safety of rosuvastatin versus atorvastatin, simvastatin, and pravastatin across doses (STELLAR* trial). Am J Cardiol. 2003;92:152–60.
10. Bonaca MP, Nault P, Giugliano RP, Keech AC, Pineda AL, Kanevsky E, et al. Low-density lipoprotein cholesterol lowering with evolocumab and outcomes in patients with peripheral artery disease: insights from the FOURIER trial (further cardiovascular outcomes research with PCSK9 inhibition in subjects with elevated risk). Circulation. 2018;137:338–50.

11. Bezafibrate Infarction Prevention (BIP) study. Secondary prevention by raising HDL cholesterol and reducing triglycerides in patients with coronary artery disease. Circulation. 2000;102(1):21.
12. AIM-HIGH Investigators, Boden WE, Probstfield JL, Anderson T, Chaitman BR, Desvignes-Nickens P, Koprowicz K, McBride R, Teo K, Weintraub W. Niacin in patients with low HDL cholesterol levels receiving intensive statin therapy. N Engl J Med. 2011;365(24):2255; Epub 2011 Nov 15.
13. ASCEND Study Collaborative Group, Bowman L, Mafham M, Wallendszus K, Stevens W, Buck G, Barton J, Murphy K, Aung T, Haynes R, Cox J, Murawska A, Young A, Lay M, Chen F, Sammons E, Waters E, Adler A, Bodansky J, Farmer A, McPherson R, Neil A, Simpson D, Peto R, Baigent C, Collins R, Parish S, Armitage J. Effects of n-3 fatty acid supplements in Diabetes Mellitus. N Engl J Med. 2018;379(16):1540; Epub 2018 Aug 26.
14. Thomas KH, Martin RM, Knipe DW, et al. Risk of neuropsychiatric adverse events associated with varenicline: systematic review and meta-analysis. BMJ. 2015;350:h1109.
15. Anthenelli RM, Benowitz NL, West R, et al. Neuropsychiatric safety and efficacy of varenicline, bupropion, and nicotine patch in smokers with and without psychiatric disorders (EAGLES): a double-blind, randomised, placebo-controlled clinical trial. Lancet. 2016;387(10037):2507–20. https://doi.org/10.1016/S0140-6736(16)30272-0.
16. Merten GJ, Burgess WP, Gray LV, et al. Prevention of contrast-induced nephropathy with sodium bicarbonate: a randomized controlled trial. JAMA. 2004;291(19):2328–34.
17. Weisbord SD, Gallagher M, Jneid H, Garcia S, Cass A, Thwin SS, Conner TA, Chertow GM, Bhatt DL, Shunk K, Parikh CR, EO MF, Brophy M, Ferguson R, Wu H, Androsenko M, Myles J, Kaufman J, Palevsky PM, PRESERVE Trial Group. Outcomes after angiography with sodium bicarbonate and acetylcysteine. N Engl J Med. 2018;378(7):603.

5 Hemodynamics, Atherosclerosis, Intimal Hyperplasia, and Wound Healing

Neha Sheng and Brittany Mead

Hemodynamics

1. Basic Principles of Arterial Hemodynamics

   (a) Energy[1]
   - Hemodynamics is the study of pressure and flow within the circulatory system.
   - Blood moves from point A to point B based on difference in fluid energy.
     - **Total Fluid Energy (E)** = potential energy + kinetic energy (total fluid energy remains constant).
     - **Potential Energy** = intravascular pressure (P) + gravitational potential energy (ρgh), where ρ is equal to blood density (~1.056 g/cm[2]), g is the

N. Sheng (✉)
Division of Vascular Surgery, Department of Surgery, Cook County Health, Chicago, IL, USA

B. Mead
Division of Vascular Surgery, Department of Surgery, Cook County Health, Chicago, IL, USA

Rush University Medical Center, Chicago, IL, USA
e-mail: Brittany_s_mead@rush.edu

A. Murga et al. (eds.), *The Vascular Surgery In-Training Examination Review (VSITE)*,
https://doi.org/10.1007/978-3-031-24121-5_5

acceleration blood due to gravity (980 cm/s^2), and h is distance above a reference point.
  - **Kinetic Energy** = $\frac{1}{2}\rho v^2$ Work done by blood secondary to its motion. Where ρ = blood density (~1.056 g/cm^2) and v is the velocity.
  - **Total Fluid Energy (*E*)** = $P + \rho g h + \frac{1}{2}\rho v^2$

(b) **Bernoulli's Principle** [1]
- In a frictionless system, when fluid flow is steady, total energy is conserved.
  - $P_1 + \rho g h_1 + \frac{1}{2}\rho v^2{}_1 = P_2 + \rho g h_2 + \frac{1}{2}\rho v^2{}_2$
- Increasing cross-sectional area of a tube results in decreased velocity.
- This is theoretical, and not achieved in human circulation secondary to friction and energy losses.

(c) **Poiseuille's Law** [1, 2]
- $P_1 - P_2 = V\frac{8L\eta}{r^2} = Q\frac{8L\eta}{\pi r^4}.$
  - Where $P_1 - P_2$ represents change in potential energy (dyn/cm^2) between a distance L (cm), Q is the flow (cm^3/s), and V is the mean flow velocity (cm/s). η is the viscosity coefficient (dyn/s/cm^2).
  - Used to describe the pressure differential between fluid flowing in different areas in a tube.

(d) Blood flow patterns [1–3]:
- Mechanical energy is lost as heat in the movement of fluid.
- Energy loss in blood circulation is related to both the viscosity of the blood as well as inertia.
- **Viscosity:** Friction between interacting layers of fluid (in blood, viscosity is mostly determined by hematocrit).
- Poiseuille's law describes flow in an idealized system with **laminar flow**, where every molecule of blood moves parallel to the wall of the vessel.

  - Velocity of a fluid is highest at the center of a tube and becomes progressively slower as it moves peripherally into contact with a wall.
- **Turbulent Flow:** Flow pattern that results in reduction in fluid energy secondary to random velocity vectors (all flow is NOT parallel to the vessel wall) (e.g. turbulent flow may occur distal to an arterial stenosis).
  - Bruits are heard in areas of turbulent flow.
- **Boundary Layer**: The layer of blood adjacent to the vessel wall.
  - Boundary layer separation (outer layer of blood flows slower; it is even possible to have reversal of flow at branch point, such as the carotid bifurcation) may contribute to plaque formation.
- **Reynolds Number (Re)**: The point at which flow changes from laminar to turbulent.
  - $\mathrm{Re} = \frac{dV\rho}{\eta}$, where d is the diameter of the tube, ρ is the density of blood, V is the mean flow velocity, and η is viscosity.
  - $\mathrm{Re} > 2000$ = turbulence develops.
  - $\mathrm{Re} < 2000$ = predominantly laminar flow.

(e) Stress [3]

- Mechanical forces acting on the vessel wall.
- Normal stress
  - Forces working perpendicular to the surface.
- Shear stress
  - Shear stress is a perpendicular frictional drag force imposed by blood flow on the endothelium that subsequently modulates endothelial structure and gene expression.
  - **Shear stress** $(\tau) = \frac{4\mu Q}{\pi r^3}$. Where μ is the viscosity, Q is the flow, and r is the radius of the vessel lumen.
  - **La Place's law** states that **tangential stress** (T) on the vessel wall is proportional to pressure (P) and radius (r): $T = Pr$.

    Hence, the higher risk of aneurysm rupture in the hypertensive patient with a larger aneurysm.
  - Vascular endothelium is constantly exposed to physiologic ranges of shear stress which promotes anti-inflammatory and antithrombotic characteristics to maintain normal endothelial function.
  - Disruption of laminar flow and reduction of shear stress causes disruption of normal endothelial cell behavior, which increases the risk of developing atherosclerosis.
- Tensile stress
  - Circumferential tension generated in the vessel wall by blood pressures.
  - **Tensile stress** (σ) = $\frac{r}{h}$ Δp, where h is vessel wall thickness, r is the vessel radius, and Δp is the change in pressure.

2. Mechanical Properties of Vessel Walls [2]
   (a) The artery wall is a layered structure that generates mechanical strength to resist forces created by blood pressure.
   (b) Three layers:
   - Intima (inner layer)
     - Endothelial cells.
     - Basement membrane.
   - Media
     - Smooth Muscle Cells: Contractile properties essential for regulation of blood flow.
     - Arrangements of collagen and elastin.
   - Adventitia (outer Layer)
     - Elastin and collagen as structural elements.
     - Nerves.
     - Vasa vasorum: Small blood vessels that supply the artery wall.

       Hypoxia in atherosclerotic segment → neovascularization → vasa vasorum supply nutrients to the plaque.

       Implicated in plaque hemorrhage.
     - Connects the artery with surrounding tissues.

(c) Pulse propagation.
  - Compliance with arterial walls results in pulse pressure being propagated as a traveling wave through the arterial system.

3. Hemodynamics of Arterial Stenosis [1]
   (a) Hypertension increases tensile force in the arterial wall.
   (b) Energy losses.
     - Most energy loss in an arterial system results from stenosis of the vasculature.
     - Determinants of energy loss in circulation:
       – Shape of the stenosis (irregular or smooth).
       – Number of stenoses.
       – Angulation of the vessel.
       – Number of branches.
   (c) According to Poiseuille's law, the extent of the stenosis as it relates to the vessel lumen is more significant than the length of that stenosis.
   (d) Critical stenosis.
     - The amount of narrowing at which noticeable changes to flow and pressure are observed is call "critical stenosis."
     - Generally, changes are not appreciable until the vessel lumen (diameter) has been reduced by approximately 50%.
     - Critical stenosis varies with downstream resistance.
       – Low resistance systems (e.g. coronary, renal, and carotid systems), can achieve critical stenosis with much less narrowing than would be required in a high resistance system (e.g. extremities).
       – Lowering peripheral resistance with exercise can reveal critical stenosis which is not observed at rest.
       – Autoregulation may allow for compensation for stenosis.
   (e) Poststenotic dilatation:
     - Dilation of arteries distal to a stenosis may occur due to increased pressure on the wall of the artery, turbulence, change in shear stress.
     - A bruit may be auscultated.

4. Hemodynamics Associated with Anastomosis [1, 2]
   (a) A change in the direction of blood flow increases energy losses.
   (b) End-to-end anastomosis is more physiologic and hemodynamically efficient than end-to-side anastomosis.
      - The greater the angle between graft and the native vessel, the greater the energy loss.
      - Flow disturbance through an anastomosis causes turbulence, stagnation, and flow separation.
         – This results in decreased shear stress.
      - Ultimately, the result is endothelial thickening and risk of thrombus formation, which increase, the risk of graft failure.

Intimal Hyperplasia [4]

1. Background
   (a) Intimal hyperplasia is the vasculature's biologic response to injury.
   (b) Primary pathology for restenosis of any open or endovascular procedure = intimal hyperplasia.
2. Pathophysiology.
   (a) Hyperacute phase (minutes to hours after injury):
      - Initial response for hemostasis:
         – Following injury, there is activation of platelet membrane receptors (GPIb, GPIc/GPIIa, GPIIA, GPIa/GPIIa).
         – Subendothelial collagen reacts with platelet membrane receptors.
         – Release of Von Willebrand Factor and fibronectin.
      - Injured/dying smooth muscle cells release basic fibroblast growth factor (bFGF).
      - Angiotensin II has a role in stimulating vascular smooth muscle vasoconstriction, proliferation, and production of the extracellular matrix [5].

(b) Acute phase (hours to weeks after injury).
    - Smooth muscle cell migration.
        - Higher levels of ICAM and VCAM on endothelium.
        - Chemokines and cytokines regulate inflammatory process.
        - Platelet derived growth factor (PDGF), bFGF, vascular endothelial growth factor (VEGF), and others → smooth muscle cell proliferation and migration.
    - Matrix metalloproteases and proteases are released by inflammatory cells to break up/remodel the surrounding matrix.
    - SMCs move into the intima where they replicate and deposit matrix.
    - SMCs in the intima are no longer capable of developing organized matrix which results in a histologically disordered layer.

(c) Chronic phase (weeks to months after injury).
    - Reendothelialization → stabilization of the SMC proliferation/migration process.
    - Intima continues to accumulate over time and results in stenosis.
        - Intima is most narrow at 1 month after injury.
        - Regulation of intimal expansion and remodeling by integrins and cytokines (e.g. transforming growth factor—beta, TGF-β).

3. Modulating Factors.
    (a) Genetic Factors.
        - Single nucleotide polymorphisms in IL-10 genes associated with higher rates of restenosis.
        - Some loci on chromosome 12.
    (b) Immune Influences.
        - Solid organ transplants increased rate or restenosis 2/2 HLA mismatch and T-cell response.

(c) Shear Stress.
  - Vessels with laminar blood flow release antithrombotic, anti-inflammatory factors.
  - Vascular intervention often causes disordered flow which induced endothelial cell activation and pro-inflammatory cytokines that result in intimal thickening.

4. Prospects for Control of Intimal Hyperplasia.
   (a) Surgical Technique: Smallest angle possible in end to side anastomosis. End-to-end anastomosis is preferable.
   (b) Promoting reendothelialization (granulocyte-colony stimulating factor, G-CSF).
   (c) Pharmacologic control of smooth muscle cell activity (including systemic and local drug delivery techniques).
     - Drug eluting stents:
       - Secrete immunosuppressive agents (i.e. paclitaxel, sirolimus, rapamycin).
       - Decrease SMC proliferation but also decrease rate of reendothelialization.
       - The FDA warned clinicians about data suggesting increased late mortality in paclitaxel coated devices in 2019. Further study is needed to evaluate this.
     - Drug eluting balloons—similar concerns as above.
   (d) Radiation therapy.
     - Can be effective by inhibiting rapidly dividing cells and can therefore prevent cell proliferation in neointimal hyperplasia.
     - May slow down reendothelialization.
     - Can result in luminal narrowing at the edges of the areas of treatment.
   (e) Cryoplasty.
     - Cold therapy with angioplasty.
     - Small trials, limited evidence.
   (f) Antithrombotic and statin therapy:
     - Aspirin and other antiplatelet therapies are widely given to patients with atherosclerosis.
     - Statin therapy helps reduce risk of stenosis.

   (g) Diabetes and smoking result in more intimal hyperplasia.
   (h) Autologous grafts are preferred over prosthetic grafts. Ongoing new technology in prosthetic and bioprosthetic grafts in hopes of reducing intimal hyperplasia.
5. Future Directions.
   (a) antibodies to growth factors,
   (b) antisense nucleotides,
   (c) gene therapy.

Atherosclerosis [6]

1. Risk Factors.
   (a) HTN.
   (b) Dyslipidemia.
   (c) Smoking.
   (d) Diabetes.
   (e) Age.
   (f) Gender (Male >Female).
   (g) Race (AA>Hispanic>Asian>White).
   (h) Hypercoagulability.
   (i) Elevated CRP.
2. Theories of Pathogenesis.
   (a) Lipid Hypothesis:
      - Cholesterol transportation is facilitated by lipoproteins.
      - The density of the lipoprotein (very low-density lipoprotein [VLDL], low-density lipoprotein [LDL], high-density lipoprotein [HDL]) makes a difference.
      - 3-hydroxy-3-methyl-glutaryl-coenzyme A reductase (HMG-CoA reductase) is regulated by LDL.
      - Familial hypercholesterolemia: patients lack cellular LDL receptors causing HMG-CoA to be insensitive to normal LDL feedback regulation, resulting in grossly elevated cholesterol levels.
   (b) Thrombogenic Hypothesis:
      - Arterial injury and inflammatory response lead to formation of mural thrombus. Subsequent organization of the mural thrombus leads to a fibrous plaque.

(c) Mesenchymal Hypothesis:
   - Proteoglycan and collagen based.
   - Shear stress, vasoactive agents, repetitive injury, hypertension, and tachycardia implicated in plaque formation.

(d) Monoclonal Hypothesis:
   - Unregulated smooth muscle proliferation (like a cancer) results in stenosis.
   - There may be clonal proliferation of a single smooth muscle cell, leading to atherosclerotic plaque.

(e) Response to Injury Hypothesis:
   - Injury can be sustained from infections, toxin exposure, systemic inflammation, mechanical injury (e.g. clamp injury).
   - Injury to the endothelium initiates.
     - Platelets release platelet derived growth factor (PDGF) which eventually leads to smooth muscle cell proliferation.
   - Injury causes retention of inflammatory lipids in the intima. The inflammatory response results in building atheromatous plaque.

3. Plaque Formation.

(a) Endothelium activated (toxins, infections, inflammation, mechanical injury, etc.)
   - Hemostatic Response: Subendothelial collagen interacts with platelet membrane receptors, Von Willebrand factor and fibronectin are released.

(b) Increased production of leukocyte adhesion molecules.

(c) Increased adhesion of leukocytes and macrophages.

(d) Increased permeability of the endothelium to lipoproteins.

(e) Chemokine production → recruit leukocytes and smooth muscle cells (SMC) into the subendothelial space.

(f) Subendothelial lipoproteins are modified, taken up by cell adhesion molecules (CAMs), and SMCs to form foam cells.

(g) Central foam cells (lipid filled macrophages) become necrotic and form the lipid core.
   - A **fatty streak** can be seen, even in youth, and represents the beginnings of atherosclerotic plaque.

(h) Activated SMCs produce growth factors (PDGFs, TGF-β) that stimulate matrix and collagen production to form the **fibrous cap**.
  - As the plaque progresses, the lipid core increases, and the fibrous cap becomes thinner.

(i) Complicated plaque and plaque disruption:
  - Complicated plaque has associated ulceration or thrombosis.
  - Plaque rupture can proceed to remodeling of the tissue resulting in occlusion or stenosis.
  - Four mechanisms of plaque disruption:
    – Complete disruption of the fibrous cap—most common cause of coronary artery thrombosis.
    – Intra-plaque hemorrhage—proliferation of friable local microvascular network.
    – Superficial plaque erosion—creates in-situ thrombus. Common in women and diabetics.
    – Intimal erosion of a calcified nodule—particularly important in coronary and peripheral arteries.

4. Location of Plaque Development.
   (a) Plaque has a propensity to form at arterial branch points due to turbulent flow (low laminar shear stress).
   (b) Areas of high laminar shear stress produce anti-inflammatory factors (eNOS, NO) that make endothelial cells more thromboresistant.
   (c) Disruption of laminar flow results in increased particle contact time with endothelium, increased NF-kB activity favoring proliferation, and entry of LDL into the vessel wall.

Wound Healing

1. Phases of wound healing [7, 8].
   (a) Inflammatory (Days 1–10):
     - Vascular injury results initially in local vasoconstriction followed by vasodilation.

- Increased vascular permeability allows RBCs and platelets to bind damaged endothelium and form platelet plug.
- Migration of cells by chemotaxis: primarily PMNs, MACS, and fibroblasts.
- Secretion of Cytokines and Growth Factors: CXCL1, IL-8, TNF-a, IL-1, PDGF.
- Epithelial cell migration:
  - Begins within hours of injury.
  - Keratinocytes at the basal layer of surrounding epidermis migrate to cover the wound.

(b) Proliferative (Day 5–Week 3).

- Angiogenesis:
  - New blood vessel formation to support tissue growth.
  - Primarily mediated by VEGF family—induced by cell disruption and hypoxia.
- Fibroplasia:
  - Quiescent fibroblasts are activated and undergo TGF-B stimulated replication and proliferation.
  - Fibroblasts migrate to site of inflammation and produce extracellular matrix and collagen (predominantly Type III).

(c) Epithelialization:

- Occurs at a rate of 1–2 mm/day.
- Keratinocytes detach, migrate, proliferate, differentiate and stratify.
- Faster if basement membrane is intact.

2. Maturation/Remodeling (Week 3–Year 1).

(a) Wound Contraction.

- Complex interaction of fibroblasts with ECM.
- Results in reduction of disorganized scar tissue.

(b) Remodeling.

- Type I collagen cross linking (Type III collagen replaced by Type I).
- Tensile strength increases rapidly from week 1–6 (maximum at 8 weeks) and then reaches a plateau.
  - Tensile strength never returns to normal.

3. Risk factors for reduced wound healing [7, 8].
    (a) Ischemia: Decreased O2 delivery and circulation of pertinent cell lines.
    (b) Steroids: Inhibits MACs, PMNs, fibroblast collagen synthesis = Decreased tensile strength.
    (c) Malnutrition: Hypoalbuminemia (goal albumin >3).
    (d) Diabetes: Hyperglycemia impedes leukocyte chemotaxis.
    (e) Necrotic Tissue: Decreased wound granulation potential.
    (f) Infection: Presence of bacteria prolongs inflammatory response.
    (g) Immunosuppression: AIDS, immunosuppressant therapy, active chemotherapy (blunts inflammatory response of wound healing; VEGF important regulator of malignancy often targeted in chemotherapy).
    (h) Nicotine: Multifactorial. Vasoconstriction, decreased inflammatory response, reduced bactericidal mechanism, alters collagen synthesis.
4. Abnormal scarring [7, 8].
    (a) Hypertrophic Scarring—Excess collagen deposition within the context of the original scar.
        - Result of prolonged local inflammation (i.e. burns).
        - Tx: steroid injections.
    (b) Keloids—Scars tissue that extends outside of the borders of the original wound.
        - More common in pts. with dark skin.
        - Occur in 15–20% of AA, Hispanic and Asian pts.
        - Tx: Steroid injection.
5. Wound management [7–9].
    (a) Negative Pressure Dressings (Wound Vac).
        - Continuous suction applied to wound bed to enhance wound closure and enhance wound environment. Can be used with non-adherent dressing over intact skin.
        - Multiple RCT demonstrate improved rate of healing when compared to moist dressings.
    (b) Hyperbaric Oxygen (HBO).
        - Improved O_2 delivery, reduction of inflammation, prevents infection.
        - 1–2 tx/day for total of 20–40 treatments.

    - May be useful in diabetic foot ulcers, necrotizing fasciitis and flap healing.
    - Poor evidence in ischemic patients and is NOT a substitute for revascularization.
    - HBO is costly.
6. Suture removal.
    (a) Face: Remove after 1 week.
    (b) Trunk and extremities: Generally removed after 1 month.
7. Supplements to wound healing [7, 8, 10].
    (a) Vitamin C: Important for collagen synthesis (500–2000 mg BID).
        - Indicated to treat deficiencies, high dose supplementation has not been shown to improve wound healing in replete patients.
    (b) Zinc: Co-enzyme in many reactions required for wound healing (40–200 mg QD for 10–14 days to prevent acute toxicity).
    (c) Vitamin A: Reduces the harmful effects of steroids on wound healing (25,000 IU PO QD over 10–14 days to prevent acute toxicity).

Questions

1. Which of the following are not part of the phases of wound healing?
    (a) Inflammatory.
    (b) Proliferative.
    (c) Epithelialization.
    (d) Desquamation.
2. Which of the following are not risk factors for the development of atherosclerosis?
    (a) Smoking.
    (b) Hypertension.
    (c) Dyslipidemia.
    (d) Elevated CRP.
    (e) Abdominal aortic aneurysm.

3. Which of the following are not risk factors for delayed wound healing?
   (a) Infection.
   (b) Smoking.
   (c) Ischemia.
   (d) HBO therapy.
   (e) Steroids.

Answers:

1. (d)
2. (e)
3. (d)

References

1. Zierler RE, Sumner DS. Arterial physiology. Rutherford's vascular surgery. 8th ed. Elsevier Saunders; 2014. p. 132–49.
2. Secomb TW. Hemodynamics. Compr Physiol. 2016;6(2):975–1003.
3. Cunningham KS, Gotllieb AI. The role of shear stress in the development of atherosclerosis. Lab Investig. 2005;85:9–23.
4. Jiang Z, Ozaki CK. Intimal hyperplasia. Rutherford's vascular surgery. 8th ed. Elsevier Saunders; 2014. p. 78–86.
5. Osgood MJ, Harrison DG, Sexton KW, Hocking KM, Voskresensky IV, Komalavilas P, Cheung-Flynn J, Guzman RJ, Brophy CM. Role of the renin-angiotensin system in the pathogenesis of intimal hyperplasia: therapeutic potential for prevention of vein graft failure? Ann Vasc Surg. 2012;26(8):1130–44.
6. Owens CD. Atherosclerosis. Rutherford's vascular surgery. 8th ed. Elsevier Saunders; 2014. p. 66–77.
7. Leong M, Phillips LG. Wound healing. Sabiston textbook of surgery: the biological basis of modern surgical practice. 20th ed. Philadelphia: Elsevier Saunders; 2016. p. 152–77.
8. Marston WA. Wound care. Rutherford's vascular surgery. 8th ed. Elsevier Saunders; 2014. p. 1222–40.
9. Raffetto JD, Eberhardt RT. Chronic venous disorders: general considerations. Rutherford's vascular surgery. 8th ed. Elsevier Saunders; 2014. p. 842–57.
10. Kogan S, Sood A, Granick M. Zinc and wound healing: a review of zinc physiology and clinical applications. Wounds. 2017;29(4):102–6.

6 Imaging/Vascular Laboratory

Kenneth R. Ziegler and Alyssa Pyun

General

Duplex Ultrasound (US)

- High frequency sound waves (2–10 mHz) have weaker tissue penetration and vice versa.
  - Corollary: use lower frequency probes for abdominal vessels.
- Duplex ultrasound functional modes.
  - B-mode: 2D imaging for soft tissue characteristics.
  - Color mode: visualizes directional flow.
  - Power mode duplex: more sensitive to low flow in small vessels. No directionality due to squared transform calculation.
- Increasing Doppler gain amplifies both signal and noise.
- If imaging angle is perpendicular (90 degrees) to the direction of motion, no velocity information will be captured.
- Acoustic shadowing does not affect PSV itself.

Disclosures: None.

K. R. Ziegler (✉) · A. Pyun
Division of Vascular Surgery, Department of Surgery, University of Southern California, Los Angeles, CA, USA
e-mail: Kenneth.Ziegler@med.usc.edu; Alyssa.Pyun@med.usc.edu

A. Murga et al. (eds.), *The Vascular Surgery In-Training Examination Review (VSITE)*,
https://doi.org/10.1007/978-3-031-24121-5_6

Intravascular Ultrasound (IVUS)

- Muscular arteries: media appears as echolucent layer between echodense intima and adventitia.
- Larger vessels (aorta): cannot see three layers due to increased elastin content.
- Four plaque components.
  - echolucent = lipid,
  - soft echoes = fibromuscular and intimal proliferation,
  - bright echoes = collagen rich fibrous tissue,
  - bright echoes with acoustic shadowing = calcified tissue,
- Virtual histology: identify four tissue components using color code system.
  - fibrous = green,
  - fibrofatty = light green,
  - calcium = white,
  - necrotic core = red,
  - visualize plaque to predict how it will react to different treatments,
- Uses: aid in PTA balloon sizing, atherectomy, EVAR, stent deployment/enfolding/apposition evaluation.
  - can reconstruct images to get longitudinal images, like angiography, but include wall morphology,
- Advantages:
  - Improves long term patency of stents.
  - Real time evaluation (e.g. stagnant flow in false lumen can mean covered entry tear).
  - Can see if stent is improperly deployed.

    not well apposed = bright with acoustic shadowing or comet tailing at stent struts,

    well apposed = difficult to differentiate stent from wall,
  - Can help mitigate contrast use in preoperative and intraoperative EVAR planning.
  - Surpasses angiography in detecting BTAI after equivocal CTA.

Computed Tomography (CT)

- Contrast agent: iodinated contrast.
  - Non iso-osmolar contrast = least nephrotoxic iodinated contrast.
- Advantages:
  - Excellent spatial resolution.
  - Rapid imaging acquisition.
  - Can reconstruct images.
- Limitations.
  - Reactions to Iodinated Contrast.

    Vasovagal = Hypotension + *bradycardia*.
      - Tx = IVF, leg raise, atropine.

    Allergy.
      - Mild allergy (itchy skin and sore throat).
      - Moderate allergy (urticarial, throat tightness).
      - Severe allergy (anaphylaxis) = laryngeal edema, bronchospasm, urticarial, refractory to albuterol. Hypotension + *tachycardia*.
        - Tx = epi.

    Contrast induced nephropathy.
      - Little evidence that IV iodinated contrast is independent risk factor for AKI if GFR > 30.
  - Calcium artifact.

Magnetic Resonance (MR)

- Magnetic resonance angiography (MRA) uses T1-weighted imaging.
  - Can be non-contrast or contrast.
  - Time-of-flight (TOF) imaging = non-contrast, use when contrast contraindicated, utilizes saturated versus unsaturated protons.

    Blood can be bright.

  - Contrast agent = Gadolinium.

    Decreases T1 relaxation time → high intravascular signal intensity.

    Need less contrast in MRA compared with CTA.
  - T1 fat is bright, muscle/organs intermediate, blood is black (gray if not moving fast eg. aneurysms).
  - T2 water is bright (e.g. tumors, organs, inflammation). Blood appears black.
- Advantages:
  - Noninvasive, no radiation.
  - Calcium does not appear on MRA → less artifact.
  - Can detect flow to differentiate stenosis versus occlusion.
- Limitations.
  - Reactions to gadolinium contrast.

    Nephrogenic systemic fibrosis (NSF): seen in patients already with CKD. Involves skin, subcutaneous tissue, and less commonly internal organ systems → contractures, immobility, hyperpigmentation.
    - Ok to use if GFR > 40.
    - Pretreat if GFR 30–40.
    - Do not use if GFR < 30.
  - Inferior spatial resolution for lower extremity.
  - Long acquisition times.

Angiography

- Contrast types (4).
  - ionic monomers, ionic dimers, nonionic monomers, nonionic dimers,
  - nonionic contrast agent has decreased incidence of renal injury, especially in high risk/diabetic patients,
- CO_2: alternative to iodinated contrast if renal insufficiency concerns exist.
  - Do not use for thoracic aorta, coronaries, cerebral.
- Access:
  - Common femoral: allows for arteriotomy compression against femoral head. Risk of retroperitoneal bleed.

  - Radial: use with antispasmodic.
  - Brachial: sole arterial supply for upper extremity so increased risk of ischemia with complications.
- Advantages:
  - Gold standard for lower extremity.
  - Best resolution for lower extremity.
  - Allows treatment in same setting.
- Limitations.
  - Same as CT iodinated contrast limitations.

    If normal renal function: 700 cc iodine up to 300 mg/cc can be tolerated.
  - Wire can create artifact appearing as stenosis.
  - Contrast induced AKI.

    High risk pre-procedural regimen: *mucomyst* (600–1200 mg PO BID ×2 doses before and ×2 doses after) + *sodium bicarb* 1 h before, continue for 6 hrs after.

    Allergy pre-procedural regimen: *prednisone* 50 mg PO Q6hr ×3 doses ending 1 h before procedure + *diphenhydramine* 50 mg IV with *ranitidine* 150 mg IV at 1 h before.

    - If emergency, *hydrocortisone* 200 mgIV Q4hr during procedure.

Cerebrovascular

Duplex Ultrasound

- Velocity and waveform morphology correlated to angiographic stenosis.
  - Angiographic measurement of stenosis based on NASCET, ECST trials.

    NASCET: stenosis is in relation to distal normal ICA. NOT linearly related to stroke risk.

    ECST: stenosis is in relation to carotid bulb. Linearly related to stroke risk.

  - Contralateral stenosis, carotid kinking, AVM, carotid body tumors can over estimate stenosis.
  - Recent stroke, aneurysm, tandem plaques, arrhythmias can underestimate stenosis.
- Limitations:
  - Older patients have tortuosities that preclude all vessels and the bulb from being visualized in single plane.
  - Left vertebral more difficult to visualize versus right due to depth.
- Normal.
  - ICA: low peripheral resistance, continuous forward flow through diastole.

    ECA: high peripheral resistance, zero flow during diastole.

    Carotid Bifurcation: complex helical flow pattern.

    Consider using ratios if PSV inaccurate, e.g. arrhythmias.
- Abnormal.
  - Stenosis: increased velocity with distal turbulence. Graded using B-mode, Doppler and diameter (see Table 6.1) [1].

    Commonly at areas of flow separation such as carotid bifurcation or vertebral artery origin.

    Turbulence = spectral broadening.

    Plaque characteristics (Sensitivity (SN) 85–87%, Specificity (SP) 89–97%).

    - Calcification can cause acoustic shadowing.
    - Homogenous vs heterogenous.
    - Smooth vs irregular surface.
  - Trauma/Dissection.

    Tapering of ICA distal to bulb.

    Intimal flaps or dual lumens.

    High resistance Doppler waveforms.
- Intra-op (carotid endarterectomy):
  - Evaluate for thrombus, dissection, stricture.

    Velocity > 130 or ratio > 2.4 with clinical suspicion →consider re-exploration.

Table 6.1 Ultrasound criteria for the diagnosis of ICA stenosis using NASCET and ECST criteria. Taken with permission from Duplex scanning and spectral analysis of carotid bifurcation atherosclerotic disease. Current Therapy in Vascular and Endovascular Surgery 5th

Stenosis (%)		Duplex velocity criteria				Plaque and Lumen
NASCET	ECST	PSVic	EDVic	PSVic/PSVic	PSVic/EDVcc	
Normal	Normal	<125	<40	<2	<8	Absent
<50	<70	<125	<40	<4	<8	Present
50–59	70–76	125–230	40–100	2–4	8–10	Narrowing
60–69	77–82	125–230	40–100	2–4	11–14	Narrowing
70–79	83–89	230–400	100–125	5–5	15–20	Narrowing
80–89	90–94	230–400	>125	>4.0	21–30	Narrowing
90–99	95–99	>400°	>125°	>4.0°	>30°	Narrowing

Intimal flaps 3 mm or less in CCA or ECA can be left uncorrected.

Intimal flaps 1 mm or less in ICA can be left uncorrected.

- Advantages:

  Superior to angiogram in detecting flaps and intraluminal thrombi.

  Equal for strictures.

- Limitations:

  Inferior for visualizing distally.

  Requires operator skill and knowledge.

- Postop:
  - recurrence rate of ICA stenosis is 5–32% with >50% diameter reduction, with substantial portion occurring in the early postop period,

    Consider early postop study as baseline with follow up evaluations.

CT

- Good for carotid, but not vertebrobasilar evaluation: diminished resolution due to surrounding bone (MRI better).
- Patients with stroke should get CTA with nonionic contrast on admission.
  - CT does not show large cortical infarcts for first 3 h.
  - Possibly early signs of MCA infarct: lentiform nucleus obscuration and loss of insular ribbon (far from ACA/PCA collaterals).
  - Positive early CT contraindicates intervention secondary to hemorrhage risk.

    Can see 60% by 24 h.

    100% by 7 days
- Immediate (15–30 min) neurologic deficits after endarterectomy → re-explore for carotid endarterectomy (CEA) site thrombus.
  - Do not obtain CT (risk for delay in diagnosis).

Angiography

- Uses: intracranial hemorrhage, ischemic disease, aneurysms, AVMs, dural AVFs, vasospasm.
- Technique:
  - Five views (Carotid bifurcation at C4-C5) [1–3] (see Fig. 6.1).

    Townes: posterior circulation, structures aligned are petrous ridge and superior orbital rim.

    Caldwell: carotid siphon circulation, structures aligned are petrous ridge and inferior orbital rim.

    Posteroanterior: anterior circulation, structures aligned are petrous ridge and lower third of orbits.

    Waters: anterior/posterior circulation, 35–45 degrees caudal to cranial angulation.

    Lateral: anterior/osterior circulation, structures aligned are external acoustic meatus.

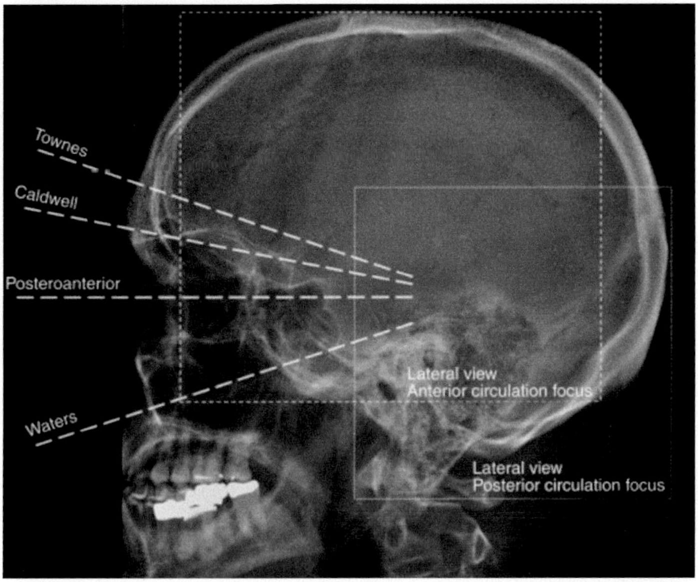

Fig. 6.1 Typical angiographic views. (Taken with permission from Arteriographic evaluation of cerebrovascular disease. Current Therapy in Vascular and Endovascular Surgery 5th)

- Advantage: high spatial resolution (200–300 μm).
- Limitations:
  - Neurologic Complications: stroke, ~1.3% (clinically evident stroke).
  - Clinically silent higher, unknown.
  - Associated with cardiovascular disease, increased fluoro time, age > 55.
  - Non-Neurologic complications: groin hematoma (most common, 0.4%). Associated with female, age > 75, diabetes, hypertension, low BMI, location/size, procedure duration, antithrombotic agents.
  - No real time analysis, risks associated with contrast use, risk of stroke, risk of anaphylaxis.

MR

- Accuracy 90%, SP 95% for carotid bifurcation stenosis, SN 95% for intracranial aneurysms.
- Gadolinium can help see plaque, plaque inflammation, plaque vascularity.
- DWI most sensitive imaging technique for acute infarction (over T1 and T2).
- Limitation: NSF (nephrogenic systemic fibrosis).

Positron Emission Tomography (PET)

- Use 18F-FDG (uptake by macrophages).
- Higher uptake in symptomatic/unstable plaques versus asymptomatic.
- Limitations: low resolution, ionizing radiation, cost, short life of tracers.

Intracranial TCD

- Uses:
  - Evaluate for acute cerebral ischemia.

    greatest yield closer in time to onset of symptoms. Higher yield for anterior circulation over posterior circulation,
  - Assess collaterals.

    Normal collaterals are dormant but open with occlusions (SN 86%, SP 92%). Can evaluate for hyperperfusion syndrome after CEA.
  - Eval for vasomotor reactivity (ability of brain to maintain perfusion despite changes in BP, pressure gradient, positioning).

    CO_2 alters tone. Hold breath → hypercapnia → watch MCA for vasomotor reactivity.

  - Detect, localize, and quantify cerebral embolism.
    Monitor during CEA, CABG, carotid angioplasty/stenting.
      - Number of microembolic signals in patients with asymptomatic carotid stenosis correlates with stroke risk.
  - Detect vasospasm, which may indicate hemorrhage (SAH).
    Spasm causes ischemic brain damage in up to 25% SAH patients.
  - Evaluate need for blood transfusion in sickle cell disease (higher mean velocities in ICA/MCA).
    Most common sickle cell cerebral infarct location is distal (intracranial) ICA and proximal MCA.
  - Confirm brain death.
  - Functional TCD used for higher cognitive function evaluation (language, memory).
  - Use with rtPA to increase thrombolytic effect.
- Technique:
  - Four US windows for transcranial Doppler evaluation with patient supine [4].
    Trans-temporal: evaluates intracranial circulation.
    Trans-orbital: evaluates ophthalmic artery and ICA siphon.
    Sub-mandibular: evaluates proximal intracranial ICA.
    Sub-occipital: evaluates basilar and vertebral circulation.
- Limitations:
  - operator dependent,
  - 15% rate of inadequate imaging through temporal windows especially in African-Americans, Asians, and females,
- Intraoperative TCD considerations.
  - 20 mHz pulsed device as accurate as arteriography for detecting ICA defects

Abdomen

Duplex Ultrasound

Aorta

- Measurement accurate within 3–5 mm.
- Ruptured AAA appears hypoechoic with retroperitoneal fluid around dilated aorta.
- Advantages:
  - US with contrast is NOT nephrotoxic (gas bubbles in phospholipid shell).
  - Can be used with non-contrasted CT in renal insufficiency patients for surveillance.
  - Post-EVAR - can detect type 1 and 3 endoleaks, less so type 2.
- Limitation: underestimates size up to 5 mm vs. CT.

Renal Arteries

- Use lower frequency transducers (2–3.5 mHz), B-mode pulsed Doppler waveforms, at 60 degree angle, transabdominal view to evaluate proximal renal artery.
- RAR = PSVrenal:PSVaorta ratio.
- Normal: low resistance, monophasic forward flow throughout cardiac cycle (similar to ICA).
- Abnormal: (stenosis often at origin).
  - Elevated PSV and RAR (see Table 6.2) [1, 5].

Table 6.2 Ultrasound criteria for the diagnosis of renal artery stenosis. Taken with permission from Duplex scanning in the Evaluation of Renal Arterial Occlusive Disease. Current Therapy in Vascular and Endovascular Surgery 5th

Renal Artery Status	Renal Artery PSV	RAR
Normal	<180 cm/s	<3.5
<60% stenosis°	≥180 cm/s	<3.5
≥60% stenosis°	≥180 cm/s	≥3.5
Occlusion	No signal	No signal

  - Decreased kidney size.
    Difference in kidney size by 1 cm between two kidneys may indicate disease.
    Atrophied kidney (6 cm or less) less likely to respond to intervention.
    Bigger kidney with low RRI (<0.8) preferred for intervention.
  - Renal parenchyma resistance quantified by EDR and RRI.
    End Diastolic Ratio (EDR) = EDV:PSV ratio.
    - Normal 0.3–0.47.
    - Abnormal <0.3.
      - Associated with decreased potential for reversible disease.

    Renal Resistive Index (RRI) = (PSV-EDV)/PSV [5].
    - Normal 0.7–0.8.
    - RRI > 0.8: highly unlikely to recover.
    - Associated with age, heart disease, diabetes, GFR, hypertension, renal allograft rejection, and failure of renal artery treatment.
- Limitations:
  - RAR unreliable if aorta is not normal (normal aorta PV 50–100) because RAR is based on ratio.
  - Regular criteria can overestimate stenosis if applied after stent placement.

Visceral Arteries

- Use 2–5 mHz transducer at <70% angle while patient fasted and head of bed elevated to 30 degrees.
- Inferior mesenteric artery hard to visualize.
- Normal.
  - Celiac: low resistance, continuous diastolic flow, no reverse flow component.
  - SMA: high resistance (PSV125–170), no spectral broadening, has reverse flow component, triphasic.
    biphasic with replaced R hepatic artery,

- Postprandial: only SMA PSV and EDV increase after meals; no reverse flow component.
- Occlusive.
  - Celiac:
    70% stenosis = PSV > 200 cm/s
    50% stenosis = EDV > 55 cm/s
  - SMA:
    70% stenosis = PSV > 275 cm/s or EDV > 45 cm/s
    Fasted: delayed PSV upstroke and prolonged EDV through diastole, PSV and EDV both elevated, spectral broadening present.
    Postprandial: blunted postprandial increase (PSV increases but not significantly).
  - In-stent stenosis during postoperative surveillance:
    PSV decreased after stent placement but still >275 despite pressure gradients and angiogram appearing normal.
- Aneurysm.
  - SMA: consider surgical intervention if 2 cm or greater.
- Dissection.
  - SMA: consider surgical intervention if 2 cm or greater and symptomatic, compressed true lumen, aneurysmal degeneration.
- Limitations:
  - bowel gas and body habitus limitations,
  - accessory branches often missed,

CT

- Gold standard for aortic postop surveillance.
  - no restrictions with body implants,
  - more resistant to metallic artifact,
  - allows aortic reconstruction views,

MR

- Useful for renal artery evaluation.
  - Look at differential flow: slower filling kidney concerning for stenosis.
  - Look at 3D gadolinium images and 3D phase images.

no stenosis on both, normal,
no stenosis on one, mild stenosis,
stenosis on both equally, borderline stenosis,
stenosis on both but worse on 3D phase, hemodynamically significant stenosis,

Angiography

- Technique:
  - 15–20 cc contrast or CO2 per second, 3 frames per second
  - Selective CA or SMA angiogram: 5 cc/s × 6–8 s.
  - Selective IMA angiogram: 2 cc/s × 6–8 s.
  - Delay by 10 s to see venous phase.
- Interpretation:
  - IMV filling but no portal vein filling during portal venous phase may indicate cirrhosis.
  - Evaluate for medial arcuate ligament.
    View lateral aortogram on inspiration and expiration.
    Expiration exacerbates compression.

Peripheral Arterial

Duplex Ultrasound

- Can identify location, length, severity of arterial lesion.
- Waveform reflects the vessel proximal to the point studied.
  - Normal = triphasic (forward systolic flow, short reverse flow, forward diastolic flow which declines to near 0).
  - Abnormal.
    Stenosis proximally eliminates the reversal of flow leading to biphasic waveforms (50% stenosis).
    Severe stenosis blunts the systolic upstroke leading to monophasic waveforms.
    More stenosis → more spectral broadening, increased PSV.
- Lower extremity (LE) [5–7].
  - Occlusion: compare ratio of PSV at tightest part of stenosis to normal portion of same artery – "step-up" [5–7].
    Stenosis >50%- >2 PSV stenosis: PSV normal.
    Stenosis >75%- >4 or PSV >400 or EDV >100.

  - Postop infrainguinal bypass graft surveillance:
    - Consider reintervention if PSV > 300 cm/s and or velocity ratio > 3.5.
  - Pseudoaneurysm.
    - Turbulent "to and fro" or "yin yang" flow.
    - Hematoma = echogenic without flow.
- Upper extremity (UE).
  - Occlusion.
    - Proximal SCA stenosis → early systolic deceleration.
    - Occluded SCA, subclavian steal→ vertebral reversal of flow on affected side, monophasic flow downstream.
    - Augmented findings with arm exercise.
- Arteriovenous Fistula (AVF).
  - Maturity assessment: flow volume, size, depth.
  - Failure associated with vein diameter <3 and artery <2.
    - Minimum AVG outflow vein diameter 4 mm.
  - Surveillance duplex improves detection of stenosis but increases number of fistulograms with unclear impact on patency.
    - Limitations: difficult to identify targets at cubital level.

Pressure-Based Noninvasive Evaluation [8–12]

- first screening for LE occlusive disease,
- Higher flow volume requires less narrowing to create hemodynamically significant stenosis.
  - Systolic pressure more affected than diastolic.
  - 60% stenosis is hemodynamically significant at rest
  - 40% stenosis is hemodynamically significant at exercise
- Limitations:
  - Calcification and improper cuff size can distort data.
  - Cannot use for profunda and hypogastric evaluation.
  - Collaterals can falsely decrease segment-segment pressure difference in the presence of adequate distal perfusion.
- ABI.
  - Detect presence and severity of disease.
  - Technique:
    - Appropriate cuff size = 40% arm width and 2× arm length.

Supine position, rested at least 15 min, cuff pressure at ankle, 8–10 mhz continuous Doppler.

Inflate cuff to 30–40 mmHg over SBP, then slowly deflate 2–4 mmhg/s. Note pressure when flow detected.

ABI – Highest ankle pressure (PTA vs ATA vs Peroneal) divided by higher of two brachial pressures (right vs left) [8, 13].

- ABI: >0.9 normal.
- ABI: 0.5–0.9 claudication.
- ABI: 0.4 Rest pain.
- ABI: <0.3 Tissue loss gangrene.

Surveillance: decrease in ABI of 0.15 or more is significant (more than expected CI/intraobserver error).

Uses:

- indicate presence of disease.
- Absolute ankle pressure >60 mmHg may indicate healing potential.

Limitations:

- tibial calcifications (diabetics, ESRD) can falsely elevate ABI. Suspect if ABI > 1.3, nonpalpable pulse.
- Does not localize disease.

- Stress testing.
  - Application: patients with claudication symptoms and suspicion for vascular etiology but normal resting ABI.
  - Treadmill Test: Exercise → increases flow to accentuate hemodynamic effect of stenosis.

    decreased vascular resistance of leg with increased resistance at lesion,

    Technique:

    - Obtain baseline ABI.
    - 1.5–2.5 mph at 10–12% grade for 5 min or until symptoms force patient to stop. Note time to symptoms
    - Obtain ABI Q30s ×2 min for × 5–10 min or Q2min ×10 min or until recovers while patient supine.

    Measure the magnitude of ABI drop as well as recovery time (correlates to severity of disease).

    - Abnormal if >0.2 ABI drop or drop >20% from baseline ABI, >25 mmHg ankle pressure drop, >2 min recovery, or.
        - 2–6 min to recover = single lesion
        - 6–12 min = multiple segments.

    Limited by patient's cardiopulmonary function.
  - Hyperemia Test: if treadmill test not practical.

    Technique:
    - Inflate thigh cuff above SBP to cause local circulatory arrest which leads to hypoxia and local vasodilatation.
    - Release cuff to cause transient increase in flow.

    The duration of increased blood flow correlates to period of ischemia.

    Measure the magnitude of ABI drop similar to treadmill test (which correlates to post exercise ABI of treadmill test).

    Recovery more rapid than that of treadmill test.

- Segmental Pressure Measurements (3 or 4 cuff technique).
  - BP readings at brachial, thigh (upper and lower if 4 cuff technique), upper calf, and above ankle.
  - Abnormal:

    Difference of 30 mmHg or more between two cuffs suggestive of stenosis of interval segment.
    - 30 mmHg difference between two thigh cuffs suggests SFA outflow disease.

    40 mmHg or more suggests complete occlusion of interval segment

    Abnormally elevated high thigh cuff (4 cuff technique) suggests aortoiliac inflow disease OR severe SFA and profunda disease.
  - Limitations.

    12 cm thigh cuff will have an elevated 20–30 mmHg artifact

    Up to 25% diagnostic error rate.

    3 cuff technique cannot differentiate aortoiliac inflow disease versus femoral/popliteal outflow disease
    Severe SFA and PFA disease can cause high thigh pressure.

- Plethysmography/PVR.
  - Technique: inflate cuff enough to occlude venous flow but not arterial flow so there is incremental change in volume of limb with each cardiac cycle → translates into waveform mimicking arterial waveform.
  - Volume in extremities vary during the cardiac cycle.
    Systole: Increase in total volume.
    Diastole: Return to resting volume.
  - Normal: brisk sharp rise to systolic peak with prominent dichrotic notch.
  - Abnormal:
    Early disease: no dichrotic notch. More gradual prolonged downslope.
    Moderate disease: rounded systolic peak.
    Severe disease: flattened wave.
- Toe Pressures/TBI.
  - Uses:
    Evaluate for wound healing potential.
    Helpful when tibial vessels are non-compressible.
  - Technique:
    Cuff size: width should be 20% of toe diameter.
    Otherwise same as ABI.
  - Normal.
    20–30 mmHg gradient between ankle and toe
    Great toe pressure roughly equals 60% ankle pressure.
    TBI 0.6 and up.
  - Abnormal.
    Claudication: TBI 0.3–0.6.
    Ischemic rest pain/tissue loss: <30 mmHg, almost never >40 mmHg.
    <30 mmHg: 95% failure rate for ulcer/amputation healing

    >30 mmHg: 15% failure rate for ulcer/amputation healing

- TcPO2.
  - Use: Assess wound healing potential.
  - Technique:

    Place small sensory on skin of interest, heat to 44 °C to induce hyperemia → decreased flow resistance.

    TcPO2 approximates true arterial oxygen pressure at that area.

    Readings in supine more predictive than readings in dependent position or during supplemental oxygen breathing.
  - Accuracy 87–100%.
  - Interpretation:

    TcPO2 > 40 mmHg associated with healing.

    TcPO2 < 30 mmHg associated with failure to heal.

    gray zone in 30–40 mmHg range,
  - Limitations: readings can be altered by infection, inflammation, edema.

Digital Subtraction Angiography

- Gold standard for lower extremity imaging.
- Advantages:
  - Diagnostic modality can be immediately followed by intervention.
  - Can obtain trans-stenotic pressure measurements.

    Hemodynamic significant = peak systolic pressure gradient >10 mmHg or mean > 5 mmHg or 10–15 after vasodilator given.
  - Can do on table 3D cone beam CT and reconstruction in technologically equipped imaging rooms.
- Limitation: invasive procedure, access site complications, contrast nephropathy.
  - Can use CO_2 in CKD patients.

CTA

- Traditionally considered limited in evaluation of lower extremities versus aortoiliac segment; newer multigated scanners with better resolution.
- Advantage:
  - "Noninvasive," fast, easily available
  - Diagnostic only.
  - Uniform enhancement of vessels allows for evaluation of arterial wall disease, collaterals.
- Limitations:
  - Radiation.
  - suboptimal imaging of calcified vessels,

MRI/MRA

- Imaging of choice for vascular anomalies (AVM, AVF): Can evaluate soft tissue extent.
- Both time-of-flight (TOF) and contrast MRA equal diagnostic accuracy versus DSA/conventional angio.
  - Can visualize low flow areas better than DSA.
  - MRA equals DSA accuracy from aorta to knee.
  - Contrast MRA less accurate versus DSA for below knee due to venous contamination.
  - TOF MRA more accurate versus DSA for below knee.
  - Contrast MRA equal or worse versus DSA for pedal vessels.

Peripheral Venous

Duplex

- Deep Venous Thrombosis.
  - Examine while head elevated.
  - Normal.
    - Continuous wave with respiratory variation.
    - Valsalva/breath holding/proximal compression decreases or abolishes flow.
    - Transient augmentation with release.

  - Abnormal.

    Thrombosed segments have no color flow.

    Non-compressible veins with probe.

    Adjacent collaterals have high pitched signal.

    Distal to occlusion: continuous flow without respiratory variation.

    Proximal to occlusion: respiratory variation present but no change with distal compression.
  - Thrombus characteristics.

    Acute = hypoechoic, homogenous, distended vein, floating tail at upper end of thrombus.

    Chronic = echoic, heterogenous, smaller vein, collaterals present.
  - Limitations.

    Cannot distinguish acute from chronic thrombus reliably.

    Fresh thrombus may not be distinguishable from flowing blood.

    False positives with late pregnancy, morbid obesity, ascites, IVC compression by intraabdominal masses.
  - Accuracy.

    89% in calf veins, 93% in proximal veins

    SN and SP ~95% with experienced sonographers.

- Venous Insufficiency.
  - Technique: Examine while patient standing to recreate maximum stimulus for reflux. Valsalva maneuver, foot flexion or compress proximal to probe to replicate calf function. Reverse velocity of 30 cm/s needed for consistent valvular closure.
  - Most common manifestation is varicose veins (varicose = >3 mm).
  - Normal.

    Compress proximal to probe or valsalva maneuver → no flow.

    Valves close in 2 s or less, and 0.5 s or less if standing.

    Femoral-popliteal valve closure time 1000 ms, saphenous system 500 ms, perforating veins 350 ms.
  - Abnormal = incompetent valves → retrograde flow → augmented flow during compression proximal to probe.
- Plethysmography.
  - Noninvasive method to estimate changes in volume → evaluate DVT and venous insufficiency.
  - General Technique:

    Supine, leg elevated 20–30 degrees, knee flexed 10–20 degrees to prevent popliteal venous outflow obstruction.

    Thigh occlusion cuff inflated to above venous pressure (50–60 mmHg) with sensor until limb volume increases to stable level.

    Release cuff rapidly – watch tracing go back to baseline.
    - Calf Venous Volume (VV) = rise to plateau.
    - Venous outflow (VO) = fall of tracing after rapid deflation.
    - VV and VO are reduced in VO obstruction or venous insufficiency.
  - Four types.

    Strain-gauge plethysmography (SGP).
    - Change in calf volume measured by stretches in mercury filled silastic tube.

    Impedance plethysmography (IPG).
    - Measures changes in electrical resistance using electrodes on calf.

    Photoplethysmography (PPG).
    - Uses light absorbance by hemoglobin as reflections of blood volume.
    - Resting recording obtained → patient does ankle flexion exercise to empty veins (tracing drops) → venous refill time (VRT) is measured (time taken to recover to 90% of baseline tracing).
    - Normal: 20–60 s.
    - Abnormal: <20 s.
    - Limitations: VRT may be reduced with PAD despite no venous reflux.

Air plethysmography (APG).

- Uses air filled cuff to measure changes in size in large sample area.
- Inflate cuff snuggly to leg and obtain baseline resting tracing while patient supine → inflate thigh cuff to 80 mmHg → patient stands and tracing increases (increases VV) → measure time to achieve 90% VV (aka 90% venous filling time) → patient tip toes (contracts muscle) causing venous emptying.
- VFI = venous filling index = rate of increase in volume on standing (ml/sec).
  - Normal: <2 ml/s.
  - Severe reflux: 30 ml/s. More reflux, higher VFI.
  - Accurate and can predict recurrence of ulcers.
- EF = percentage of volume removed from leg with one calf contraction. Measures efficacy of calf muscles to pump blood.
- RVF = residual volume fraction = volume expression as percentage of baseline volume of leg.
  - Lower is better.
- Limitations: requires patient cooperation. Less reliable to differentiate superficial versus deep reflux.

- Venography.
  - Ascending venography.

    Distal access at dorsal foot.

    Uses: Evaluate when duplex nondiagnostic or technically not feasible.
  - Descending venography.

    Uses: Evaluate for incompetent valves.
  - Other uses:

    Evaluate or venous stenosis, anatomic entrapment, venous malformations, tumor involvement.
  - No absolute contraindications.
  - Relative contraindications: cellulitis, iodine allergy, renal insufficiency.

Questions

1. A 58-year-old male with a history of diabetes presents with worsening exertional right calf pain over the last seven 7 months. Right ABI is 0.95 and left ABI is 1.01. What is the next most appropriate diagnostic test to confirm the diagnosis?
   (a) Digital subtraction angiography.
   (b) **Ankle pressure measurement with exercise treadmill.**
   (c) MRI of lumbar spine.
   (d) Pelvic X-ray.
2. On duplex evaluation of celiac artery compressions by median arcuate ligament is best evaluated during what phase of respiration?
   (a) **Expiration.**
   (b) Inspiration.
   (c) Valsalva.
3. A patient begins to have hypotension and bradycardia after IV iodinated contrast administration. What reaction is this patient having, and what agent should be administered?
   (a) **Vasovagal. Leg raise, IVF, atropine.**
   (b) Allergic. Epinephrine.
   (c) Iatrogenic. Fluid bolus.
   (d) Acute nephrotoxic reaction. Dialysis.

References

1. Nicolaides AN, Griffin M, Labropoulos N. Duplex scanning and spectral analysis of carotid bifurcation atherosclerotic disease. In: Stanley JC, Veith FJ, Wakefield TW, editors. Current therapy in vascular and endovascular surgery. 5th ed. Philadelphia, PA: Elsevier/Saunders; 2014.
2. Harrigan MR, Deveikis JP. Handbook of cerebrovascular disease and neurointerventional technique. New York: Springer Science & Business Media; 2009.
3. Pellerito JS, Revzin MV. Ultrasound assessment of native renal vessels. In: Pellerito JS, Polak JF, editors. Introduction to vascular ultrasonography. 6th ed. Philadelphia: Elsevier Saunders; 2012.
4. Nabavi DG, Ritter MA, Otis SM, Ringelstein EB. Ultrasound assessment of the intracranial arteries. In: Pellerito JS, Polak JF, editors. Introduction

to vascular ultrasonography. 6th ed. Philadelphia: Elsevier Saunders; 2012.
5. Cossman DV, Ellison JE, Wagner WH, et al. Comparison of contrast angiography to arterial mapping with color-flow duplex imaging in the lower extremities. J Vasc Surg. 1989;10:522–9.
6. Kohler TR, Nance DR, Cramer MM, et al. Duplex scanning for diagnosis of aortoiliac and femoropopliteal disease: a prospective study. Circulation. 1987;76:1074–80.
7. Gonsalves A, Bandyk DF. Duplex scanning for lower extremity arterial disease. In: AbuRhama A, Bergan J, editors. Noninvasive Vascular Diagnosis. New York: Springer-Verlag; 2000.
8. Pellerito JS, Polak JF, editors. Introduction to vascular ultrasonography. 6th ed. Philadelphia: Elsevier Saunders; 2012.
9. Baker JD. The noninvasive laboratory. In: Moore WS, editor. Vascular and endovascular surgery: a comprehensive review. 8th ed. Philadelphia: Elsevier Saunders; 2013.
10. Gomes AS. Principles of imaging in vascular disease. In: Moore WS, editor. Vascular and endovascular surgery: a comprehensive review. 8th ed. Philadelphia: Elsevier Saunders; 2013.
11. AbuRhama AF. Clinical and vascular laboratory evaluation. In: Cronenwett JL, Johnston KW, editors. Rutherford's vascular surgery. 8th ed. Philadelphia: Elsevier Saunders; 2014.
12. Blankensteijn JD. Vascular imaging. In: Cronenwett JL, Johnston KW, editors. Rutherford's vascular surgery. 8th ed. Philadelphia: Elsevier Saunders; 2014.
13. Kohler TR, Sumner DS. Vascular laboratory: arterial physiologic assessment. In: Cronenwett JL, Johnston KW, editors. Rutherford's vascular surgery. 8th ed. Philadelphia: Elsevier Saunders; 2014.

7 Vascular Medicine

Agustin Sibona, Alexander M. Schurman, and Christian Bianchi

Atherosclerosis

- Buildup and deposit of cholesterol into the vessel wall is the primary pathophysiology for the great majority of cardiovascular disorders.
- Classically divided into 6 types of lesions.
  - Type I: “initial lesion”; microscopic lipid deposits in infants and children.
  - Type II: includes “fatty streaks”.
  - Type III: “intermediate”; transition between indolent to subsequent clinically significant lesions.
  - Type IV: first of the “advanced lesions”; intra and *extra*cellular lipid accumulation form a lipid core known as atheroma.

A. Sibona (✉)
General Surgery, Loma Linda University Health, Loma Linda, CA, USA
e-mail: asibona@llu.edu

A. M. Schurman
Department of Surgery, University of California-Riverside/Riverside University Health System, Moreno Valley, CA, USA
e-mail: alexander.schurman@ruhealth.org

C. Bianchi
Vascular Surgery, Loma Linda University, Loma Linda, CA, USA
e-mail: cbianchi@llu.edu

A. Murga et al. (eds.), *The Vascular Surgery In-Training Examination Review (VSITE)*,
https://doi.org/10.1007/978-3-031-24121-5_7

  - Type V: fibrous tissue and smooth cells replace lipid distorted tissues and form fibroatheroma.
  - Type VI: type IV or V lesions which have been complicated by fissure, hematoma, and/or thrombus.
- Atherosclerosis is now considered a chronic inflammatory disease.
- Plaques tend to form in arterial areas with turbulent shear stress (i.e. carotid bifurcation).

Smoking

- Smoking produces between 440,000 and 480,000 deaths per year in the United States.
- 20% of the US population are active smokers
- Prevalence is higher in middle age males with lower social-economic status.
- Smoking is a known major risk factor for vascular disease mainly by three mechanisms:
  - Impairs normal vasomotor autoregulation by inhibiting the production of nitric oxide. Vessels do not dilate as they wound normally do after endothelial mechanical stress increases.
  - Smoking is a strong prothrombotic factor: platelets are hyperactivated and aggregate easily, plasminogen activation is decreased.
  - Inflammation: most of inflammatory markers are elevated in smokers. Leukocyte adhesion, activation, and migration are stimulated.
- Nicotine: increases HR, BP, and myocardial contractility.
- The body produces more RBC in response to carboxyhemoglobin, increasing the viscosity of blood.
- Strongest risk factor for claudication.
- Smoking cessation strategies: start with 5 A's.
  - Ask about tobacco use.
  - Advice tobacco user to quit.

  - Assess willingness to quit.
  - Assist with smoking cessation.
  - Arrange follow up.
- if patient is *not* willing to quit: use the 5 **R**'s,
  - explain the **R**elevance of quitting,
  - clearly delineate the **R**isks of smoking and,
  - pinpoint the **R**ewards of smoking cessation,
  - ask the patient to identify **R**oadblocks to quit smoking,
  - **R**epeat the intervention on each visit.
- Tx: nicotine replacement therapy: gum, inhaled, lozenge, nasal spray, transdermal patch, and/or meds:
  - Bupropion (Zyban): 150 mg daily for 3 days and then 150 mg BID.
  - Verenicline (Chantix): day 1–3: 0.5 mg daily; day 4–7 0.5 mg BID; >day 8 1 mg BID.
  - both medications should be started 1–2 weeks prior to quit date and are associated with neuropsychiatric side effects.

Hypertension

- SBP > 140 mmHg or DBP > 90 mmHg.
- Roughly 1/3 of the US population has hypertension (>60 yo: 65%).
- SBP has stronger association with PAD than DBP.
- Management: goal is <140/90 in age 30–59; < 150/90 in >60 yo.
  - Lifestyle modifications: for patients with pre-HTN (120–139/80–89): weight loss (DASH diet), limit sodium intake, aerobic physical activity 30 min/day, etc.
  - Medications.

    First line: thiazide diuretic.

    BP > 160/90: combination therapy (*diuretic + ACE inhibitor or ARB or beta blocker or CCB*).

    HTN + DM: use ACE inhibitor or ARBs.

    HTN + CHF: use beta blockers.

Dyslipidemia

- LDL-Cholesterol: most predictive for atherosclerotic risk.
  - Goal: <100 mg/dL in high risk (PAD) patients; <70 mg/dL in very high risk patient (i.e. CAD + PAD) [1].
- non-HDL-Cholesterol (total cholesterol *minus* HDL),
  - Useful in patients with elevated TG (triglycerides).
  - Secondary target after LDL goals have been met.
  - Goal: 30 mg/dL more than LDL goal.
- Management.
  - Lifestyle modifications: saturated fats <7%; cholesterol <200 mg/day, exercise.
  - Statins: first line; all patients with PAD should be on statin therapy.

    Reduce LDL and TG and increase HDL. Improve pain free walking time in claudication.

    Adverse reaction: mild elevation of LFTs (common but self-limiting; check labs at 6–8 weeks) and rhabdomyolysis (rare).
  - Niacin: most effective agent for increasing HDL levels.
  - Fibrate: mainly to treat hypertriglyceridemia.

Diabetes

- Type 1 (5–10%): absolute deficiency of insulin. Autoimmune destruction of beta cells.
- Type 2 (90–95%): insulin resistance + inadequate secretion. Stronger genetic component than type 1.
- Diabetes and cerebrovascular disease.
  - Stroke has two- to threefold higher incidence in DM, independent of other factors.
  - Small vessel lacunar infarct: most common manifestation.
- DM and PAD.
  - Distal arteries (popliteal, tibial, etc.) more commonly involved.

  - Most common cause of non-traumatic lower extremity amputation.
  - All patients with DM should have an ABI done at 50 years of age.
- Diabetic foot.
  - Prevention is the clue.
    - Mandatory annual foot exam.
    - Diabetic neuropathy evaluation.
    - Patient education.
    - Custom footwear for high risk patients.
- Management.
  - HbA1c goal: 6.5–7% [2].
  - Glucose target in hospital: 140–180 mg/dL for ICU patients; <140 mg/dL (fast) and <180 mg/dL (random) for ward patients [3].
  - Metformin—first line in general—has benefits on pts. with CV disease (independent of glycemic lowering properties).
  - If Hc A1c target still not met → add insulin or sulfonylurea.

Preoperative Assessment

Cardiovascular

- All major vascular procedures are high risk.
- The fundamental aspect of preoperative cardiovascular risk evaluation is to determine the patient's functional status:
  - Moderate or greater (>4 METs) → no further testing necessary [4].
  - Poor (<4 METs) or unknown → Pharmacologic stress testing (with subsequent coronary revascularization strategies is indicated).
- Revascularization generally reserved for patients with *unstable* angina.
- Beta-blockade has been associated with less perioperative cardiac events but increased stroke rate and bradycardia.

  - Medication should be continued on patients who have been on beta-blockade chronically [4].
  - Initiate therapy only on patients at high risk for cardiac ischemia.
- Antiplatelet therapy perioperative management:
  - General rule of thumb: evaluate risk of stopping vs risks of bleeding.
  - For patients with recent PCI and DAPT.

    Elective surgery should be delayed 30 days after BMS implantation and ideally 6 months after DES implantation [5].

    For urgent surgery, continue DAPT if possible or stop Plavix and restart as soon as possible after surgery.
- Warfarin: stop 5 days prior to surgery and restart 12–24 h after [6]; bridge with heparin on high risks patients (mechanical valve prosthesis, AFib with high CHADS2, etc.) (Fig. 7.1).

Pulmonary

- There is role for *routine* CXR and labs.
- Pa02 < 60 mmHg or PaCO2 > 45 mmHg: increased perioperative morbidity.
- Of all pulmonary toilet strategies, only lung expansion exercises (spirometry) have demonstrated clear benefits [7].
- Continue chronic bronchodilator therapy.

Renal

- Obtain baseline creatinine and GFR in all patients.
- Ideally dialysis the day before surgery.
- Contrast induced nephropathy.
  - Strongest predictor factor: previous renal disease.
  - Other factors: volume of contrast, other nephrotoxins, and dehydration.
  - Prevention: most of the guidelines support the use of perioperative IV normal saline or sodium bicarbonate, but none has shown to be superior to the other [8].
  - Consider using N-acetylcysteine.

ASA PS Classification	Definition	Examples, including, but not limited to:
ASA I	A normal healthy patent	Healthy, non-smoking, no or minimal alcohol use
ASA II	A patient with mild systemic disease	Mild diseases only without substantive functional limitations. Examples include (but not limited to): current smoker, social alcohol drinker, pregnancy, obesity (30 < BMI < 40), well-controlled DM/HTN, mild lung disease
ASA III	A patient with severe systemic disease	Substantive functional limitations: One or more moderate to severe diseases. Examples include (but not limited to): poor, controlled DM or HTN. COPD, morbid obesity (BMI ≥ 40), active hepatitis. alcohol dependence or abuse, implanted pacemaker, moderate reduction of ejection fraction. ESRD undergoing regularly scheduled dialysis, premature infant PCA < 60 weeks. history (>3 months) of MI. CVA, TIA. or CAD/stents.
ASA IV	A patient with severe systemic disease that is a constant threat to life	Examples include (but not limited to): recent (< 3 months) MI, CVA, TIA, or CAD/stents. ongoing cardiac ischernia or severe valve dysfunction, severe reduction of ejection fraction, sepsis, DIC, ARD or ESRD not undergoing regularly scheduled dialysis
ASA V	A moribund patient who is not expected to survive without the operation	Examples include (but not limited to): ruptured abdominal/thoracic aneurysm, massive trauma, intracranial bleed with mass effect, ischemic bowel in the face of significant cardiac pathology or multiple organ/system dysfunction
ASA VI	A declared brain-dead patient whose organs are being removed for donor purposes	

**The addition of "E" denotes Emergency surgery: (An emergency is defined as existing when delay in treatment of the patient would lead to a significant increase in the threat to life or body part)*

Fig. 7.1 ASA classification. Excerpted from the ASA Physical Status Classification System (1991) of the American Society of Anesthesiologists. A copy of the full text can be obtained from ASA, 1061 American Lane Schaumburg, IL 60173–4973 or online at www.asahq.org

Intraoperative Management

Cardiovascular

- ECG, Pulse oximetry, End-Tidal CO_2.
- Use arterial line in cases when hemodynamic instability from blood loss, fluid shifts, or significant cardiopulmonary disease is anticipated [9].
- CVP monitoring and PA catheter have fallen out of favor (replaced by TTE or TEE).
- TEE (Transesophageal echocardiography).
  - Better than TTE to evaluate thoracic aorta and aortic arch.
  - For non-cardiac surgery, its use is recommended for patient's known or suspected cardiovascular that might result in severe hemodynamic, pulmonary, or neurologic compromise [10].

Neurologic Monitoring

- CNS monitoring.
  - Regional anesthesia: neurologic monitor done by physical exam.

    Reliable in predicting the need for shunting but cannot use in patients with communication difficulties.
  - General anesthesia.

    Electroencephalogram: widely used but high rate of false positives.

    Transcranial Doppler: can detect micro emboli.
- Spinal Monitoring: done by Somatosensory and/or Motor Evoked Potentials.

Perioperative Antibiotics

- For vascular procedures: Cefazolin is the agent of choice (Vancomycin or Clindamycin for the β-lactam allergic) [11].
  - Administer antibiotics within 1 h from incision, adjust dose based on weight and re-dose if necessary.
- For endovascular procedures: routine administration of prophylactic antibiotics is only recommended when endografts are used [12].

Intraoperative Anticoagulation

- Heparin: classically given prior to arterial clamping (50–100 IU/kg). Repeat dose every 45–60 min.
- Monitor anticoagulation level with ACT or anti-Xa levels [13].

Blood Transfusions

- Generally accepted blood transfusion threshold → Hb < 7 mg/dL (8–10 for acute cardiac disease).
- Perioperative transfusion is independently associated with increased 30-day morbidity and mortality [14].
- Most common intraoperative strategy to reduce blood transfusion: IAT (Intraoperative blood recovery and transfusion).

Anesthesia Considerations in Vascular Surgery

- For open thoracic and/or abdominal surgeries, consider epidural analgesia:
  - Has shown superior postoperative analgesia [15].
  - Essential part of most of ERAS protocols.
- For ruptured aneurysms: prep and drape patient prior to anesthesia induction → high risks of rapid hemodynamic decompensation.

Postoperative Care and Management of Complications

Fluid Homeostasis

- Lactated ringer's is preferred over normal saline.
- Colloids are often used but have not demonstrated clear survival benefit [16].
- Goal directed strategies (toward HR, BP, or urine output) are preferred over established maintenance rates.

Nutrition

- Goal is to start *enteral* nutrition as soon as possible.
- Malnutrition: significantly poorer outcomes.
  - Low albumin and weight loss are better predictors for mortality than age [17].

  - Hypoalbuminemia is an independent risk factor for increased length of stay and wound complications.
- Most guidelines recommend goal of 25 kcal/kg/day.
- Consider TPN if more than 5–7 days of NPO are anticipated.

Colonic Ischemia
- Occurs in about **2%** of AAA repairs (5.2% for open repair and 1.8% for EVAR) [18].
- High mortality: 40%.
- Diagnosis: sigmoidoscopy or colonoscopy.
- Management: Hydration/Antibiotics → surgical exploration, possible reimplantation of IMA.

Hypertension
- "Acute on chronic" - Most commonly due to failure to restart regular antihypertensives
- Hypertensive crisis (urgency): >179 mmHg (SBP) or >119 mmHg (DBP).
- Hypertensive emergency: hypertensive crisis + signs of end organ dysfunction.
  - Management: reduce BP slowly (<25% during the first hour) *except* aortic dissection or stroke [19].
  - Typical drugs used: IV labetalol, IV nicardipine, IV esmolol, IV sodium nitroprusside.

Hypotension
- Most common cause: hypovolemia.
- First cause to rule out: hypovolemia secondary to bleeding.
- In vascular surgery patients, think about cardiogenic shock.

Postoperative Myocardial Infarction
- Myocardial *injury*: elevated cardiac troponin values with at least one value above the 99th percentile upper reference limit [20].
- Myocardial *infarction*: myocardial injury + symptoms, EKG changes, imaging evidence of wall motion abnormality or demonstration of thrombus on angiography.

  - Type I: due to coronary thrombosis.
  - Type 2: imbalance between myocardial oxygen supply and demand.
- Management: oxygen, afterload reducing agents (β-blocker/ACE-I), antiplatelet therapy, anticoagulation +/− PCI.

Arrhythmia

- Ventricular arrhythmia: SVT (incidence 4–13%), mono/poly VT, V Fib.
  - Etiologies: hypokalemia, hypomagnesemia; hypocalcemia, MI.
  - Treatment: β-blockers, calcium channel blockers, IV amiodarone.

    Unstable VT/Vfib: Electrical defibrillation.

    Polymorphic VT w/ prolonged QT - IV magnesium.
- Atrial fibrillation: most common arrhythmia in the post-op period.
  - Treatment: β-blocker, amiodarone, digitalis, calcium channel block.
  - If >48 h: need to evaluate for intracardiac thrombus.
  - UFH before cardioversion.
- Bradyarrhythmia: MI (most common cause), increased vagal tone.
  - Treatment: Atropine, Dopamine, Transcutaneous pacing.

Questions and Answers

1. What is the blood pressure goal for the management of hypertension in vascular surgery patients?
   (a) SBP > 140 mmHg or DBP > 90 mmHg.
   (b) SBP > 120 mmHg or DBP > 80 mmHg.
   (c) SBP < 140 mmHg or DBP < 90 mmHg.
   (d) SBP < 120 mmHg or DBP < 80 mmHg.
2. What is the ideal level of LDL-cholesterol in vascular surgery patients?
   (a) Less than 100 mg/dL.
   (b) Less than 70 mg/dL.

(c) Less than 70 mg/dL in high risk (PAD) patients; less than 100 mg/dL in very high risk patient (i.e. CAD + PAD).
(d) Less than 100 mg/dL in high risk (PAD) patients; less than 70 mg/dL in very high risk patient (i.e. CAD + PAD).

3. How long should elective surgeries be delayed after placement of a coronary drug-eluting stent?
   (a) 6 months
   (b) 6 weeks
   (c) 18 months
   (d) 2 years.
4. What is the stronger predictor factor for the development of contrast induced nephropathy?
   (a) Contrast allergy.
   (b) Baseline renal disease.
   (c) Dehydration.
   (d) Use of ACE inhibitors.
5. What is the perioperative antibiotic of choice for vascular procedures?
   (a) Cefoxitin (Vancomycin or Clindamycin for the β-lactam allergic).
   (b) Ertapenem (Clindamycin for the β-lactam allergic).
   (c) Cefazolin (Vancomycin or Clindamycin for the β-lactam allergic).
   (d) Ciprofloxacin – Metronidazole.

Answers: 1(c), 2(d), 3(a), 4(b), 5(c).

References

1. Grundy SM, Stone NJ, Bailey AL, et al. AHA/ACC/AACVPR/AAPA/ABC/ACPM/ADA/AGS/APhA/ASPC/NLA/PCNA guideline on the management of blood cholesterol. J Am Coll Cardiol. 2019;74:e285–350.
2. Arnett DK, Blumenthal RS, Albert MA, Michos ED, Buroker AB, Miedema MD. ACC/AHA guideline on the primary prevention of cardiovascular disease. J Am Coll Cardiol. 2019;140(11):e596–646. https://doi.org/10.1161/CIR.0000000000000678.
3. American Diabetes Association. Standards of medical care in diabetes--2014. Diabetes Care. 2014;37(Suppl 1):S14–80.

4. Fleisher LA, Fleischmann KE, Auerbach AD. ACC/AHA guideline on perioperative cardiovascular evaluation and management of patients undergoing noncardiac surgery: executive summary: a report of the American College of Cardiology/American Heart Association task force on practice guidelines. Circulation. 2014;130:2215–45.
5. Levine GN, Bates ER, Bittl JA, et al. ACC/AHA guideline focused update on duration of dual antiplatelet therapy in patients with coronary artery disease: a report of the American College of Cardiology/American Heart Association task force on clinical practice guidelines. J Am Coll Cardiol. 2016;68:1082–115. https://doi.org/10.1016/j.jacc.2016.03.513.
6. Douketis JD, Spyropoulos AC, Spencer FA, et al. Perioperative management of antithrombotic therapy: antithrombotic therapy and prevention of thrombosis, 9th ed: American College of Chest Physicians Evidence-Based Clinical Practice Guidelines. [published correction appears in Chest. 2012;141(4):1129]. Chest. 2012;141(2):e326S–50S.
7. Lawrence VA, Cornell JE, Smetana GW. Strategies to reduce postoperative pulmonary complications after noncardiothoracic surgery: systematic review for the American College of Physicians. Ann Intern Med. 2006;144:596–608.
8. Weisbord SD, Gallagher M, Jneid H, et al. Outcomes after angiography with sodium bicarbonate and acetylcysteine. N Engl J Med. 2018;378:603–14. https://doi.org/10.1056/NEJMoa1710933.
9. Gelb AW, Morriss WW, Johnson W, et al. World Health Organization-World Federation of Societies of Anaesthesiologists (WHO-WFSA) international standards for a safe practice of anesthesia. Can J Anaesth. 2018;65:698.
10. American Society of Anesthesiologists and Society of Cardiovascular Anesthesiologists Task Force on Transesophageal Echocardiography. Practice guidelines for perioperative transesophageal echocardiography. An updated report by the American Society of Anesthesiologists and the Society of Cardiovascular Anesthesiologists Task Force on transesophageal echocardiography. Anesthesiology. 2010;112:1084–96.
11. Bratzler DW, Dellinger EP, Olsen KM, et al. Clinical practice guidelines for antimicrobial prophylaxis in surgery. Am J Health Syst Pharm. 2013;70:195–283.
12. Chehab MA, Thakor AS, Tulin-Silver S, et al. Adult and pediatric antibiotic prophylaxis during vascular and IR procedures: a Society of Interventional Radiology practice parameter update endorsed by the cardiovascular and interventional radiological Society of Europe and the Canadian Association for Interventional Radiology. J Vasc Interv Radiol. 2018;29(11):1483–501.
13. Dieplinger B, Egger M, Luft C, Hinterreiter F, Pernerstorfer T, Haltmayer M, et al. Comparison between activated clotting time and anti-activated factor X activity for the monitoring of unfractionated heparin therapy in patients with aortic aneurysm undergoing an endovascular procedure. J Vasc Surg. 2018;68:400–7.

14. Obi AT, Park YJ, Bove P, Cuff R, Kazmers A, Gurm HS, et al. The association of perioperative transfusion with 30-day morbidity and mortality in patients undergoing major vascular surgery. J Vasc Surg. 2015;61(4):1000–9.e1. https://doi.org/10.1016/j.jvs.2014.10.106.
15. Wu CL, Cohen SR, Richman JM, Rowlingson AJ, Courpas GE, Cheung K, Lin EE, Liu SS. Efficacy of postoperative patient-controlled and continuous infusion epidural analgesia versus intravenous patient-controlled analgesia with opioids: a meta-analysis. Anesthesiology. 2005;103:1079–88; quiz 109-10.
16. Perel P, Roberts I, Ker K. Colloids versus crystalloids for fluid resuscitation in critically ill patients. Cochrane Database Syst Rev. 2013;28:CD000567.
17. Jabbour J, Abou Ali AN, Rabeh W, Al-Shaar L, Avgerinos ED, Habib RH. Role of nutritional indices in predicting outcomes of vascular surgery. J Vasc Surg. 2019;70(2):569–79.
18. Moghadamyeghaneh Z, Sgroi MD, Chen SL, Kabutey NK, Stamos MJ, Fujitani RM. Risk factors and outcomes of postoperative ischemic colitis in contemporary open and endovascular abdominal aortic aneurysm repair. J Vasc Surg. 2016;63:866–72.
19. Whelton PK, Carey RM, Aronow WS, et al. ACC/AHA/AAPA/ABC/ACPM/AGS/APhA/ASH/ASPC/NMA/PCNA guideline for the prevention, detection, evaluation, and management of high blood pressure in adults: a report of the American College of Cardiology/American Heart Association task force on clinical practice guidelines. Hypertension. 2018;71(6):e13–e115.
20. Thygesen K, Alpert JS, Jaffe AS, et al. Fourth universal definition of myocardial infarction. J Am Coll Cardiol. 2018;72:2231–26.

8 Cerebrovascular Disease

Beatriz Valdovinos Leong
and Christian Bianchi

Diagnosis and Management (Including Surgical and Endovascular) of Carotid Artery Occlusive Disease

Atherosclerotic Carotid Artery Disease: *Asymptomatic*

1. *Screening*: The United States Preventive Services Task Force (USPSTF) published screening for asymptomatic carotid artery stenosis and recommends against routine screening for asymptomatic carotid artery stenosis in the general population (Grade D) [1]. The Society of Vascular Surgery (SVS), however, recommends carotid screening with ultrasound in asymptomatic patients who are candidates for intervention in the following settings: multiple atherosclerotic risk factors, clinically significant peripheral arterial disease (PAD), clinically

B. V. Leong (✉)
Loma Linda University, Loma Linda, CA, USA
e-mail: beleong@llu.edu

C. Bianchi
Vascular Surgery of Loma Linda, Loma Linda University, Loma Linda, CA, USA
e-mail: cbianchi@llu.edu

A. Murga et al. (eds.), *The Vascular Surgery In-Training Examination Review (VSITE)*,
https://doi.org/10.1007/978-3-031-24121-5_8

significant coronary artery disease (CAD), presence of a bruit, patients undergoing coronary artery bypass grafting (CABG), and patients with weak radial pulses [2].

2. *Diagnosis*:
   (a) *Duplex ultrasound*: Ultrasound examination is considered first line imaging for carotid artery disease screening given its cost-effectiveness, high penetrance, and robust analysis. Consensus criteria for the grading of carotid artery stenosis, based on these ultrasound findings have been developed and summarized below (Table 8.1):
   (b) *MRA*: Rivals angiography as the gold standard for diagnosis of carotid artery stenosis. MRA is highly sensitive and accurate; however, there is no role for MRI in screening.
   (c) *CT*: Readily available, rapid, cheaper than MRA, offers submillimeter resolution, in addition to being relatively easy to interpret it also offers more anatomic detail compared to ultrasound. CTA has no role in screening; however, is it necessary if planning an endovascular intervention as well as in trauma and atypical presentations. Intracranial lesions and kinks are often missed on ultrasound and more clearly detailed on CT.
   (d) *Angiography*: Previously considered "gold standard" for diagnosis of carotid disease, catheter directed angiography is an invasive procedure with inherent procedural risks. As reported in Asymptomatic Carotid

Table 8.1 Consensus criteria for ultrasound based carotid artery stenosis

Degree of Stenosis	ICA PSV (cm/s)	Plaque estimate (%)	ICA/CCA PSV ratio	ICA EDV
Normal	<125	None	<2.0	<40
<50	<125	<50	<2.0	<40
50–69	125–230	>50	2.0–4.0	40–100
70–99	>230	>50	>4.0	>100
Near occlusion	High, low, or undetectable	Visible	Variable	Variable
Total occlusion	Undetectable	Visible, no detectable lumen	N/A	N/A

Atherosclerotic Study (ACAS) study, approximately 50% (2.6% of patients) of the procedural morbidity incurred during angiography was attributable to embolic strokes; permanent strokes also occurred at rate of 0.2%; additional complications include hematoma 4%, anaphylaxis 0.03%, and death 0.06%. While angiography is not indicated for screening or first line for diagnosis it is highly valuable in certain clinical scenarios.

3. *Management*
   (a) *Best Medical Therapy (BMT)*: Aimed at reducing risk factors is first line therapy for all patients with carotid stenosis, including those who will undergo surgical intervention. The American Heart Association (AHA) has published perioperative cardiovascular guidelines [3]. Management of comorbidities such as HTN, DM, HLD and reducing patient factors such as smoking is essential.
   - *Beta-Blockade*: BP control is critical for primary stroke reduction. POISE trial supporting SVS guidelines of goal heart rate 60–80 in patients with carotid stenosis [4]. There is a 33% reduction in stroke risk for every 10 mmHg reduction in blood pressure.
   - *Antiplatelet*: Significantly reduces the risk of stroke in high risk patients with overall 25% reduction in stroke [5]. Use of plavix has also been investigated, and studies show decreased preoperative embolization without increased risk of bleeding.
   - *Heparin*: There is no reported benefit of routine heparin administration for acute stroke due to increased risk of hemorrhagic conversion. In crescendo TIA the use of IV unfractionated heparin has been described to control the risk of thrombosis/embolic phenomena prior to surgical intervention.
   - *Protamine*: General anesthesia versus local anesthesia for carotid surgery (GALA) looked at protamine use and found it to be safe, with no association with increased thrombosis leading to stroke [6].
   - *Statin*: The use of statins offers several benefits to carotid artery stenosis patients, including reducing

cholesterol level which confers an overall protective effect for the patient, satins are associated with reduced carotid artery intimal-media thickness in addition to lower rate of cardiovascular events [7]. Statin use has also been shown to have protective effects when it comes to developing recurrent carotid artery stenosis, as well as late anatomic failures after carotid endarterectomy (CEA) as shown in the SPARCL trial [8].

(b) *Surgical*
  - Indications for carotid endarterectomy are well delineated; evidence based guidelines are published by the SVS, according to these guidelines CEA should be considered for patients who are asymptomatic and have 60–99% carotid stenosis, if the perioperative risk of stroke and death is less than 3% *AND* the patient has at least a 3–5 year life expectancy. Two landmark trials ACAS and ACST have demonstrated the efficacy of CEA in asymptomatic patients who have at least 60% carotid artery stenosis.
    - *Asymptomatic Carotid Artery Stenosis (ACAS)* [9] multicenter randomized controlled trial, enrolled 1662 patients with carotid stenosis of greater than or equal to 60%.

      Stroke with BMT: 11% at 5 years.

      Stroke with CEA: 5.1% at 5 years.
    - *Asymptomatic Carotid Surgery trial (ACST)* [10] multicenter randomized controlled trial enrolling 3120 patients with asymptomatic carotid stenosis of greater than or equal to 60%.

      Stroke with BMT: 11.8% at 5 years.

      Stroke with CEA: 6.4% at 5 years.

(c) *Endovascular*: While there is a paucity of data regarding asymptomatic patients and carotid artery stenting, data from the Stenting and Angioplasty with Protection in Patents at High Risk for Endarterectomy (SAPPHIRE) [11] trial included asymptomatic patients and determined carotid stunting was not inferior to CEA when looking at the primary outcome of 30-day incidence of death, stroke, MI; this occurred in 5.4% of asymptomatic patients who underwent carotid artery stenting (CAS) and 10.2% of those who underwent CEA. This trial has been met with many criticisms, however, primarily the high incidence of postoperative complications for patients who are asymptomatic, conferring a minimal benefit of intervention at all. The Carotid Stenting versus Endarterectomy for Treatment of Carotid Artery Stenosis (CREST) [12] trial randomized 2502 patients, of which 1181 patients were asymptomatic, to CAS versus CEA and analyzed their outcomes for combined stroke or death. Among asymptomatic patients the risk of stroke or death was 4.5% for CAS, and 2.7% for CEA. Peri-procedural ipsilateral stroke occurred in 2.5% of CAS patients and only 1.4% of CEA patients. Importantly these large trial results have not been replicated, thus real life CAS results may be considerably different. The upcoming CREST 2 trial may better elucidate some unanswered questions when it comes to modern BMT compared to CEA and CAS. Additionally, new technology of trans carotid arterial revascularization (TCAR) newly approved in the US, eliminates the need to cross the arch with wires and catheters reducing the ipsilateral embolic stroke risk as well as providing a proprietary flow reversal system which additionally protects the brain from emboli. Early adoption of TCAR shows promising results with currently available registry data.

- SVS currently does not recommend CAS for asymptomatic patients.

Atherosclerotic Carotid Artery Disease: *Symptomatic*

1. *Diagnosis*: stroke and TIA workup typically includes a hyperacute CT and CTA of the head and neck which gives an accurate degree of stenosis and amount of contralateral disease. Duplex US still provides valuable information, provides

information about accessibility of lesions, physiologic information regarding inflow stenosis; in addition, carotid US is the preferred modality for surveillance after intervention.

2. *Management*
   (a) *Surgical*: CEA is recommended as first-line treatment for all patients who have symptomatic carotid stenosis of 50–99% stenosis. North American Symptomatic Carotid Endarterectomy Trial (NASCET) demonstrated that CEA was not beneficial compared to maximum medical therapy in symptomatic patients with less than 50% carotid artery stenosis, however, was highly beneficial in those patients with >50% stenosis.
      - *NASCET 1 trial* [13] 659 patients with acute strokes (within 120 days), and ipsilateral carotid artery stenosis of 70–99% was randomized to BMT and CEA; primary outcomes of death or stroke. The study was terminated early due to the clear benefit of CEA over BMT.
        – Stroke with BMT: 24.5% at 2 years.
        – Stroke with CEA: 7% at 2 years.
      - *NASCET 2 trial* [14] 858 patients with symptomatic carotid artery stenosis of 50–69% were randomized to BMT and CEA.
        – Stroke with BMT 15% at 2 years (22.2% at 5 years).
        – Stroke with CEA 9% at 2 years (15.7% at 5 years).
      - *European Carotid Surgery Trial (ECST)* [15] demonstrated that CEA is superior to BMT.
        – Stroke in BMT 26.5% at 3 years.
        – Stroke with CEA 7% at 3 years.
   (b) *Endovascular*: SVS recommends CAS be performed in symptomatic patients with 50–99% carotid artery stenosis who are high risk for CEA. High risk criteria generally fall into two categories anatomic and physiologic, a summary of the high risk criteria is depicted in Table 8.2. The CREST trial demonstrated a lower incidence of non-fatal MI in patients undergoing CAS compared to CEA.

Table 8.2 Anatomic and physiologic factors affecting perioperative morbidity with carotid intervention. *Reproduced with permission from Rutherford's Vascular Surgery and Endovascular Therapy*

Favors CEA	Favors Stenting	Favors Medical Management
Age > 70	Prior neck radiation	Life expectancy <3 years
Severe aortic arch calcification	Prior radical neck dissection or laryngectomy	Asymptomatic patient with: CHF w/ EF <30% Severe uncorrectable CAD Oxygen dependent COPD
Type III arch	Patent tracheostomy	
Carotid artery tortuosity	History if cranial nerve injury	
Circumferential heavy plaque/calcification	Proximal common carotid artery stenosis below clavicle	
Ulcerated/soft plaque	Distal ICA stenosis above C2	
Near occlusive lesion	Symptomatic carotid stenosis with: CHF w/ EF <30% Severe uncorrectable CAD Oxygen dependent COPD	
Extensive plaque >15 mm		

- Anatomic.
  - Location: Lesions extending above C2, or below the clavicle can be difficult to access.

    Maneuvers for high carotid lesions:
    - Division of digastric muscle.
    - Mandible subluxation (required Nasotracheal intubation).
    - Mandible division.

    - Re-operative field: i.e., repeat carotid stenosis after prior CEA, prior neck/lymph node resection/neck surgery.
    - Cervical stoma.
    - Neck radiation.
  - Physiologic.
    - Renal: ESRD on dialysis.
    - Cardiac: CHF (NYHA III or IV), EF <30%, left main coronary disease, aortic valve dysfunction.
    - Pulmonary disease (oxygen dependence or steroid dependence).
    - Contralateral carotid occlusion.

Carotid Artery Fibromuscular Dysplasia (FMD)

1. Background
   (a) Incidence ~3.4% of all cases undergoing operations. With bilateral FMD in 35%–85%, predominantly affects women 40–60 years old.
   (b) Four types of FMD, type 2 affects carotid most (medial fibroplasia) appearing as a string of beads on an angiogram (Fig. 8.1).
   (c) Concomitant disease:
   - Carotid bifurcation occlusive disease 20%.
   - Extracranial carotid artery aneurysms 20%.
   - Carotid artery dissection 5–15%.
   - Vertebral artery FMD 7–38%.
   - Intracranial aneurysms and occlusive disease 10–50%.
   - Renal Artery FMD 8–40%.
2. *Diagnosis*: Patients who are symptomatic may present with a range of symptoms from TIA (31–42%), to stroke (12–27%), and amaurosis fugax (22–28%). They may have dizziness, headache, altered mentation, pulsatile tinnitus, or neck pain; and usually lack the typical risk factors of atherosclerosis.
   (a) *Duplex*: Useful for screening, for evaluating an incidental finding on physical exam, and for long term surveillance.

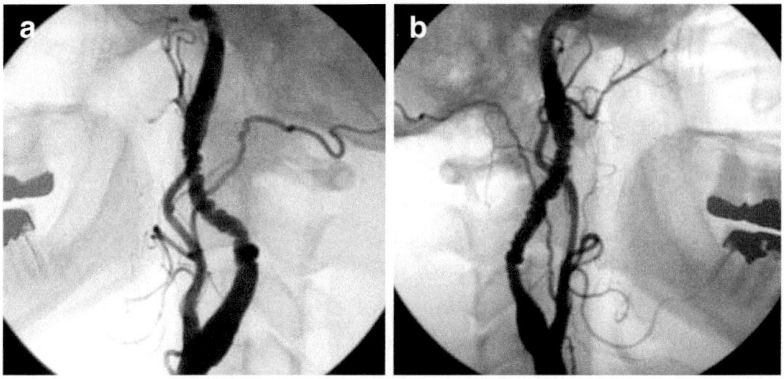

Fig. 8.1 (**a**) Carotid angiogram demonstrating the classic appearance of fibromuscular dysplasia in the usual locations opposite C1-C3 vertebral bodies and intervening disks. Note the low bifurcations in the ICA. (**b**) The carotid bifurcation is typically spared as the internal carotid artery is elongated, tortuous, and often demonstrates kinks. (Reproduced with permission from Rutherford's Vascular Surgery and Endovascular Therapy)

(b) *Arteriography*: Ideal study to identify locations and number of stenosis, tortuosity, kinks, of carotid arteries, as well as dissections (which may best benefit from stenting and minimal dilation), aneurysm (which should be managed with surgical approach).
(c) *CTA*: May replace traditional use of angiography in FMD, also has the added benefit of delineating contralateral and intracranial lesions.
(d) *MRA*: Not useful in carotid FMD due to signal dropout with tight lesions, also gives beaded appearance to normal arteries.

3. *Management*: Although there is a paucity of data regarding ideal management for carotid artery FMD, the accepted management for asymptomatic patients is typically with medical management including antiplatelet therapy for primary stroke prevention, statin, and comorbidity management.
   (a) *Surgical*: Few series describe surgically dilating the carotid artery stenosis under direct visualization, with acceptable peri-operative and long term outcomes. Kinks, coils, and aneurysms also benefit from surgical correction.

Surgically inaccessible lesions may also be treated with open-access balloon dilation where the length of the carotid artery is manually dissected and balloon dilated, the open access allows the operator the ability to back-boned the artery minimizing embolization.

(b) *Endovascular*: Percutaneous intervention is the preferred approach in more proximal carotid FMD. Angioplasty is offered to patients with intractable symptoms; these interventions carry similar risks to carotid angiography with interventions. Distal embolic protection should be considered, the use of stents has not been investigated in this setting although extrapolating from renal artery FMD data stents is typically not indicated. The endovascular angioplasty technique is pictured below (Fig. 8.2).

Carotid Artery Radiation Injury

1. *Background*: Radiation injury to the carotid leads to damage to the artery and acceleration of atherosclerosis. Post-radiation patients have an increased prevalence of carotid artery stenosis, and in addition to increased prevalence the disease can present at a much younger age. Neck radiation is associated with an increased risk of cerebrovascular events (OR 9.0) [16], highest among head and neck cancer patients.
2. *Diagnosis*: Starts with a detailed history and physical examination. Duplex US is indicated after radiotherapy however there are no guidelines regarding timing or frequency. If ultrasound detects a stenosis, this should be followed by cross-sectional imaging either MRA or CTA due to difference in lesions. Radiation induced stenosis tends to affect the common carotid, distal internal carotid artery than typical atherosclerotic disease and can often present with more diffuse stenosis as well.
3. *Management*: Decision regarding therapy should be a multi-specialty decision, considering each patient's disease individually. Revascularization in any patient who is symptomatic and has a stenosis of >50%, or in asymptomatic patients with ste-

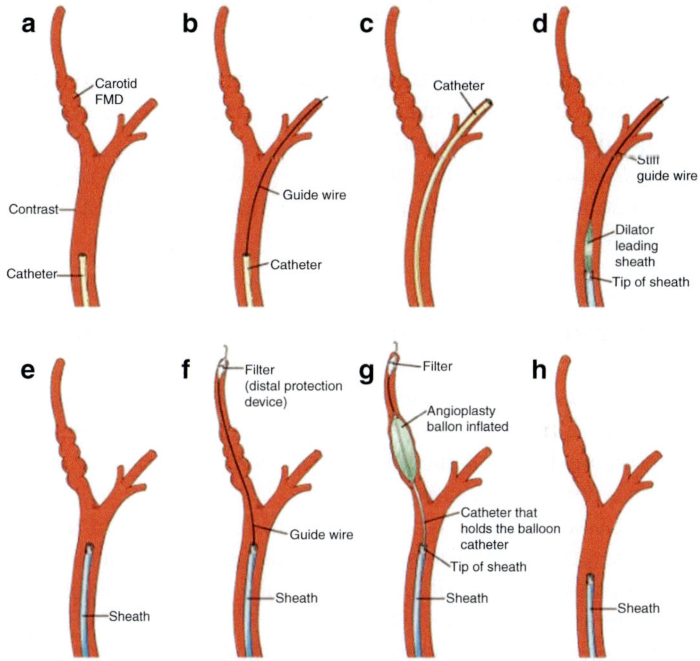

Fig. 8.2 Fibromuscular dysplasia endovascular technique. (**a**) Internal carotid artery narrowed by fibromuscular dysplasia. An arteriogram was performed through a carotid catheter. (**b**) guidewire placed in the external carotid artery through the use of road-map arteriogram of the carotid bifurcation. (**c**) Cerebral catheter advanced into the external carotid artery. (**d**) Stiff guidewire advanced into the external carotid artery. The carotid artery access sheath is advanced over the exchange guidewire. (**e**) Carotid sheath in place with the tip of the sheath in the distal common carotid artery. (**f**) Cerebral protection device in place in the distal internal carotid artery. (**g**) Balloon angioplasty of the fibromuscular lesion in the internal carotid artery. (**h**) After balloon angioplasty, the lumen improves significantly. (Reproduced with permission from Rutherford's Vascular Surgery and Endovascular Therapy)

nosis of >70% is recommended. Prior radiation is identified as a risk for open surgical therapy, and thus stenting should be considered. Patients who are at high risk for both procedures, or have an estimated life expectancy that is low are best managed with medical therapy.

4. *Surgical*: Preferred in *younger* post-radiation patients due to stenting being associated with higher rates of recurrent stenosis as well as in patients who are not eligible for carotid stents or have allergies to material used in stents or have contrast allergies or contraindications.
5. *Endovascular*: Carotid stenting is preferred for most post-radiation patients since it eliminates the risk of cranial nerve injury.

Uncommon Carotid Condition: Carotid Body Tumor

1. *Background*: Carotid body tumors are rare paragangliomas that arise from the chemoreceptors at the carotid bifurcation, most are benign although can be locally destructive and a small percentage can be malignant.
2. *Diagnosis*: Patients typically present for work-up of a neck mass, a thorough history and physical may identify a pulsatile mass although the differential is quite broad. Radiographic imaging is critical, usually starting with a duplex US, and is the most important noninvasive method of identifying and characterizing carotid body tumors. CTA and MRA offer much of the same details as gold standard angiography. *Percutaneous biopsy is contraindicated.* The Mayo group developed a classification system based on neurovascular involvement.
   (a) Shamblin Classification (Fig. 8.3).
      - Group I: smaller, can be easily dissected off walls of the carotid arteries.
      - Group II: larger, more adherent to adventitia, partially surround carotid.
      - Group III: intimately adherent to the vessels, encasing the carotid arteries.
3. *Management*: Surgical resection remains the primary treatment for carotid body tumors, smaller tumors are easier to remove, most tumors become locally invasive or destructive. There are no effective chemotherapeutic agents for these

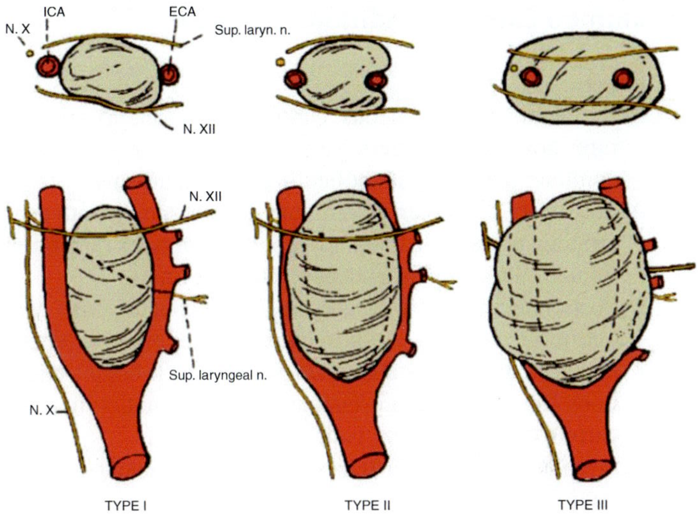

Fig. 8.3 The Shamblin classification describes the staging of carotid body tumors and can assist in preoperative planning. Type I tumors are smaller and can be easily dissected from the walls of the carotid arteries in the periadventitial plane. Type II tumors are larger, more adherent to the adventitia, and partially surround the carotid vessels. Type III tumors have more intimate adherence to the vessels and encase the internal and external carotid arteries. (Reproduced with permission from Rutherford's Vascular Surgery and Endovascular Therapy)

tumors, and radiation therapy is only used as a treatment adjunct.

(a) *Surgical*: Careful preoperative work-up to determine extent of tumor, adjacent structures involved including nerves, and distal synchronous lesions such as pheochromocytomas should be ruled out.
(b) *Endovascular*: Preoperative embolization of mass remains controversial, and selectively used by surgeons in particular with Shamblin II and III tumors; embolization of the ECA branches feeding the mass with the goal of reducing intraoperative blood loss.

Uncommon Carotid Condition: Aneurysm

1. *Etiology*
   (a) Extracranial spontaneous carotid artery aneurysms are rare; however, degenerative (atherosclerosis) is the most common pathology identified in these aneurysms.
   (b) Secondary carotid aneurysms are due to trauma; both penetrating trauma (leading to pseudoaneurysm) and blunt trauma (dissection may degenerate over time).
   (c) Post-endarterectomy aneurysms/pseudoaneurysms: second most common. Additionally, degeneration of venous patches can lead to aneurysm formation. Indolent infections can also lead to pseudoaneurysm formation in post-carotid endarterectomy patients.
   (d) Dysplasia (such as FMD) can also lead to aneurysm formation.
2. *Diagnosis*: Duplex US is the first line diagnostic modality of choice or evaluation of carotid artery aneurysm, CTA and MRA may be used if the aneurysm is not entirely visualized on ultrasound, or to gain information regarding adjacent anatomy and structures. Angiography is no longer considered critical in the diagnosis of carotid aneurysms however is still employed rarely, in particular if aneurysm ligation is being entertained a test balloon occlusion is done to evaluate physiologic effect of such ligation.
3. *Management*: Indications for intervention include patients who are symptomatic due to the aneurysms, an aneurysm size of >2 cm, mycotic etiology, presence of thrombus in the aneurysm due to risk of embolization, and enlargement over time; although medical management with antiplatelet or anticoagulation and serial imaging has been shown to be effective in patients with small aneurysms <2 cm, or those who are exceedingly high risk for surgery.
   (a) *Surgical*
      - Ligation.
      - EC to IC bypass.
      - Resection and reconstruction.

(b) *Endovascular*: Offers the advantage of avoiding a potentially difficult dissection in the neck, also essential in surgically inaccessible lesions.
   - Bare Metal Stent with trans-stent coiling of the aneurysm.
   - Percutaneous thrombus injections.

Carotid and Vertebral Artery Dissection: Traumatic Vs Spontaneous

1. *Etiology*: Extracranial cervical arteries are mobile and adjacent to fixed bony structures, thus are susceptible to dissections. Minor trauma usually preceded by a minor trauma, chiropractic manipulation, although 25% of patients have a connective tissue disorder such as fibromuscular dysplasia, Ehlers-Danlos syndrome, cystic medial necrosis, Marfan syndrome, autosomal dominant polycystic kidney disease, and osteogenesis imperfecta type I.
2. *Diagnosis*: Patients may describe an antecedent small traumatic event, and present with lateralizing symptoms, or evolving symptoms (headache, neck pain, hemiparesis, hemiplegia, dysphagia, aphasia, Horner syndrome, TIA, or stroke). There is no consensus recommending routine evaluation with imaging; however, the level of suspicion must be heightened in certain clinical scenarios such as high impact head and neck trauma. Carotid US is readily available; however, four vessel selective angiography is still considered "gold standard" for diagnosis and allows the possibility of intervention and surgical planning; although invasive procedures are not without risk (1–2% of access related complication, 1–2% contrast nephropathy, 1% risk of stroke) [17]. CTA and MRA allow a noninvasive means of detection as well as give additional anatomic details. Both are superior to conventional angiography in this way in addition to being more sensitive for intramural hematoma [18].

3. Management.
   (a) *Medical*: Antithrombotic therapy aimed at protection against micro emboli coming from intimal tear; full anticoagulation is also thought to be protective; however, this increased the risk of hemorrhage (intracranial hemorrhage 0.5% compared to 0% without antiplatelet therapy alone) [19].
      - CADISS trial-prospective multicenter RCT looking at carotid and vertebral artery dissections treated with antiplatelet alone vs. anticoagulation for 3 months. Outcomes included ipsilateral stroke, TIA, major bleeding, and residual stenosis. CADISS trial showed no statistically significant difference in the recurrence of stroke (2% antiplatelet vs 1% for anticoagulation $p = 0.63$). There was one patient who developed a major bleeding complication in the anticoagulation group which was not observed in the antiplatelet alone group [20].
   (b) *Surgical*
      - Acute Indications [21].
         (a) deteriorating neuralgic symptoms despite medical treatment,
         (b) compromised intracranial blood flow,
         (c) contraindications to antithrombotic therapy,
         (d) rapidly expanding or symptomatic aneurysm,
      - Chronic indications (<6 months).
         (e) Persistent high-grade stenosis.
         (f) New aneurysmal degeneration (>2x size of ICA).
   (c) *Endovascular*: indications same as above, endovascular procedures tend to have less morbidity and less mortality compared to surgical interventions. Carotid artery stenting requires dual antiplatelet therapy (DAPT) with aspirin and Plavix prior to intervention, and for at least 6 weeks postoperatively. Strategies include bare metal stenting, covered stenting, aneurysm coiling, stent assisted coiling, embolization of vessels [22]. *There is no data supporting surgical or endovascular treatment of asymptomatic patients with carotid artery dissections.*

Diagnosis and Management Including Surgical and Endovascular of Brachiocephalic and Vertebrobasilar Arterial Disease

Brachiocephalic Artery Disease

Brachiocephalic disease can present in a variety of ways, TIA, stroke, upper extremity ischemia with the most common etiology being atherosclerotic disease, however dissection, embolic phenomena, and trauma. Knowing the patient's anatomy is critical to understanding symptomatology. Aortic arch anatomy and incidence vary widely (Fig. 8.4). Variations include a normal anatomy in 70–74% (Fig. 8.4a), a bovine arch with a common origin of left common carotid and innominate arteries (Fig. 8.4b), or directly off the innominate artery (not pictured) in 13–20% of patients, an aberrant left vertebral artery (Fig. 8.4c) in 2–6% of patients, as well as an aberrant right subclavian artery (Fig. 8.4d) occurring in 0.5–2% of patients, additionally aberrant left subclavian which is not pictured in <0.5% patients and right aortic arch, not pictured, occurring in <0.1% patients. The course of an aberrant right subclavian artery has been further delineated to occur behind esophagus 80%, between esophagus and trachea in 15%, or anterior to trachea 5%.

Brachiocephalic Occlusive Disease

1. *Diagnosis*: A careful history and physical examination including bilateral upper extremity pulse and blood pressure checks is important. Carotid US allows evaluation of subclavian and vertebral arteries for reversal of flow alluding to subclavian proximal disease. CTA has largely replaced conventional angiography when it comes to diagnosis of arch vessel disease.
2. *Management*: Indications for interventions largely depend on the symptomatology of the patient. As atherosclerotic disease is multifocal, identifying symptoms and chronicity to guide interventions is important. Intervention is clearly indicated in

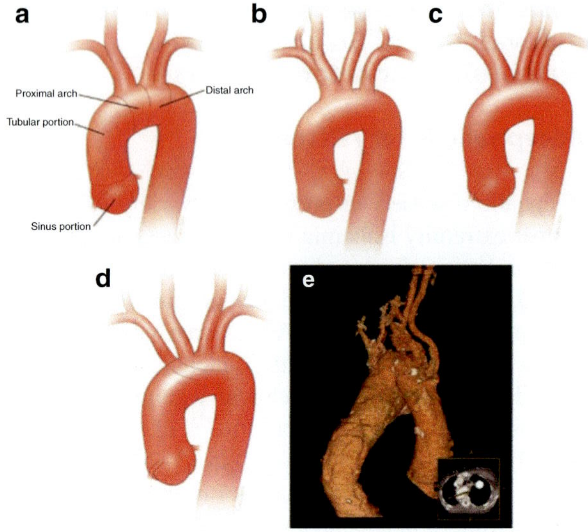

Fig. 8.4 Normal and Variant Aortic Arch Anatomy (**a**) The normal aortic arch configuration (70–74% prevalence) consists of three great vessels originating from the arch of the aorta. The first branch is the innominate artery which branches into the right subclavian artery and right common carotid artery. The second branch is the left common carotid artery. The third branch is the left subclavian artery. (**b**) the "bovine arch" subtype II (13–20% prevalence) consists of the innominate and left common carotid arteries sharing a common origin (more common in African Americans 25% vs 8% in whites). In type I "bovine arch" the left common carotid artery originated from the innominate artery, usually within 1 cm of the aortic arch (more common in African Americans 10% compared to whites 5%). (**c**) The aberrant left vertebral artery (2–6% prevalence) arising directly from the aortic arch, most frequently between the left common carotid and left subclavian arteries. (**d**) The aberrant right subclavian artery (0.5–2% prevalence) occurs as the last branch of the aortic arch, arising distal to the left subclavian artery. It typically courses posterior to the esophagus (80%), between the esophagus and trachea (15%) or anterior to the trachea or mainstem bronchus (5%). The aberrant left subclavian artery occurs less frequently (<0.5% prevalence) and manifests as the second branch off the aortic arch arising proximal to the left carotid artery. (**e**) The right-sided aortic arch is a rare variant (<0.1% prevalence) whereby the arch vessels originate in the following order: left common carotid, right common carotid, right subclavian, left subclavian artery. The last image is a three dimensional reconstruction of a contrast-enhanced computed tomography scan depicting a patient's right sided aortic arch. (Reproduced with permission from Rutherford's Vascular Surgery and Endovascular Therapy)

patients with stroke, TIA, subclavian steal, upper limb ischemia or thromboembolic phenomena, however asymptomatic lesions (>75% of patients) should be medically managed, except in patient with severe subclavian stenosis in the presence of patent internal mammary-coronary bypass, in presence of patent and functional ipsilateral arteriovenous graft/fistula, planned sternotomy for repair of other intrathoracic lesions. Other indications for intervention include infections, penetrating trauma, blunt trauma with pseudoaneurysm or rupture, traumatic occlusions/thrombosis, symptomatic dissections, arterial thoracic outlet syndrome, aneurysm formation (which should be repaired regardless of size).

(a) *Surgical*: transthoracic revascularization is preferred in patients with multi-vessel disease, extra-anatomic configuration may be necessary depending on the indication for revascularization (Fig. 8.5). Total arch replacement may be necessary in the setting of ascending or arch disease. Extra-anatomic revascularization may also be necessary depending on the indication for repair.
    - *Subclavian-Carotid Transposition*: (Fig. 8.6) Avoids the need for use of prosthetic material. The subclavian-carotid transposition involves dissection of the subclavian artery centrally, and transection of the LSCA proximal to the vertebral, thyrocervical trunk, and internal mammary arteries. Complications are rare with 2.2% mortality, 1% stroke, and patency is excellent at 99% [23].
    - *Carotid-Subclavian Bypass*: (Fig. 8.7) avoids excessive dissection of proximal subclavian artery, requires a reinforced conduit (typically prosthetic due to higher patency); also carries overall low complications with mortality <2%, 2.1% stroke, 94% 5 year patency [24].
    - *Carotid-Carotid Bypass*: Occasionally necessary depending on arch anatomy and disease being addressed. Carotid-carotid bypasses are done with reinforced prosthetic and carry a slightly higher rate of stroke ranging from 4–6% [25].

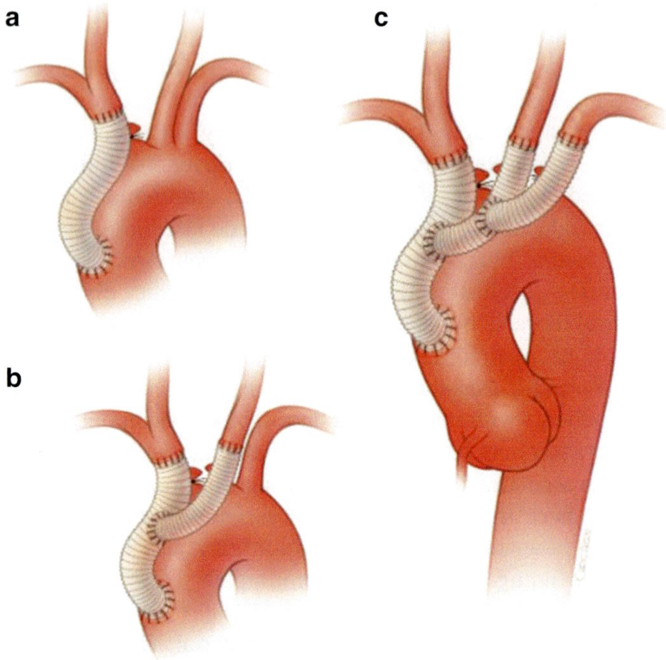

Fig. 8.5 Technical approach for transthoracic revascularization. (**a**) Creation of an aorto-innominate bypass. (**b**) Sidearm bypass graft to the left carotid artery. (**c**) Sidearm bypass graft to the left subclavian artery. (Reproduced with permission from Rutherford's Vascular Surgery and Endovascular Therapy)

- *Axillo-axillary and subclavian-subclavian bypass*: Requires longer prosthetic material, carries increased risk of skin erosion, graft infection, graft thrombosis, complicates access to sternum if future sternotomy is needed; despite these issues reported mortality is lowest at 0.5% and stroke at 1.1% [26].

(b) *Endovascular*: Endovascular management of brachiocephalic occlusive disease requires meticulous pre-procedure planning, as well as detailed knowledge about concomitant disease. The degree of stenosis, lesion characteristics,

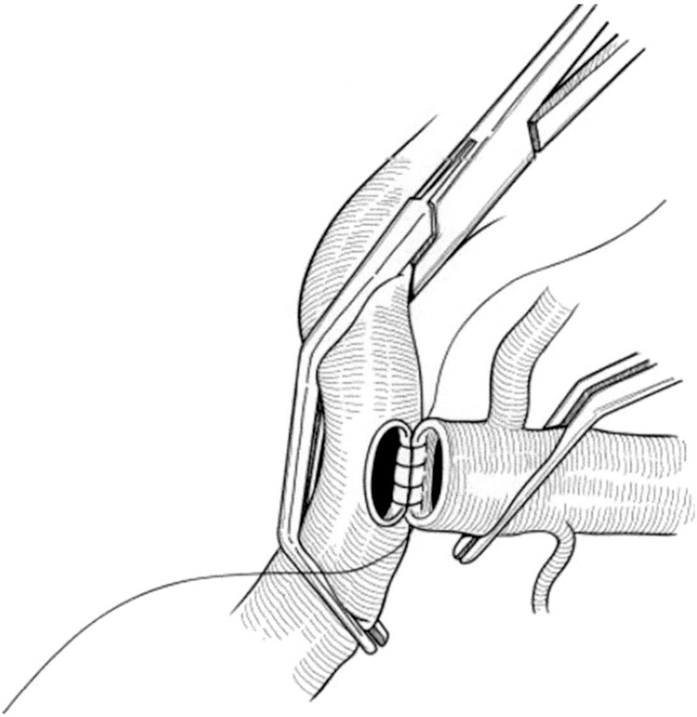

Fig. 8.6 Left subclavian to carotid transposition: end-to-side anastomosis of the left subclavian artery to the common carotid artery. (Reproduced with permission from Atlas of Vascular Surgery and Endovascular Therapy)

and anatomic landmarks are best determined with axial imaging, although conventional angiography is still employed. Endovascular treatment options include balloon angioplasty alone with reported immediate technical success rates of >90%, balloon angioplasty with primary stenting, angioplasty with rescue stenting. Stents designed to be used in occlusive disease have changed the trends from rescue stenting in this setting to primary stenting in recent years with improved technical success rates of 90–100% and up to 2 year patency ranging up to 77–100 [27]. Drug coated balloon angioplasty is generally

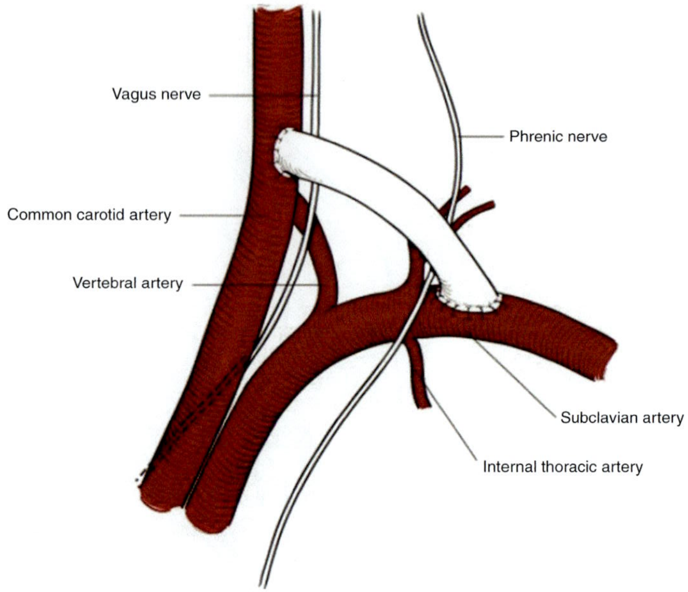

Fig. 8.7 Carotid to subclavian bypass to the third portion of the LSCA. The anastomosis on the subclavian artery lies inferior to the divided anterior scalene muscle, with preservation of the phrenic nerve. (Reproduced with permission from Atlas of Vascular Surgery and Endovascular Therapy)

reserved for recurrent stenosis, or in stent restenosis. Preprocedural planning, in particular access planning, is vital to success with the endovascular management of brachiocephalic artery occlusive disease.

Vertebral Artery Disease

1. *Stenotic Vertebral Artery Disease*: The vertebral artery is classically divided into four segments based on the anatomic location of disease (Fig. 8.8). Ischemia affecting the temporo-occipital areas of the cerebral hemispheres, brain stem, or cerebellum classically leads to bilateral symptoms described as vertebrobasilar ischemia where patients have dizziness, vertigo and drop attacks, diplopia, peripheral numb-

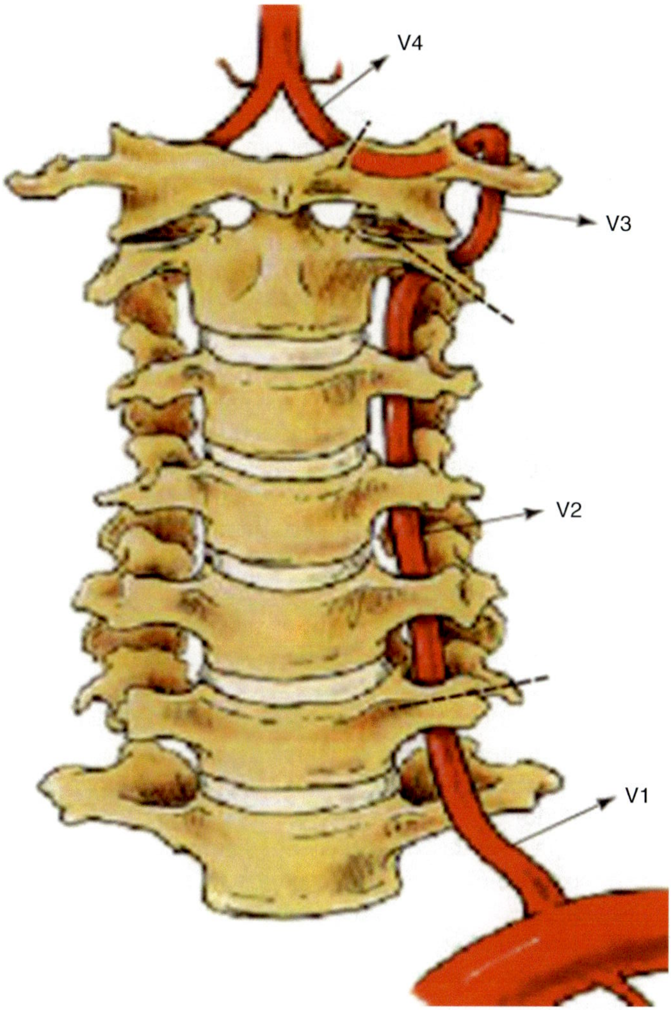

Fig. 8.8 The four segments of the vertebral (V) artery. (Reproduced with permission from Rutherford's Vascular Surgery and Endovascular Therapy)

ness, alternating paresthesias, tinnitus, dysphagia, dysarthria, or ataxia. Posterior circulation strokes are either hemodynamic or embolic; culprits being occlusive disease in 32%, cardiac embolic source 24%, arterial embolic source 18%. The V1 segment is most commonly affected by atherosclerosis. V2 is most commonly affected by extrinsic compression by bone or tendon (osteophytes) and symptoms are triggered by neck rotation; as well as the most common location of traumatic arteriovenous fistulas (AVF), but can also be affected by traumatic dissections, occlusions and source of emboli. V3 segment is susceptible to traumatic and spontaneous dissections, occlusions, AVF, and pseudoaneurysms; even minor traumas that cause excess rotation at C1/C2, chiropractic manipulation, etc. can lead to injury. V4 is prone to AVF formation and aneurysmal degeneration.

   (a) *Low flow*: Results in transient symptoms affecting basilar artery, these usually produce symptoms if there is *inadequate* compensation from the carotids (due to either severe carotid stenosis or incomplete circle of Willis). Additionally, patients may have subclavian artery stenosis and symptoms with ipsilateral arms leading to vertebral artery steal.
   (b) *Embolic*: Generally due to microembolization from cardiac etiology, arch vessels, or subclavian artery. Embolic etiologies are more likely to cause permanent ischemia or fatal strokes.

2. *Management*: reconstruction is indicated in symptomatic patients in the following scenarios:
   (a) 60% diameter reduction in both vertebral arteries (if symmetric)
   (b) In the setting of a stenotic dominant artery with an occluded or hypoplastic contralateral vertebral artery.
   (c) Diseased vertebral artery with an occluded contralateral vertebral artery.
3. *Surgical*: Reconstruction options vary based on the location of disease:
   (a) V1:
      - Transposition of proximal vertebral artery to the adjacent carotid artery.
      - Bypass from the carotid (CCA) or subclavian (SCA).
      - Subclavian-vertebral endarterectomy.

(b) V2: interosseous location, usually not surgically accessible, and interventions are avoided, except in the setting of hemorrhage.
  - Proximal and distal ligation in setting of hemorrhage.

(c) V3: usually performed at C1-C2 level.
  - Bypass from CCA, SCA, or proximal vertebral artery (saphenous or radial artery conduit).
  - Transposition of the vertebral to the external carotid or occipital artery.

4. *Endovascular*: Vertebral interventions are both safe and technically feasible. Access is femoral (93%), brachial (3%), or radial (5%) with the use of coronary balloons (smaller sizes available) with or without embolic protections devices used to treat stenosis, there is no data to support the use of stents in this location and stents tend to have high rates of fracture and restenosis [28].
   (a) Vertebral Artery Disease: FMD,
     - Vertebral artery FMD is seen in 7–38% of patients with carotid lesions but can be an isolated finding as well. FMD in the vertebral artery usually affects the C2 segment of the artery.
     - Vertebral artery dissection (see section for carotid artery dissection).

Subclavian Steal Syndrome

1. Diagnosis: Subclavian steal (Fig. 8.9) is due to a flow restricting lesion in the subclavian artery or innominate artery that can produce relative hypo perfusion of the posterior circulation. Subclavian steal occurs when a stenosis in the proximal left subclavian artery (proximal to the vertebral artery) is stenotic or occluded leading to reversal of flow in the vertebral artery. These findings may be asymptomatic in some patients, but may present with symptoms related to, or exacerbated by ipsilateral arm use. Diagnosis should include an ultrasound of the carotid artery which will determine the degree of concom-

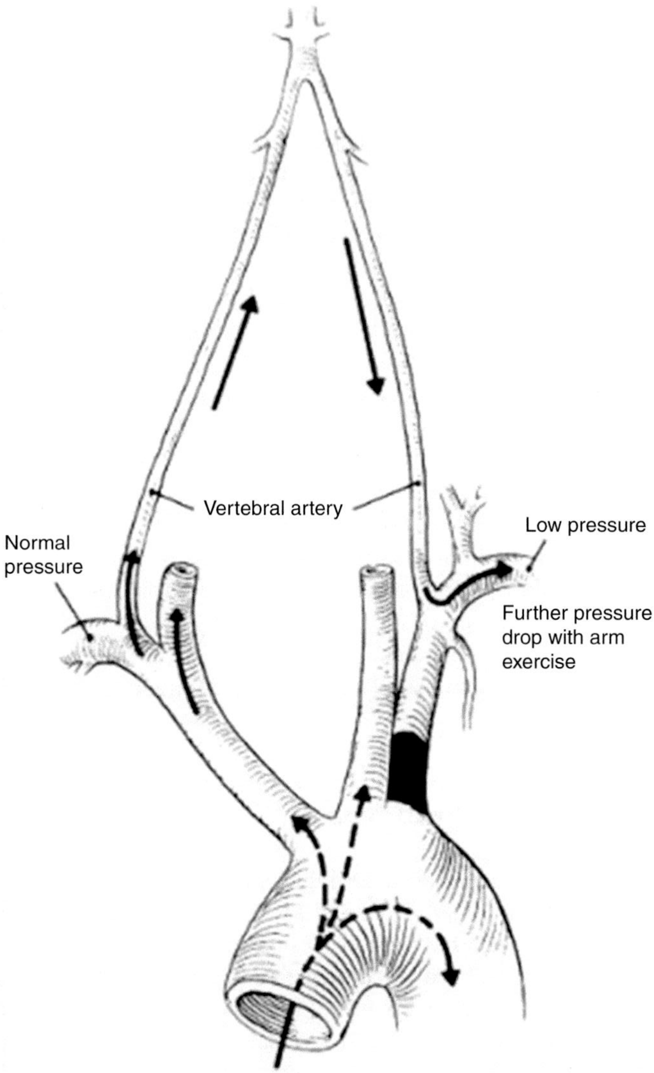

Fig. 8.9 Mechanism of subclavian artery steal syndrome. Note the occlusion in the origin of the left subclavian artery. This produces a pressure gradient with reversal of blood flow in the left vertebral artery, producing a siphoning of steal from the basilar artery. (Reproduced with permission from Vascular and Endovascular Vascular Surgery: A comprehensive Review)

itant carotid artery disease as well as directionality of flow in the vertebral arteries. Reversal of flow in the vertebral arteries indicates a proximal subclavian stenosis. Further work-up should include CTA of the arch vessels and the affected extremity for a detailed anatomic characterization of the disease.

2. *Management*
   (a) *Surgical*: Indicated in symptomatic patients, patients with LIMA bypass, and those with functional ipsilateral AV access. Surgical repair options include Subclavian-carotid transposition, carotid subclavian bypass, as well as other extra-anatomical bypasses (Figs. 8.5, 8.6, 8.7, 8.8, and 8.9 in Brachiocephalic Disease section).
   (b) Endovascular:
      - *Angioplasty*: Initial success ranges from 80–95%, with up to 25% recurrence.
      - *Stents*: Mainstay of therapy since their introduction, success rate 91–100% and patency 77–100% at 2 years. Primary stenting is preferred including complex stenosis (i.e. occlusions that are recanalized).

References

1. LeFevre M, et al. Screening for asymptomatic carotid artery stenosis: US preventive services task force recommendation statement. Ann Intern Med. 2014;161:356–62.
2. Rocotta JJ, et al. Updated Society for Vascular Surgery guidelines for management of extracranial carotid disease. J Vasc Surg. 2011;52(3):e1–31.
3. Fleischer LA, et al. ACC/AHA 2007 guidelines on perioperative cardiovascular evaluation and care for non-cardiac surgery: a report of the American College of Cardiology/American Heart Association task force on practice guidelines. Circulation. 2007;116:e418–99.
4. Devereaux PJ, et al. Effects of extended-release metoprolol succinate in patients undergoing non-cardiac surgery (POISE trial): a randomized controlled trial: POISE study group. Lancet. 2008;371(9627):1839.
5. Fleisher LA, et al. ACCF/AHA focused update on perioperative beta blockade incorporated into the ACC/AHA 2007 guidelines on perioperative cardiovascular evaluation and care for non-cardiac surgery: a report of the American College of Cardiology Foundation/American Heart

Association task force on practice guidelines. Circulation. 2009;120:e169–276.
6. Paty PSK, et al. The use of low-dose heparin is safe in carotid endarterectomy and avoids the use of protamine sulfate. Cardiovasc Surg. 1999;7:39–43.
7. Amarenco P, et al. Statins of stroke prevention and carotid atherosclerosis: systemic review and up-to-date meta-analysis. Stroke. 2004;35:2902–9.
8. The Stroke Prevention by Aggressive Reduction in Cholesterol Levels (SPARCL) Investigators. High-dose atorvastatin after stroke or transient ischemic attack. N Engl J Med. 2006;355:549–59.
9. Endarterectomy for asymptomatic carotid artery stenosis; Executive Committee for the Asymptomatic Carotid Atherosclerosis Study. JAMA. 1995;(273):1421–8.
10. Halliday A, et al. Prevention of disabling and fatal strokes by successful carotid endarterectomy in patients without recent neurological symptoms: randomized controlled trial. Lancet. 2004;363(9420):1491–502.
11. Yadav JS, et al. Protected carotid-artery stenting versus endarterectomy in high risk patents. NEJM. 2004;351:1493–501.
12. Brott TG, et al. Stenting versus endarterectomy for treatment of carotid-artery stenosis. NEJM. 2010;363:11–23.
13. North American Symptomatic Carotid Endarterectomy Trial Collaborators (NASCET). Beneficial effect of carotid endarterectomy in symptomatic patients with high-grade carotid stenosis. N Engl J Med. 1991;325:445–53.
14. Barnett HJ, et al. Benefit of carotid endarterectomy in patients with symptomatic moderate or severe stenosis. North American Symptomatic Carotid Endarterectomy Trial Collaborators. NEJM. 1998;339:1415–25.
15. Randomized trial of endarterectomy for recently symptomatic carotid stenosis final results of the MRC European Carotid Surgery Trial (ECST). Lancet. 1998;351:1379–87.
16. Scott AS, et al. Risk of cerebrovascular events after neck and supraclavicular radiotherapy: a systematic review. Radiother Oncol. 2009;90:163–5.
17. Bliff WL. Diagnosis of blunt cerebrovascular injuries. Curr Opin Crit Care. 2003;9:530–4.
18. Eastman AL, et al. Computed tomographic angiography for the diagnosis of blunt cervical vascular injury: is it ready for primetime? J Trauma. 2006;60:925–9.
19. Lyrer P, et al. Antithrombotic drugs for carotid artery dissection. Cochrane Database Syst Rev. 2003;(3):CD000255.
20. CADISS trial investigators, et al. Antiplatelet treatment compared with anticoagulation treatment for cervical artery dissection (CADISS): a randomized trial. Lancet Neurol. 2015;14(4):361–7.

21. Muller BT, et al. Surgical treatment of 50 carotid dissections: indications and results. J Vasc Surg. 2000;31:980–8.
22. Pham MH, et al. Endovascular stenting of extra cranial carotid and vertebral artery dissections: a systematic review of literature. Neurosurgery. 2011;68:856–66.
23. Edwards WH, et al. Subclavian revascularization. A quarter century experience. Ann Surg. 1994;219:673–7.
24. Takach TJ, at. Contemporary relevance of carotid-subclavian bypass defined by an experience spanning five decades. Ann Vasc Surg. 2011;25:895–901.
25. Ozsvath KJ, et al. Carotid-carotid crossover bypass: is it a durable procedure? J Vasc Surg. 2003;37:582–5.
26. Aziz F, et al. Endovascular and open surgical treatment of brachiocephalic arteries. Ann Vasc Surg. 2011;25:569–81.
27. Ahmed AT, et al. Comparing percutaneous trans luminal angioplasty and stent placement for treatment of subclavian arterial occlusive disease: a systematic review and meta-analysis. Cardiovasc Intervent Radiol. 2016;39:652–67.
28. Jenkins JS, et al. Endovascular stenting for vertebral artery stenosis. J Am Coll Cardiol. 2010;55(6):538–42.

9 Upper Extremity, Medical Surgical, and Endovascular Management

Shayna Brathwaite and Olamide Alabi

Upper Extremity Ischemia: Acute-Embolization, Iatrogenic and Chronic

Acute-Embolization

- Represents 10–20% of acute limb ischemia (ALI)
- Ulnar artery > radial artery
- 2:1 female:male ratio [1]
  - Secondary to smaller caliber vessels
- Physical Exam:
  - 6Ps—pulselessness, pain, pallor, paresthesia, poikilothermia, and paralysis

S. Brathwaite
Department of Vascular Surgery, Emory University, Atlanta, GA, USA
e-mail: sabrath@emory.edu

O. Alabi (✉)
Department of Surgery, Emory University School of Medicine, Atlanta, GA, USA
e-mail: olamide.alabi@emory.edu

A. Murga et al. (eds.), *The Vascular Surgery In-Training Examination Review (VSITE)*, https://doi.org/10.1007/978-3-031-24121-5_9

- Rarely results in tissue loss secondary to dense collateral network
  - Axillary artery occlusion—<10% limb loss
  - Brachial artery occlusion distal to deep brachial artery—<5% leads to digital gangrene (Fig. 9.1)
- Etiology:
  - Eighty percent related to cardiac embolus secondary to atrial fibrillation
  - Other etiologies:
    - Native and prosthetic valvular disease
    - Septic emboli from endocarditis
    - Cardiac mass such as myxoma or fibroelastoma
    - Left ventricular thrombus
    - Right to left shunt such as patent foramen ovale
    - Aortic diseases such as mural thrombus in aneurysm or unstable plaque
- Treatment:
  - Anticoagulation
  - Open versus percutaneous mechanical thrombectomy

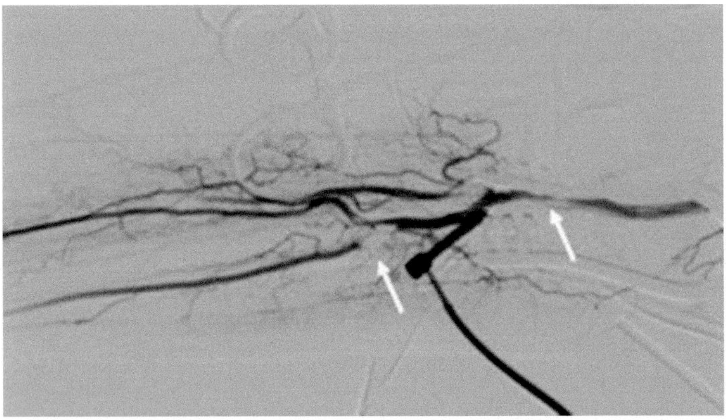

Fig. 9.1 Digital subtraction angiography of upper extremity highlighting a brachial artery embolus. Filling defects indicated by white arrows

- +/– thrombolysis
- +/– fasciotomies [2]

Iatrogenic Injury

- Radial Artery Injury
  - Increased rates with the increased incidence of coronary and peripheral intervention via radial access
  - Complications after radial artery cannulation include thrombosis, pseudoaneurysm, infection, hematoma, and perforation [3]
  - Rates of occlusion range from 3 to 10%, but clinical hand ischemia is rare due to extensive collateral network [2, 4]
  - Treatment
    - Medical: Anticoagulation and observation
    - Surgical:
      - Open thrombectomy
      - Pseudoaneurysms may require radial artery ligation or repair [5]
- Brachial Artery Injury
  - Clinically significant complications after cannulation rare (<1%): thrombosis with ischemia, hematoma with median nerve dysfunction, Volkmann's contracture, or pseudoaneurysm [6, 7]
  - Diagnosis: duplex ultrasonography or cross-sectional imaging i.e. CTA
  - Treatment:
    - Thrombosis with ischemia
      - Thrombectomy
    - Hematoma with median nerve dysfunction
      - Early evacuation to prevent median nerve neuropathy and Volkmann's contracture
    - Pseudoaneurysm
      - If small, asymptomatic—observe
      - Symptomatic—suture repair

Chronic Ischemia

- Etiology:
  - Atherosclerosis (most commonly subclavian artery disease)
  - Fibromuscular disease
  - Other etiologies: Raynaud's disease, Buerger's disease, thoracic outlet syndrome (Fig. 9.2), iatrogenic injury after arm catheterization, immediate or delayed traumatic injury, rheumatoid arthritis, collagen vascular disease, rarer causes include Takayasu, giant cell arteritis, radiation induced injury, ESRD
  - Subclavian artery is the typical locations of UE arterial atherosclerosis, left greater than right
- Clinical Manifestations:
  - Change in sensation, hand temperature, muscle pain with use, ulcers or digital gangrene, effort induced hand pain
- Physical Exam:
  - Often normal at rest
  - May have cool hands and digits and diminished pulses with activity

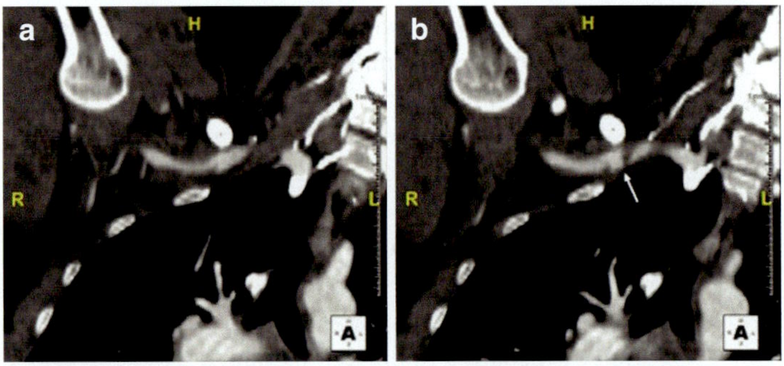

Fig. 9.2 CT Angiogram of the chest in a patient with arterial thoracic outlet syndrome. (**a**) Coronal CT angiogram image highlighting the anatomy of the thoracic outlet including the clavicle, first rib and axillosubclavian artery. (**b**) Coronal CT image. White arrow indicates the location of the axillosubclavian artery thrombosis from mechanical compression of the artery

- Diagnostic Evaluation:
  - Wrist to brachial/forearm index:
    - Normal 0.85–1.0
    - Abnormal < 0.85
  - Cross-sectional imaging with CTA or MRA
  - Arteriography
- Treatment:
  - Conservative therapy—50% of patients treated non-operatively will have ongoing symptoms
  - Surgical/Endovascular therapy
    - Angioplasty and stenting, particularly for subclavian stenosis
    - Open surgical bypass

Occupational Vascular Disease

Hypothenar Hammer Syndrome

- Etiology:
  - Digital ischemia caused by repetitive blunt trauma to hypothenar portion of the hand
  - Superficial branch of ulnar artery crosses through hypothenar muscles before penetrating palmar aponeurosis
  - Ulnar artery compressed against adjacent hamate bone
- Arteriogram Findings:
  - Digital artery occlusions with segmental ulnar artery occlusions in the palm
  - "Corkscrew" elongation with alternating stenosis and ectasia [8]
- More common in men, in dominant hand, usually occurs in occupational setting
- Treatment:
  - Ulnar Artery Aneurysm—Reversed autologous vein graft
  - Digital ischemia related to aneurysm thrombosis or embolization—thrombolytic therapy

Hand-Arm Vibration Syndrome

- Etiology:
  - Prolonged use of vibrating hand tools
- Clinical Manifestations:
  - Intermittent tingling and numbness
  - Extensive blanching and Raynaud's phenomenon
  - <1% progress to ulceration or gangrene
- Diagnosis:
  - History of vibrating tools and Raynaud's phenomenon
  - Angiogram with multiple segmental occlusions of the digits and corkscrew configuration of vessels in the hand
- Treatment:
  - Prevention is key with personal protective equipment
  - Discontinuation of tools
  - Calcium channel blockers
  - Rarely cervical or digital sympathectomy

Axillosubclavian and Brachial Artery Aneurysmal Disease

Axillosubclavian Artery Aneurysms

- One percent of all peripheral artery aneurysms
- Etiology: Blunt or penetrating trauma, atherosclerosis, congenital axillary aneurysms, related to thoracic outlet syndrome and cervical ribs
  - Blunt trauma: repetitive abduction and external rotation of the upper extremity. Circumflex humeral arteries create a tethering point
  - Penetrating trauma: Pseudoaneurysms can rupture into axillary sheath causing brachial plexus compression [2]
  - Atherosclerosis: typical etiology of proximal disease

- Congenital Aneurysms
    - Thoracic outlet syndrome and cervical ribs [9]
    - Often leads to more distal axillosubclavian disease and can have post-stenotic dilation of subclavian artery beyond a point of mechanical obstruction
- Kommerell Diverticulum
    - Aneurysmal degeneration of proximal portion of aberrant right subclavian artery [10]
    - Right subclavian artery that passes posterior to the esophagus. Aneurysm can lead to dysphagia lusoria (Fig. 9.3a–c)

- Clinical Manifestation:
    - Supra or infraclavicular pulsatile and expansile mass
    - Compression of adjacent structures
    - Distal embolization
- Treatment:
    - Distal Embolization
        - Thrombolysis versus thrombectomy

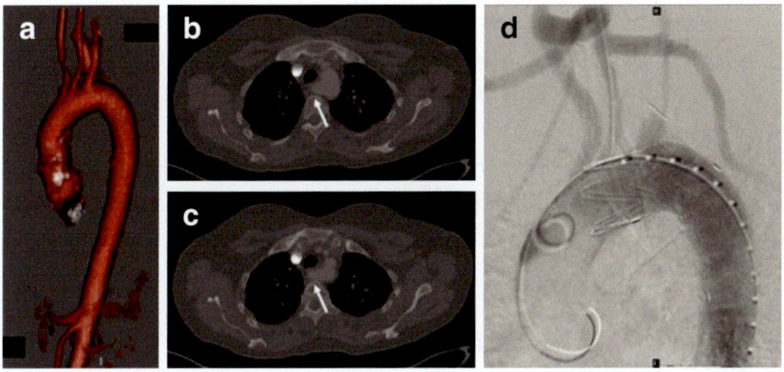

Fig. 9.3 Aberrant right subclavian artery. (**a**) 3D reconstruction of patient with aberrant right subclavian artery. (**b, c**) CT Angiogram of the chest. White arrow indicates retroesophageal right subclavian artery. (**d**) Digital subtraction angiography showing patient anatomy after prior aberrant right subclavian artery to right common carotid artery transposition with proximal ligation followed by left subclavian to left common carotid artery transposition and TEVAR several years later for persistent dysphagia symptoms

  - Aneurysm (Fig. 9.3d)
    - Resection of aneurysm and interposition graft
    - Carotid subclavian bypass with proximal ligation
    - Endovascular—stent graft exclusion
  - Consider laterality of the dominant vertebral artery—risk of stroke with ligation or endovascular occlusion

Brachial Artery Aneurysms

- Etiology:
  - Repetitive trauma, iatrogenic or idiopathic
- Clinical manifestations:
  - Pulsatile mass, median nerve compression, pain, hand or digital ischemia secondary to thrombosis or distal embolization [2]
- Diagnosis:
  - Duplex ultrasonography, cross-sectional imaging
- Treatment:
  - Resection of aneurysm with interposition graft, resection and primary anastomosis, primary repair for iatrogenic pseudoaneurysm, endovascular stent

Small Vessel Arteriopathies

Scleroderma

- Most common connective tissue disorder
- Clinical manifestations: progressive scarring and small vessel occlusions in the skin, GI tract, kidneys, lung, and heart

Rheumatoid Arthritis

- Chronic inflammatory joint disease
- May have extra-articular involvement of the skin, eyes, lungs, spleen, and arteries

Sjogren's Disease

- Characterized by dry eyes and mouth
- May be primary or secondary to another connective tissue disease that is associated with small vessel arteriopathy
- Subdivided into acute necrotizing, leukocytoclastic, and lymphocytic vasculitis

Systemic Lupus Erythematosus

- Immune complex mediated disease that causes fevers, arthralgias, skin rashes, nephritis, and Raynaud's phenomenon

Thromboangiitis Obliterans (Buerger's Disease)

- Chronic, non-atherosclerotic arteritis with segmental thrombotic occlusions of small and medium sized vessels and corkscrew collaterals [11]
- Clinical Presentation: Young, male, smoker, palpable proximal pulses, distal limb ischemia
- Characterized by relapsing episodes of digital extremity ischemia
- Treatment: Smoking cessation, Risk factor modification, and Prostacyclin analogue, surgical and endovascular treatments often fail [11]

Vasospastic and Vasoocclusive Disease

Raynaud's Phenomenon

- Prevalence 3–5% in general population
- Diagnosis: Clinical assessment with history or direct observation
- Triphasic color change: White (ischemia), blue (cyanosis), red (reperfusion)

- Triggers: Emotional stress, caffeine, cold exposure, frostbite freeze injury
- Types:
  - Primary (Idiopathic) Raynaud's
    Progression to digital ischemia rare
  - Secondary Raynaud's
    More likely to progress to severe occlusive lesions with rest pain and ulceration
    Etiology local or systemic disease:
    - **Rheumatologic** (systemic sclerosis, connective tissue disorder, systemic lupus erythematous, dermatomyositis, polymyositis, rheumatoid arthritis, Sjogren syndrome, vasculitides)
    - **Hematologic** (polycythemia vera, leukemia, thrombocytosis, cold agglutinin disease, paraproteinemia's, protein C/S deficiency, antithrombin deficiency, Factor V Leiden, Hepatitis B/C)
    - **Occlusive Arterial Disease** (external neurovascular compression, carpal tunnel, thoracic outlet syndrome, thrombosis, Buerger's disease, embolization, arteriosclerosis) [12]
- Treatment [11]
  - Medical:
    Avoid triggers
    Pharmacologic Vasodilation: Sustained release dihydropyridine-class calcium channel blocker (nifedipine, amlodipine, felodipine), second line phosphodiesterase inhibitor, topical nitrate, angiotensin receptor blocker (losartan), or an SSRI [13]
  - Surgical: Amputation and debridement for gangrene or ischemic infection, thoracic sympathectomy (rarely performed)

Questions and Answers

1. A 72-year-old male presents with the acute onset of left arm pain. The arm is insensate, pulseless and the patient is unable to move his hand. What is the most likely etiology?
   (a) Worsening of Raynaud's phenomenon
   (b) Cardiac arrhythmia
   (c) Atherosclerotic plaque
2. A 32-old otherwise healthy male smoker presents ischemia of the digits of bilateral hands. He is noted to have palpable pulses on exam. The mainstay of treatment includes:
   (a) Smoking cessation
   (b) Angiogram and balloon angioplasty of digital vessels
   (c) Initiation of calcium channel blocker
3. A 56-year-old male had a recent NSTEMI and coronary PCI via right brachial artery. Two weeks after procedure he is noted to have flexion contracture of the hand at the wrist. The most likely etiology is:
   (a) Brachial artery tense hematoma
   (b) Atherosclerotic plaque rupture
   (c) Brachial plexus injury

Answers: 1 (b), 2 (a), 3 (a)

References

1. Stonebridge PA, Clason AE, Duncan AJ, Nolan B, Jenkins AM, Ruckley CV. Acute ischaemia of the upper limb compared with acute lower limb ischaemia; a 5-year review. Br J Surg. 1989;76(5):515–6.
2. Cronenwett JL, Johnston KW, Rutherford RB. Rutherford's vascular surgery. 8th ed, 2 volumes. Philadelphia, PA: Elsevier Health Sciences. 2014.
3. Scheer B, Perel A, Pfeiffer UJ. Clinical review: complications and risk factors of peripheral arterial catheters used for haemodynamic monitoring in anaesthesia and intensive care medicine. Crit Care. 2002;6(3):199–204.

4. Valentine RJ, Modrall JG, Clagett GP. Hand ischemia after radial artery cannulation. J Am Coll Surg. 2005;201(1):18–22.
5. Garg K, Howell BW, Saltzberg SS, Berland TL, Mussa FF, Maldonado TS, et al. Open surgical management of complications from indwelling radial artery catheters. J Vasc Surg. 2013;58(5):1325–30.
6. Armstrong PJ, Han DC, Baxter JA, Elmore JR, Franklin DP. Complication rates of percutaneous brachial artery access in peripheral vascular angiography. Ann Vasc Surg. 2003;17(1):107–10.
7. Macon WL, Futrell JW. Median-nerve neuropathy after percutaneous puncture of the brachial artery in patients receiving anticoagulants. N Engl J Med. 1973;288(26):1396.
8. Ferris BL, Taylor LM Jr, Oyama K, McLafferty RB, Edwards JM, Moneta GL, et al. Hypothenar hammer syndrome: proposed etiology. J Vasc Surg. 2000;31(1 Pt 1):104–13.
9. Criado E, Berguer R, Greenfield L. The spectrum of arterial compression at the thoracic outlet. J Vasc Surg. 2010;52(2):406–11.
10. Simon RW, Lachat M, Pfammatter T, Amann-Vesti BR. Giant aneurysm of an aberrant right subclavian artery from the left aortic arch. J Thorac Cardiovasc Surg. 2006;132(6):1478–9.
11. Wu W, Chaer RA. Nonarteriosclerotic vascular disease. Surg Clin North Am. 2013;93(4):833–75. viii
12. Goundry B, Bell L, Langtree M, Moorthy A. Diagnosis and management of Raynaud's phenomenon. BMJ. 2012;344:e289.
13. Wigley FM, Flavahan NA. Raynaud's phenomenon. Rheum Dis Clin N Am. 1996;22(4):765–81.

10 Thoracic Outlet Syndromes

Sharon Kiang, Hans Keenan Boggs,
and Roger Tomihama

Statistics [1]

- True incidence is unclear given the lack of objective criteria and failure to recognize; estimated as 3–80/1000 people
- Most patients are between 20 and 50 years old
- Female to male ratio is 4:1
- nTOS most common (95%); vTOS (2–3%); aTOS (1–3%)

S. Kiang (✉)
Department of Vascular Surgery, Loma Linda University Medical Center,
Loma Linda, CA, USA
e-mail: Skiang@llu.edu

H. K. Boggs
Department of Surgery, Loma Linda University Medical Center,
Loma Linda, CA, USA
e-mail: HABoggs@llu.edu

R. Tomihama
Department of Interventional Radiology, Loma Linda University
Medical Center, Loma Linda, CA, USA
e-mail: RTomihama@llu.edu

A. Murga et al. (eds.), *The Vascular Surgery In-Training Examination Review (VSITE)*,
https://doi.org/10.1007/978-3-031-24121-5_10

Relevant Anatomy [1] (Fig. 10.1)

Boundaries of the Thoracic Outlet

- Anterior: manubrium
- Posterior: T1 vertebral body
- Laterally: first rib; costal cartilage

The thoracic outlet area includes *three anatomical spaces* where compression can occur:

Scalene Triangle—space formed between the anterior scalene and middle scalene muscles

- Contains the subclavian artery and brachial plexus
- Here, the 5 nerve roots of the plexus become 3 trunks
- Most common site of brachial plexus compression
- If present, cervical and anomalous first ribs may compress the plexus at this position

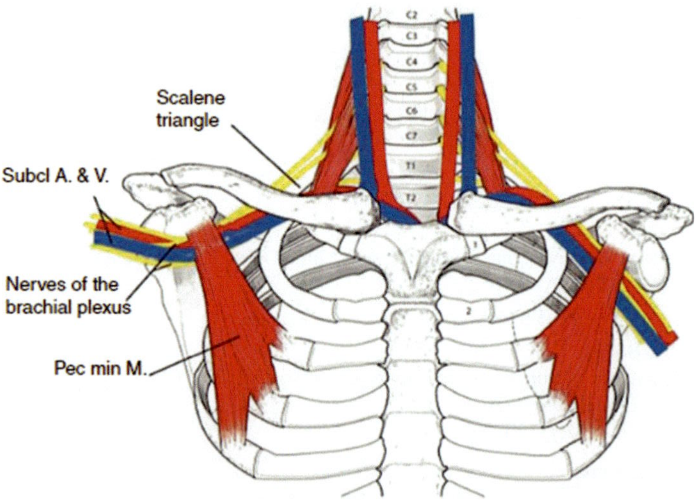

Fig. 10.1 The three anatomic spaces relevant in thoracic outlet syndrome; Scalene triangle; Costoclavicular Space; Pectoralis Minor space. (From Sanders J. Anatomy of the Thoracic Outlet and Related Structures. 2013. Springer Nature)

- Compression at this space is usually associated with occipital headaches and neck pain

Costoclavicular Space—most common site of subclavian vein compression (Fig. 10.2)

Pectoralis Minor Space—possible location of brachial plexus compression

- Typically branches of the plexus lie under the Pectoralis minor (Pm) muscle
- Axillary artery and vein pass under Pm muscle as well

Cervical rib—congenital overdevelopment of a cervical transverse process, typically C7; can have various relationships with the first rib

Anomalous first rib—congenital; thinner, often more cephalad, typically fuse with second rib

Clinically, cervical and anomalous first ribs act in identical fashion; predispose to nTOS

Fracture of the clavicle or first rib can result in thickened bony callus at healing site leading to compression

A variety of *ligaments and bands* have been classified that can act as predisposing factors

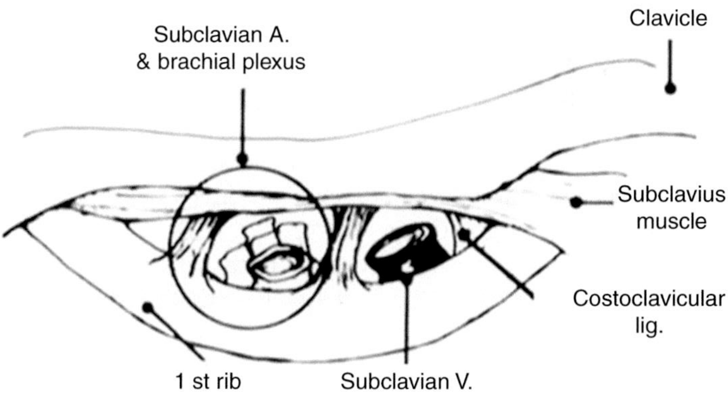

Fig. 10.2 Costoclavicular space—the subclavian vein is most often compressed in this space. (From Sanders J. Anatomy of the Thoracic Outlet and Related Structures. 2013. Springer Nature)

Thoracic Duct—empties into the *left subclavian vein*; injury → lymphatic leak

Brachial Plexus

- Arises from nerve roots C5 to T1
- Nerve roots network into 3 trunks, 6 divisions (3 anterior, 3 posterior), 3 cords, and 5 branches

Adjacent Nerves—of important surgical purpose

- Phrenic Nerve
  - Innervates diaphragm
  - Arises primarily from C4 and usually receives branches from C3 and C5
  - Can be doubled or tripled in up to 13% of individuals
  - Descends from the lateral to medial on the anterior border of the anterior scalene muscle in 84% of individuals; remains lateral in 16%
  - Injury → elevated hemidiaphragm
- Long Thoracic Nerve
  - Arises primarily from C6 and usually receives branches from C5 and C7
  - Passes through middle scalene muscle
  - Supplies serratus anterior muscle
  - Injury → "winged scapula"
- Dorsal Scapular Nerve
  - First branch of C5
  - May course close to dissection in a supraclavicular approach to thoracic outlet decompression
- Cervical Sympathetic Chain
  - Lies over the transverse processes of the cervical vertebrae
  - Close to the origins of the anterior and middle scalene muscles
  - Though usually out of the operative field, can be indirectly damaged in supraclavicular scalenectomy
  - Injury causes *Horner's syndrome* (ipsilateral miosis, ptosis, anhidrosis)

Variations in Scalene Muscle Anatomy—very common; may modify risk of TOS [1, 2]
- Narrowed "scalene triangle"
- Interdigitation of anterior and middle scalene muscles
- Adherence of scalene muscles to cervical nerve roots
- Splitting of anterior scalene around C5 and C6
- Presence of a Scalene minimus muscle—commonly found in normal cadavers, suggested as a causative factor
- Congenital bands or ligaments
- Pathway of phrenic nerve—anterior position to vein may rarely lead to compression
- Relation of subclavian vein and costoclavicular ligament, subclavius tendon—medial position of vein on first rib may lead to compression by the above structures

Skeletal Abnormalities [1, 2]
- Nearly a third of TOS patients have skeletal abnormalities
- Cervical ribs arise from transverse process of C7
  - Thirty percent are "complete" with a true joint or other direct attachment to the first rib
  - Seventy percent are "incomplete" without direct attachment to the first rib; most will have a tight fibrous band connecting the two which can also compress the outlet (Table 10.1)

Table 10.1 Description of cervical ribs by type

Cervical rib type	Description
1	Rib extends to the C7 transverse process
2	Rib extends past the transverse process but does not connect to the first thoracic rib
3	Rib extends past the transverse process and partly fuses to the first rib via cartilage or fibrous bands
4	Rib is completely fused to the first rib via a bony pseudoarticulation

Adapted from Illig et al.

- Anomalous first ribs arise from transverse process of T1
- At risk for all forms of TOS, but most commonly results in nTOS
- Cervical or anomalous first ribs are almost always present in aTOS
- Most will remain asymptomatic

Pectoralis Minor Syndrome—Pectoralis minor muscle (Pm) can also compress the thoracic outlet leading to all forms of TOS [1, 2]

- Causes compression in the Pectoralis minor space (subcoracoid space); technically outside of the thoracic outlet but structures can be compressed between Pm and ribs
- Caused by trauma or excessive exercise via hyperabduction
- Responsible for up to 75% of recurrent nTOS following outlet decompression
- *Pectoralis minor tenotomy* may be an effective primary treatment

Neurogenic TOS (nTOS) [1, 2]

- Underlying cause of the pathology thought to be compression by the scalene muscles
- Predisposing factors:
  - Various anomalies of the scalene muscles, including narrowed triangle
  - Cervical ribs
  - Congenital ligaments or bands
  - Higher origin of the cervical nerve roots, closer to scalene triangle apex
- Eighty percent will have preceding history of neck trauma, especially hyperextension injuries; e.g. *whiplash following motor vehicle accident* (most common)
- Can be caused by *repetitive stress injuries* or activities of daily living in those with predisposing anatomy

- Patients are often asymptomatic until trauma
  - Muscle is stretched and torn, leading to local swelling
  - Upper extremity pain and paresthesia result from compression of nerve bundle
  - Resolution of swelling and scar tissue formation leads to muscle fibrosis and narrowing of the scalene triangle
  - Symptoms persist
- If compression involves the lower trunk of the plexus (i.e. C8, T1) sympathetic fibers may also be compressed → unilateral Reynaud's phenomenon with temperature and color changes
- *History*
  - Classically present with cervicobrachial pain following an acute injury or cumulative work or sport-related exposure
  - Positive features include: numbness, tingling, or weakness of the upper extremity
  - Can also complain of occipital headache; pain to palpation over the scalene triangle and pectoralis minor insertion site
  - Symptoms are exacerbated with maneuvers that compromise the thoracic outlet (arms over the head) or stretch the brachial plexus (arms dangled)
  - Atrophy of the thenar and hypothenar muscles of the hand may occur in rare occasions
  - Symptoms confined to the distal forearm, hand more suggestive of carpal or cubital tunnel pathology
  - Consider previous interventions of the cervical spine or shoulder
  - May report subjective coolness and color changes in the affected limb if sympathetic nerves involved
- *Exam*
  - Often not identified by standard neurologic exam
  - Tenderness over scalene muscles or pectoralis minor insertion site
  - Provocative maneuvers—occasionally helpful but not particularly sensitive or specific

    Adson test—palpate radial artery and extend, abduct, and externally rotate limb while patient rotates and ipsi-

laterally flexes the neck → positive if pulse amplitude is decreased
    - Often positive in healthy volunteers

    Elevated arm stress test (Roos test, EAST)—patient seated with abducted arms to 90°, head neutral, while opening and closing hands for 3 min or until symptoms begin
    - High negative predictive value if for 3 min or greater
    - Thought to be the most effective test
    - EAST—identical test but for 1 min
    - Modified upper limb tension test (Elvey test)—patient abducts arms to 90° with elbows extended while progressively dorsiflexing both wrists → positive if symptoms are elicited on ipsilateral side
- Electromyography (EMG) or nerve conduction velocity tests (NCV)—usually normal or non-specific; most helpful to exclude unrelated pathologies
- Median antebrachial cutaneous nerve (MACN) conduction tests = gold standard of nerve function testing
- On pathology: significant reduction in type 2 (fast-twitch) scalene muscle fibers and increase in type 1 (slow twitch) fibers
- MRI is generally the imaging modality of choice
  - Should be done with arms neutral and in hyperabduction/external rotation
  - MR Angiography should also be considered as vascular compression may be coexisting
- *Anterior Scalene Muscle Block*—highly predictive of success following thoracic outlet decompression
  - Local anesthetic injection intended to cause temporary relaxation of muscle, decompression of outlet
  - Botulinum toxin chemodenervation targeting the scalene muscles may be helpful in patients not appropriate for surgery
- *Differential diagnosis* should include:
  - Cervical spine disorders
  - Cervical dystonia
  - Musculoskeletal injuries

  - Carpal tunnel syndrome or ulnar neuropathy
  - Chronic headache
  - Somatization or depression
  - Complex regional pain syndrome
  - Fibromyalgia
  - Opioid hyperalgesia
- *Treatment*
  - Initial treatment for most will be physical therapy (PT), focusing on biomechanics and stretching
  - Non-steroidal anti-inflammatories, muscle relaxants can be used as adjuncts
  - Most with mild symptoms or if diagnosed early will improve
  - Surgical management is reserved for persistent, disabling symptoms in patients with a confident diagnosis and who have undergone at least 8 weeks of PT
  - Surgery involves *scalenectomy* with *first rib resection* from either a transaxillary or supraclavicular approach
    - Both approaches appear to have similar results when done by experienced personnel
    - Supraclavicular approach offers better exposure and theoretical benefit of complete scalenectomy
    - Rib resection requires division of the anterior and middle scalene muscles
  - *Pectoralis minor tenotomy*: consider in:
    - Patients with recognized nerve compression at the level of the pectoralis minor
    - Patients with persistent or recurrent symptoms following scalenectomy
  - Surgical complications
    - Post-operative *pneumothorax* is common and often unavoidable in cases of rib resection as the pleura forms the posterior surface of the rib
    - Brachial plexus injury is uncommon; usually indirect (e.g. retractor injury) and temporary
    - Most common complication of transaxillary approach—injury to subclavian vessels

Complications are thought to be more common in supraclavicular approach given more extensive exposure

  - Up to 10% may have temporary phrenic nerve dysfunction; should have diaphragm evaluated prior to any contralateral procedure
  - Lymphatic leakage is not uncommon and usually from small tributaries; mostly spontaneously resolved

Vascular injury during rib resection is typically related to side branch avulsion that can often be treated with clipping or ligation

Venous TOS (vTOS) [1, 2]

- Defined as presence of compression and resultant thrombosis of the axillo-subclavian vein
  - Defined as "Primary thrombosis"
  - Synonymous with Paget-Schroetter syndrome and the older "effort thrombosis"
  - Secondary thrombosis = following injury, systemic disease (malignancy), or iatrogenic cause (e.g. catheter)
- Symptoms without thrombosis → intermittent compression or "McCleery Syndrome" (~10% of vTOS)
- Subclavian vein passes through costoclavicular space
  - Medial borders: subclavius muscle, costoclavicular ligament
  - Lateral border: anterior scalene muscle
  - Superior: clavicle
  - Inferior: first rib
- Predisposing factors:
  - Abnormally lateral insertion of the costoclavicular ligament (always present)
  - Narrowed costoclavicular space
  - Repetitive movements wherein the arm is held above the head for long periods (throwing, swimming, etc.) cause hypertrophy of ligament → repeated compression → fibrosis → stenosis → thrombosis

  - Congenital or acquired hypercoagulable state: thrombophilia, pregnancy, malignancy
- *History and Exam*
  - Most commonly young athletic individuals who perform repetitive overhead movements
  - Historically, 2:1 male predominance; however, gender ratio is likely close to equal
  - Typically asymptomatic until triggering event (e.g. exercise or labor) → acute venous obstruction → pain, arm swelling, cyanosis, paresthesia, weakness
  - Right side is most commonly affected
  - In cases of intermittent, partial or chronic occlusion, pain worsens with exercise or use of arm
  - Chronic venous obstruction → Dilated subcutaneous veins
  - Urschel's sign—venous collaterals around the shoulder → suggests total obstruction of subclavian vein
  - Must rule out secondary causes → central catheters, pacemaker wires, malignancy
  - Untreated vTOS will frequently lead to significant long-term morbidity
  - ~10% will develop pulmonary embolism; low rate likely due to narrowing of the vein which may trap thrombus
- *Duplex ultrasound* = Imaging study of choice
  - Highly sensitive and specific
  - Should include the entirety of vein
  - Will demonstrate near or complete obstruction without venous flow
  - Can be conducted with provocative maneuvers → can be helpful for diagnosis in McCleery Syndrome (intermittent compression)
- *Contrast venography*—sometimes helpful if US is negative and clinical suspicion remains high; magnetic resonance and computed tomographic venography usually not as helpful
- *Differential diagnosis* should include:
  - Thrombophilia
  - Pancoast tumors

  - Central venous stenosis (e.g. from arteriovenous fistula for dialysis)
  - Lymphedema
  - Rheumatic disorders
  - Infections or allergy
  - Metabolic causes (e.g. thyroid disease, heart failure)
- *Treatment*
  - Best results if treated within 14 days from onset, though good results have been seen up to 8 months
  - Empiric anticoagulation can be started prior to diagnostic imaging if suspicion is high
  - Initial treatment should involve thrombolysis, either *catheter-directed* or *pharmacomechanical*
  - Thrombolysis or angioplasty without operative decompression can be insufficient for complete resolution as the problem is extrinsic compression of the vein
  - First rib resection and external venolysis from a transaxillary, infraclavicular, or paraclavicular approach should follow
  - Medial claviculectomy can be considered in patients needing complex venous reconstruction (e.g. jugular turndown) to provide improved exposure
  - In chronic settings, patients may not benefit from aggressive attempts at recanalization; decompression and anticoagulation may be sufficient
  - Anticoagulation should be continued post-operatively for at least 3–6 months after surgery or longer if a clotting disorder is present
  - Angioplasty may be required adjunctively to manage venous stenosis
  - Chronic occlusion or persistent symptomatic occlusion despite treatment may need *axillosubclavian venous reconstruction* with *adjunctive arteriovenous fistula* to increase venous blood flow (generally poor outcomes)

Arterial TOS (aTOS) [1, 2]

- Least common form, 1–3%
- Related to repeated damage of the subclavian artery as it crosses the first rib
- Potential risk for aneurysm formation, embolism, and ischemic symptoms
- Of the forms of TOS, strongest indication for operative intervention
- Natural history: Arterial compression and injury → stenosis → post-stenotic dilation → aneurysmal degeneration and thrombus formation → secondary embolism → upper extremity ischemia
- Predisposing factors:
  - Cervical or anomalous first rib
  - Congenital bands
  - Clavicular fracture with bony callus
  - Anomalous insertion of anterior scalene muscle
- *History.*
  - Patients are often young, healthy and report vigorous use of their arms in occupational or recreational activities
  - Usually asymptomatic until thromboembolism occurs, resulting in digital or limb ischemia
  - Unilateral digital ischemia is one of the most common presenting problems
  - Some may present with claudication symptoms, including early fatigability, cramping, pallor or coldness, and paresthesias during exertion
  - Document constitutional symptoms suggestive of vasculitis (e.g. fever, malaise), particularly in younger patients
- *Exam*
  - Over 90% will have either a cervical rib or anomalous first rib
  - Examine supraclavicular fossa for a palpable pulsatile mass or bruit on auscultation

  - Provocative tests may elicit a bruit if not present at rest in a relaxed position
  - Bilateral brachial blood pressure should be measured
  - Attention should be paid to the hands which may show stigmata of embolic phenomenon (mottling, petechiae, gangrene, etc.)
- *Diagnosis*
  - Duplex ultrasonography should be obtained in all patients being worked up for aTOS; focus on axillary and subclavian arteries
  - Provocative maneuvers should be utilized
  - In equivocal cases, computed tomographic angiography (CTA) may be helpful and, in some cases, may be superior to conventional angiography
    - CT allows for views with (1) arms at sides and (2) hyperabducted/externally rotated to trigger compression
    - Conventional angiography has a high false negative rate in supine position
    - Helpful for surgical planning
  - Conventional angiography remains the gold standard
  - Chest X-ray may identify skeletal abnormalities like cervical ribs
- *Treatment*
  - There is no role for true conservative therapy in aTOS
  - Distal revascularization of an ischemic limb can be accomplished via arterial thrombolysis (either conventional or pharmacomechanical) or open thromboembolectomy
  - Definitive surgical treatment involves thorough anterior and middle scalenectomy with resection of any cervical or anomalous first ribs
  - Can be done through a supraclavicular, infraclavicular, or paraclavicular approach

- Aneurysm and other diseased artery segments, if present, should be resected and reconstructed with interposition grafting using reversed saphenous vein
- Focal lesions can be treated with patch angioplasty
- Stenting in this area should be approached with caution given the lack of long-term results and theoretical risk of failure
- Administration of catheter-directed vasodilators (e.g. Prostaglandin E) and thrombolytic agents (e.g. tissue Plasminogen activator) may provide benefit for patients with digital ischemia
- Duplex ultrasound is useful for routine surveillance

Questions and Answers

1. A 24-year old right-handed male professional baseball pitcher player presents with 48-h of right upper extremity pain and swelling after playing a tournament. His arm is discolored and there is non-pitting edema. Pulses are present. Duplex ultrasound identifies an obstruction of the subclavian vein. What is the best initial treatment?
   (a) Bedrest
   (b) Anticoagulation alone
   (c) Anticoagulation and thrombolysis
   (d) Second rib resection
2. Neurogenic TOS is most commonly caused by:
   (a) Cervical rib
   (b) Neck trauma
   (c) Anomalous first rib
   (d) Diabetes mellitus
3. A 42-year-old woman presents to the urgent care with a painful, pallorous thumb that has progressed over the last 6 h. She is otherwise healthy and does not use tobacco. She has palpa-

ble ulnar and radial pulses bilaterally. You note a harsh bruit over her supraclavicular fossa on the ipsilateral side. You give her an aspirin and order an urgent duplex ultrasound of her upper extremity. What would you expect to see on plain chest X-ray?
(a) Subclavian artery dissection
(b) Pneumothorax
(c) Subclavian vein obstruction
(d) Cervical rib

Answers: 1 (c), 2 (b), 3 (d)

References

1. Sidawy AN, Perler BA. Rutherford's vascular surgery and endovascular therapy, vols. 1 and 2. 9th ed. Philadelphia: Elsevier; 2018. p. 5279–443.
2. Illig KA, Thompson RW, Freischlag JA, Donahue DM, Jordan SE, Edgelow PI. Thoracic outlet syndrome. London: Springer; 2013. p. 3–653.

11 Aortoiliac Artery Aneurysms and Peripheral Artery Aneurysms

Emaad Farooqui and Sukgu M. Han

Abdominal Aorta and Iliac Artery Aneurysms

- Epidemiology and Pathogenesis
  - Definition of an *aneurysm* = dilation of all layers of a vessel wall 1.5 times their expected normal diameter [1].
  - **Risk factors:** Tobacco use, increased age, hypertension, male gender, hypercholesterolemia, and family history [2, 3]

    Tobacco use is the single strongest risk factor for AAA development and growth (7× risk of AAA compared to nonsmokers [ADAM trial])

E. Farooqui
University of Southern California/Keck School of Medicine, Los Angeles, CA, USA
e-mail: emaad.farooqui@med.usc.edu

S. M. Han (✉)
University of Southern California/Keck School of Medicine, Los Angeles, CA, USA

Division of Vascular Surgery and Endovascular Therapy, Comprehensive Aortic Center at Keck Hospital of University of Southern California, Los Angeles, CA, USA
e-mail: Sukgu.han@med.usc.edu

A. Murga et al. (eds.), *The Vascular Surgery In-Training Examination Review (VSITE)*,
https://doi.org/10.1007/978-3-031-24121-5_11

- Risk of rupture is related to the size of the aneurysm

  Location, growth rate, and morphology (saccular vs. fusiform) impact risk assessment of aneurysm rupture
- **Pathophysiology**: Underlying imbalance between proteases and anti-proteases. Can be due to degenerative processes including inflammatory, infectious, and genetic.

  Elastin and collagen are the structural proteins responsible for the integrity of the aortic wall
  - Collagen comprises 25% of the wall in a non-atherosclerotic aorta, but only 5–18% of an aneurysmal aortic wall [4].
  - Elastin fragmentation and depletion is the structural event in aneurysm formation [4].
  - Aneurysmal aortas have a *decrease in both* **collagen** and **elastin**, but there is an *increased ratio of collagen to elastin* within the walls of aneurysms

  Weakening of elastic lamellae results in decreased ability of elastin to provide retractive circumferential and longitudinal force, thus increasing aneurysm diameter and length
  - Increased levels of degenerative matrix metalloproteinases (MMPs) within the **media** of the vessel wall (most common)
    - MMP-1,2,3 most common *collagenase* within aneurysmal wall
    - MMP-9 most common *elastase* within aneurysmal wall
  - Increased antiproteases (α_1-antitrypsin)
  - Increased inflammatory infiltrate (macrophages, lymphocytes, cytokines)

  Infectious (mycotic) causes of aneurysms: results from primary infection of the arterial wall from hematogenous seeding or extension of an adjacent infectious process.
  - 0.7–1.5% of all aortic aneurysms. Tend to be saccular.
  - Usually immunocompromised (diabetes mellitus, AIDS, malnutrition, cirrhosis) but also from trauma

or luminal defects (atherosclerotic plaque/ulceration, pre-existing aneurysm)

  - *Staphylococcus aureus* is most common. *Streptococcus*, *Salmonella,* tuberculosis, syphilis, and fungal causes have all been documented as potential organisms [5].
  - Computed tomography (CT) findings of periaortic soft tissue mass, stranding/fluid, and/or destruction of surrounding tissue such as the kidney or vertebral column.
  - Repair with aggressive intravenous antibiotics, surgical repair and debridement of infected tissue
    - Extra-anatomic bypass and in situ reconstructive techniques with equal short-term mortality
    - Endovascular repair as bridge to definitive therapy or in patients unable to tolerate open surgery.

Associated with anomalous arterial structures

  - Kommerell diverticulum, persistent sciatic artery, etc.

- Aneurysm Classification
  - True vs. False Aneurysm:

    True aneurysm: Dilatation of all layers of the vascular wall

    False aneurysm (pseudoaneurysm): Locally contained hematoma by surrounding tissue resulting from disruption of the vessel wall
  - Morphology: Refer to Fig. 11.1

    Fusiform: Generalized increase in entire diameter of affected vessel
    - More common

    Saccular: Localized, eccentric outpouchings on the vessel wall
    - Results from focal weakness of the arterial wall
- **Abdominal aortic aneurysms**
  - Infrarenal aortic aneurysms represent 30% of all aortic aneurysms
  - Seventy-five percent of infrarenal AAAs are asymptomatic when first identified

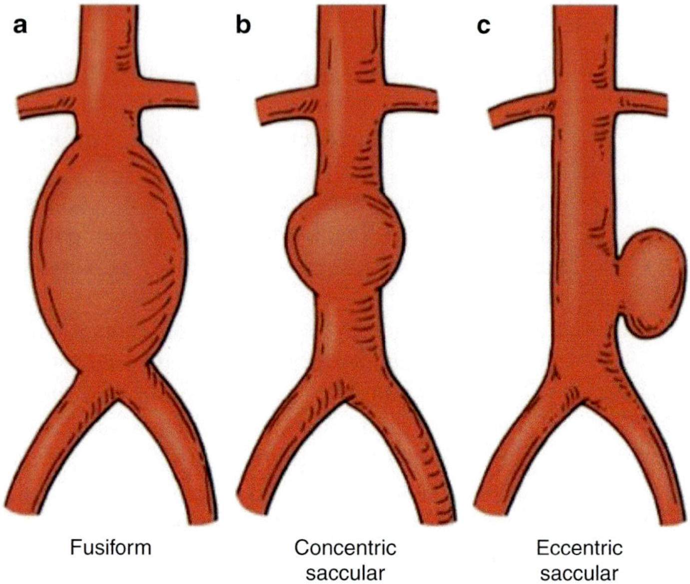

Fig. 11.1 (**a**–**c**) Fusiform and saccular aneurysm morphology. (Taken from Rutherford's Vascular Surgery and Endovascular Therapy 9th ed. Ch. 69 P.879)

Fifty percent with palpable, pulsatile abdominal mass on physical exam

Can present with any type of abdominal pain due to pressure on adjacent structures, embolization, rupture, or expansion.

- Direct correlation between incidence of AAA and smoking history
- Diabetes, African American race, and female sex are *negative risk factors* correlated with presence of aneurysms [6].
- Juxtarenal: aneurysm sac extends up to, but does not involve, the renal arteries

  Requires suprarenal clamping
- Pararenal: aneurysm involves the renal arteries and extends up to the superior mesenteric artery

Requires more extensive dissection and exposure in open aortic repair than juxtarenal aneurysms

- 5–15% extend are juxtarenal or suprarenal; 10–25% involve the iliac arteries. 12% involve the thoracic aorta [7].
- AAAs often lined with thrombus which interferes with nutrient delivery to aortic wall
- Average enlargement rate of AAA is 0.2–0.3 cm/year for small aneurysms (3–5 cm) to 0.3–0.5 cm/year for larger aneurysms (>5 cm) [8]

  Factors associated with rapid growth include larger initial size, hypertension, increased pulse pressure, tobacco use, or history of cardiac/renal transplant.

  - Aneurysms progress due to physical principles described by Laplace's law, which states that tangential wall stress (T) is equal to the radius (R) and the transmural pressure (P). $T = PR$

  Tobacco use increases rate of enlargement by 35% and is the most significant modifiable risk factor for controlling aneurysm growth

- **Rupture risk:** directly correlated with maximal AAA diameter, Refer to Table 11.1

  Females have 3× increase in rupture risk compared with males of similar aortic diameter

Table 11.1 Annual rupture risk based on AAA diameter

AAA diameter (cm)	Rupture risk (%)
3.0–3.9	0.3
4.0–4.9	0.5–1.5
5.0–5.9	1–11
6.0–6.9	11–22
>7	>30

Taken from Rutherford's Vascular Surgery and Endovascular Therapy 9th Ed. Ch. 70
AAA abdominal aortic aneurysms

Tobacco use, chronic obstructive lung disease, hypertension, female gender, transplant recipient, and AAA growth >1 cm/year all increase overall risk of rupture

- Annual rupture risk based on AAA diameter (based on UKSAT and ADAM trials):
- Saccular morphology more prone to rupture than fusiform.
- Classically, AAA rupture presents with abrupt onset of severe back, flank, or abdominal pain.

  Rupture most frequently occurs through *posterolateral aortic wall on the left side* into the retroperitoneal space, less commonly through anterior wall into peritoneal cavity. Can be contained within the retroperitoneum or freely ruptured.
- **Diagnostic methods**

  Ultrasound: both sensitive and specific but limited by body habitus and bowel gas pattern. Not good for use in emergently examined patients
  - Good for screening AAA
  - Fails to detect 50% of aneurysm ruptures

  CT with angiography (CTA): Greater reproducibility of diameter measurements than ultrasound.
  - Can provide anatomic information, vessel calcification, and thrombosis, and provides multiplanar and 3-dimensional reconstruction for both endovascular and open operative planning.
  - Downside of iodinated contrast media in patients with associated kidney disease; radiation exposure

  Magnetic resonance imaging (MRI) and angiography (MRA): Similar to CT with detecting AAAs.
  - Pros: Does not require iodinated contrast (MRA utilizes gadolinium)
  - Cons: Time consuming, limited availability, contraindicated with metallic implants/foreign bodies does not demonstrate aortic wall calcification

  Conventional angiography: Only required when further characterization of aneurysm is required or for intervention purposes.

- **Screening and Surveillance**

  Society for Vascular Surgery (SVS) guidelines 2018

  - Screening: One-time AAA ultrasound screening for men *and* women ages 65–75 with history of tobacco use [9].
  - Surveillance: Based on aortic size and risk factors. Ultrasound should be used for surveillance unless other imaging modalities specifically indicated [9].
  - Based on AAA diameter
    - 3–4 cm: several years
    - 4–4.9 cm: Annually
    - 5–5.4 cm: Every 6 months
  - Surveillance ultrasound every 5 years after open aortic repair
- **Medical therapy**

  There is *no* definitive evidence to suggest any specific medical management strategy that slows the growth rate of AAAs.

  - Statins, ACE inhibitors, beta-blockers, antibiotics (tetracycline/doxycycline), antiplatelets, and exercise have been shown in animal models to slow aneurysm progression, but have *not* been demonstrated in humans.
- **Indications for elective intervention of AAAs**

  Men: *5.5 cm* or growth rate >*1 cm/year*

  Women: *5 cm* or growth rate >*1 cm/year*

  - **No** survival benefit to early elective repair (before recommended size criteria)
  - Surveillance of aneurysms between 4 and 5 cm is safe with compliant patients based on UK Small aneurysm trial and U.S. Veterans Administration: ADAM trial, though 80% of these patients eventually progress to needing repair [10, 11].

- **Open Repair of AAAs**
  - More durable long-term data with open repair, but associated increased morbidity and mortality in the perioperative period as compared to endovascular aneurysm repair (EVAR). Additionally, given the advancements in endovascular technology there are no absolute indications for open repair.

- Indications for open repair of AAA:
  Infection/mycotic aneurysm
  Horseshoe kidney
  Inferior mesenteric artery preservation required (bilateral hypogastric artery occlusion, SMA occlusion, or prior colectomy)
  Long life-expectancy, young age
  Poorly compliant with follow-up
  No aortic neck or hostile aortic neck not suitable for EVAR
  Anatomic constraints in distal aorta and iliac arteries
  Inadequate access for EVAR
- **Transperitoneal vs. retroperitoneal approach to open AAA repair: Refer to** Figs. 11.2 and 11.3
  Transperitoneal:
  - Rapid access to infrarenal aorta, better access to right renal and right internal/external iliac arteries.
    - More difficult to expose visceral aortic segments
  - Exposure: Supine position, midline incision. Cephalad retraction of omentum and transverse colon, small bowel packed into right hemiabdomen.
    - Ligament of Treitz divided and the third and fourth portions of the duodenum are reflected to patient right to expose aorta.
    - Incision is started left of the aorta at ligament of Treitz and courses to the right of the aortic midline to prevent injury to inferior mesenteric artery and autonomic venous plexus at the aortic bifurcation.
  - Pararenal aorta: Juxtarenal and pararenal aneurysms require **suprarenal clamping**, thus requiring proximal aortic exposure up to the renal veins
  - Supraceliac aorta exposure: Necessitates dividing lesser omentum. Mobilize the overlying fibers of the right crus of the diaphragm. Mobilize left lobe of liver by dividing triangular and coronary ligaments. The esophagus is retracted to the left and aorta dissected anteriorly down to the level of the celiac axis.

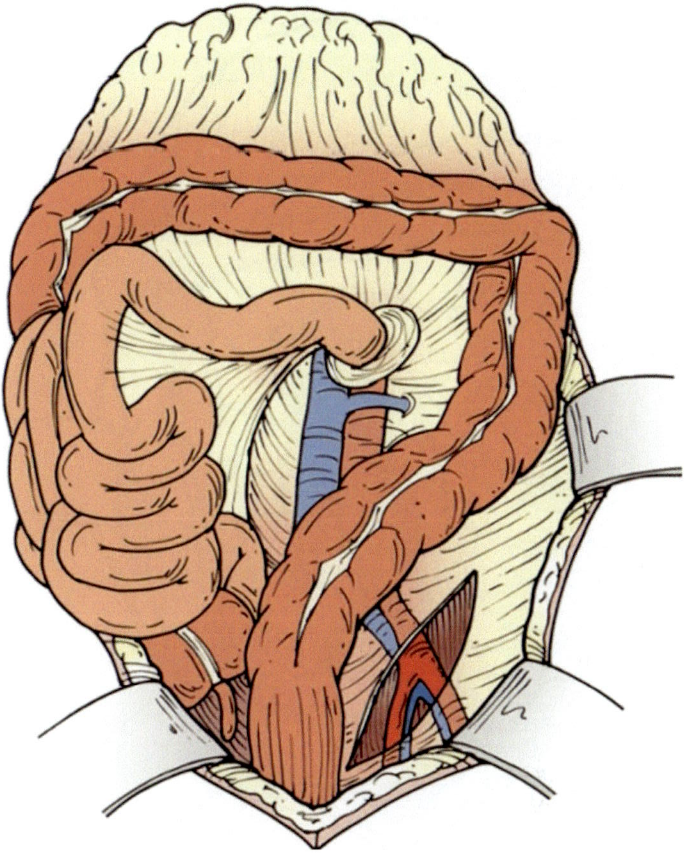

Fig. 11.2 Left iliac artery exposure accessed by mobilizing sigmoid colon medially and incising posterior peritoneum at its base. (Taken from Rutherford's Vascular Surgery and Endovascular Therapy 9th Ed. Ch.71 P.899)

- Medial visceral rotation: Left colon mobilized by incising white line of Toldt.
  - Carried cephalad through phrenocolic ligament and medially toward aortic hiatus under the diaphragm.

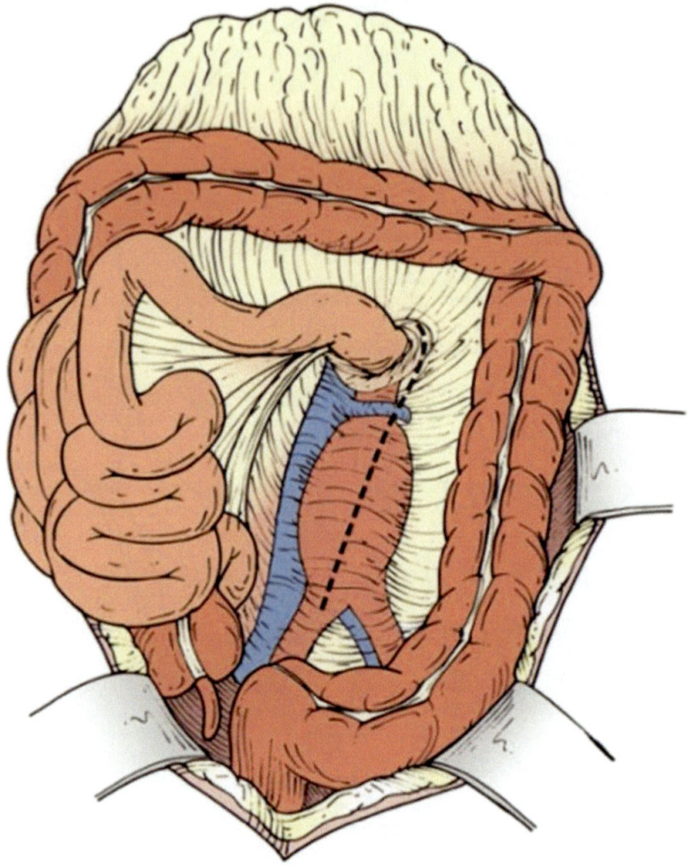

Fig. 11.3 Aortic exposure after incising overlying posterior peritoneum. (Taken from Rutherford's Vascular Surgery and Endovascular Therapy 9th Ed. Ch. 71 P.899)

- Reconstruction:
  - Distal aortic clamping first to prevent embolization
  - Longitudinal aortotomy with T shaped incision at proximal and distal ends for graft. Clear thrombus/calcium off aorta

End-to-end anastomosis with permanent suture

Closure aneurysm sac over the graft or omental coverage to prevent bowel contact with graft.

Retroperitoneal: Usually through tenth interspace incision, can allow for superior exposure of supraceliac aorta and left renal artery

- Useful in pararenal aortic aneurysms, extent IV thoracoabdominal aortic aneurysms
- Avoids hostile abdomen (adhesions, re-do laparotomy)
- Advantageous in obese patients by allowing abdominal contents to fall away from operative field

Retroperitoneal:

- Right lateral decubitus position with table flexion at iliac crest
- Incision at tenth intercostal space at posterior axillary line lateral and parallel to lateral border of left rectus muscle down to umbilicus.
- Expose anterior fascia of external oblique. Sequentially open external, internal oblique, and transversus abdominus muscles sequentially without peritoneal violation and free peritoneum from abdominal wall and diaphragm with blunt dissection
- Identify left psoas muscle and sweep peritoneal/retroperitoneal contents anteromedially
- Supraceliac exposure: Divide left crus of diaphragm

– Considerations during aortic repair

In the presence of significant superior mesenteric artery disease, bilateral hypogastric artery occlusions, or prior colectomy, then inferior mesenteric artery preservation is indicated

Venous abnormalities:

- 1–10% of population [12]
  – Retroaortic left renal vein, circumaortic left renal vein, left-sided IVC, duplicated IVC, accessory left renal veins

Renal protection:

    - Agents for renal protection during cross-clamping include furosemide, mannitol, dopamine, and acetylcysteine
      - Cold hyperosmolar crystalloid, histidine-tryptophan-ketoglutarate (HTK) solution, mannitol, and methylprednisolone have been shown to improve renal outcomes following juxtarenal aneurysm repair requiring suprarenal aortic clamping [13, 14].

        Requires perfusion circuit and cannulation resulting in prolonged ischemia time.
  - Post-operative complications

    Seventy-one percent overall complication rate in perioperative period with open repair (11% major adverse event rate) [15].

    Increased perioperative cardiac complications with aortic cross-clamping due to hemodynamic changes and increased demand on the heart.

    - Ten percent perioperative myocardial infarction rate in perioperative period [16].

    Post-operative pneumonia occurs in 17% of patients.

    Twenty percent post-operative renal insufficiency in pararenal AAAs, 3.5% dialysis dependency [16].

    0.2–6% colonic ischemia rate [17].

    Lower extremity ischemia secondary to embolic sequelae of distal cross-clamp.

    Spinal cord ischemia rare in open AAA repair (less than 1%) [17]

    3.5% overall mortality rate with open aortic repair
- **Endovascular repair of AAAs**
  - Mainstay of treatment for elective repair of anatomically suitable aortic aneurysms
  - Numerous commercially available stent grafts with variety of configurations
  - Pre-operative CTA is essential using thin (1 mm) cuts.

    Intravascular ultrasound (IVUS) can be adjunctive or used in patients with renal insufficiency.

- Endograft sizing
  - Aortic neck diameter: measured at level of lowest renal artery in multiple short segment (5 mm) increments using centerline measurements or the **minor axis of axial cuts.**
  - Endografts should be oversized **10–20%** compared to the aortic neck
    - Oversizing >20% leads to graft in-folding and creates pleats in the fabric.
  - Length measurements: CT will underestimate the length between aortic bifurcation and hypogastric arteries on axial imaging without centerline measurements.
  - For modular devices, the contralateral iliac gate should be positioned 1–2 cm from the aortic bifurcation
  - Iliac diameters: 10–20% oversizing on minor axis
- Anatomic considerations and patient selection:
  - Access vessels: free of calcium, >7 mm diameter
    - Can use iliac conduit or endoconduit for difficult femoral access
    - Hydrophilic dilators for long-segment occlusive disease in access vessels
  - Aortic neck diameter: maximum 32 mm
  - Proximal landing zone: minimum of 10–15 mm (device dependent)
  - Distal landing zone: 2 cm of healthy vessel wall
  - Angulation: less than 45–60°.
  - Vessel wall appearance: free of thrombus or calcification at landing zones
  - Accessory renal artery
    - Safe to cover in patients with normal renal function
      - Consider fenestrated approach or open repair
- Complications of EVAR in AAA repair
  - **Endoleaks:** Luminal filling around stent-grafts into aneurysm sac
    - Refer to Table 11.2 and Fig. 11.4
  - Renal artery coverage
  - Stent migration

Table 11.2 Types of endoleaks

Endoleaks			
Type I	• Inadequate seal at graft ends • Requires definitive treatment	Type Ia	• Inadequate seal from proximal end of stent-graft
		Type Ib	• Inadequate seal from distal end of stent-graft
		Type Ic	• Inadequate seal at common iliac artery
Type II	• Retrograde flow from aortic collaterals into aneurysm sac • Most common • Can be monitored with serial imaging for aneurysmal expansion, as these are often self-limiting – Otherwise requires embolization of feeding branches		
Type III	• Requires re-lining of stent-graft	Type IIIa	• Due to component disconnection between stent-graft devices
		Type IIIb	• Due to stent fabric disturbance
Type IV	• Due to graft porosity • Rare with new stent-graft devices		
Type V	• Endotension • Continued aneurysm sac growth and pressurization without evidence of sac perfusion		

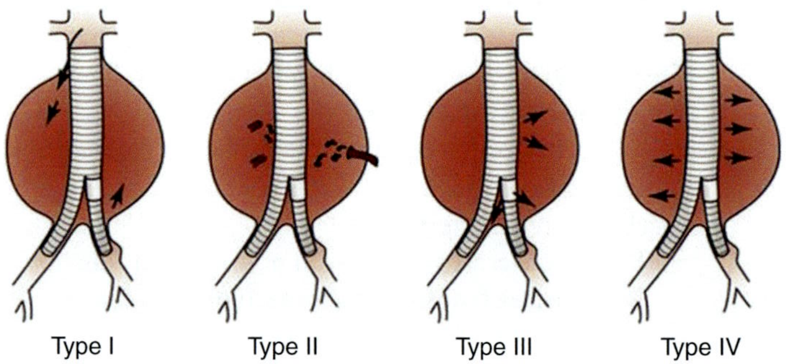

Fig. 11.4 Types of endoleaks. (Taken from Rutherford's Vascular Surgery and Endovascular Therapy 9th ed. Ch. 72)

- Management of ruptured AAAs:
  - Defined as the presence of a AAA with extraluminal blood on CT
  - Contained rupture: blood outside the aneurysm sac confined to the retroperitoneal space
  - Free rupture: bleeding into the peritoneal cavity
  - Treatment after rupture associated with 10-fold increase in mortality as compared with elective repair [18].
  - Operative mortality declining overall with use of EVAR for ruptured AAAs

    47–67% of ruptured AAAs are suitable for endovascular repair [19]

    EVAR associated with reduced mortality compared to open repair [19–21].

    - EVAR mortality 42% vs. open repair 54%. Lower length of hospital stay, improved quality of life with EVAR [21].
    - Preferred method of treating ruptured AAAs for those with suitable anatomy

    Thirty-day outcomes improved with EVAR in suitable patients compared to open repair in multiple trials.
  - Clinical presentation: triad of abdominal/back pain, hypotension, and pulsatile abdominal mass
  - Initial management of ruptured AAA:

    Permissive hypotension and judicious resuscitation

    - Intravenous fluids raise blood pressure and worsens hemorrhage by releasing tamponade, hemodilution, coagulopathy, hypothermia, and acidosis
      - Fluid resuscitation should maintain consciousness and minimize organ ischemia (systolic pressure of 70–80 mmHg) [22].
  - Operating room considerations

    Local anesthesia for EVAR reduced 30-day mortality compared with general anesthesia [21]

    Aortic occlusion balloon for endovascular management in hemodynamic instability

Maintain pelvic perfusion with at least one internal iliac artery patent

Open repair:

- Transperitoneal approach for rapid control
  - Supraceliac clamping until infrarenal aorta dissected.

    Supraceliac clamping induces ischemic injuries to liver, bowel, and kidneys and contributes to multi-organ system failure.

    Supraceliac unclamping can result in sudden hypotension
- Continuous bleeding into the open aneurysm after proximal and distal control indicates *aorto-caval fistula*.
  - Suture of fistula within the aneurysm is recommended repair

Avoidance of hypothermia due to coagulopathy and higher rate of wound infections [23].

Complications of ruptured AAA repair

- Bleeding, acute limb ischemia, thromboembolism, colonic ischemia, abdominal compartment syndrome, spinal ischemia, cardiac complications, liver failure, renal failure, multisystem organ failure
  - Colonic ischemia incidence 38% after open repair and 23% after EVAR of ruptured AAA [24].
  - Paraplegia rate 1.2% in open repair vs. 0.5–1.5% for EVAR

    Factors associated with spinal cord ischemia include pelvic blood supply interruption, embolization, prolonged cross clamping, and perioperative hypotension [25]
  - Multiorgan system failure 2 hit hypothesis: Hemorrhagic shock combined with ischemia from aortic cross-clamping

    Incidence of 3.8% after elective repair, 64% in open repair of ruptured AAA [26].

- **Isolated iliac artery aneurysms (IAAs)**
  - Prevalence of <2% of population
  - **70–90%** involve common iliac artery and 10–30% involve internal iliac artery (IIA) [27].
    - Fifty percent of common IAAs are bilateral [28]
    - Rarely involve external iliac artery (EIA) possibly due to embryonic lineage of EIA vascular smooth muscle being different from the common and internal iliac arteries [29].
- Generally asymptomatic and found incidentally
  - Symptoms are obscure and can include vague lower abdominal pain from compression of nerve roots or pelvic veins, claudication, lower extremity paresis, ureteral obstruction, or constipation [30].
    - Thromboemboli to lower extremity with resulting limb ischemia
    - Sudden onset abdominal, groin, or flank pain with shock indicates rupture
  - However, high rate of mortality from rupture secondary to asymptomatic disease progression and lack of true physical exam findings
    - **Twenty-eight percent mortality rate** during emergent repair over last 20 years compared to 5% in elective cases [31]
      - Mean size at time of rupture 6–6.8 cm.
      - Iliac artery aneurysms <4 cm are not frequently associated with rupture
- Pathogenesis is similar to AAA involving altered balance between proteolytic degradation of the extracellular matrix, mechanical integrity, inflammation, and impaired arterial remodeling [30, 31].
  - Risk factors include tobacco use and hypertension
    - Less commonly include traumatic and infectious causes
- Diagnosis of IAA:
  - Ultrasound is the primary diagnostic screening tool
    - CT angiography and MR angiography provide more detail of aortoiliac anatomy and are used in operative

planning to delineate diameter, landing zones, tortuosity and angulation, and atherosclerotic disease for endovascular planning.

  - Management of IAAs

    Consensus statements favor elective repair of asymptomatic IAAs 3–3.5 cm in diameter in healthy patients [32–34].

- Operative considerations
  - Similar to AAA repair, goal is to exclude aneurysm sac from circulation to limit expansion and induce sac thrombosis.
  - Standard open surgical treatment for isolated common iliac aneurysms is interposition graft replacement via midline or retroperitoneal approach

    External iliac artery (EIA) is almost never aneurysmal and so the operation can generally be confined to the abdomen

    Open endoaneurysmorrhaphy and grafting is possible but challenging given its deep pelvic location

    - Ligating neck of internal iliac aneurysms (IIA) alone is ineffective due to continued pressurization from extensive collaterals to the internal iliac artery
  - *EVAR has become procedure of choice* for management of iliac artery aneurysms

    Accounts for 70% of iliac aneurysm repairs

    - Survival benefit with EVAR compared to open repair within first 3 years.
    - However, open repair with better long-term survival [28].

    Requires 2 cm of proximal and distal landing zone

    Limitations of EVAR for IAA repair

    - Unsuitable anatomy for EVAR, prior failed EVARs, persistent type 1 endoleak, inadequate access, infection

    Pitfalls of EVAR include compromising internal iliac artery perfusion with stent graft

        - Unilateral internal iliac artery is associated with buttock claudication in 28% of patients. Bilateral occlusion with 41% incidence in addition to increased risks of spinal cord ischemia, colonic ischemia, erectile dysfunction, and pelvic ischemia [28, 35].
        - Iliac branched stent-grafts are now available specifically for iliac system to limit these complications in suitable patients
  - Internal iliac artery aneurysms can be treated with catheter-based coil injections, plugs, and thrombogenic materials into the aneurysmal portion and its branches.

    Direct stent graft repair is feasible if proximal and distal landing zones are appropriate

    - Can "chimney" or "sandwich" into external iliac artery for compromised proximal landing zones
    - Use of Iliac Branched Device in anatomically suitable patients

    Hybrid approaches consisting of aorto-uni-iliac endograft followed by femoral-to-femoral artery bypass with contralateral internal iliac occlusion depending on patient anatomy. Refer to Fig. 11.5

- **Peripheral arterial aneurysms**
  - Most common cause of non-mycotic peripheral arterial aneurysms is **atherosclerotic disease**

    Atherosclerotic aneurysms occur *mostly in men older than 50*

    Peripheral aneurysms in decreasing frequency

    - Popliteal → Femoral → Subclavian → Axillary → Carotid

    Distal tibial, forearm, and hand aneurysms are secondary to trauma or mycotic in origin [36, 37].

  - Frequently associated with concomitant aortic, iliac, and splanchnic aneurysms.
  - Can be asymptomatic or have clinical manifestations, but generally **do not rupture**

    Peripheral aneurysms **thrombose** or **embolize** which result in their associated morbidity

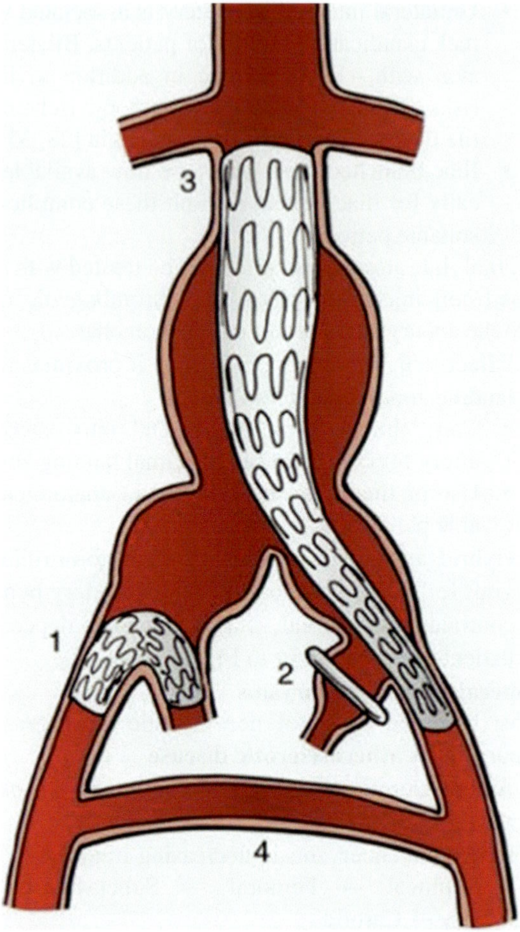

Fig. 11.5 External-to-internal iliac artery stent (1) and contralateral internal iliac artery occlusion (2). Aortouniiliac device (3) and femoral-femoral artery bypass (4). (Taken from Rutherford's Vascular Surgery and Endovascular Therapy 9th Ed. Ch 72.)

– *Popliteal artery aneurysms*

  Most common peripheral aneurysm. Account for 70% of peripheral aneurysms with a 20:1 male-to-female ratio [38].

Seventy-eight percent of patients have a second aneurysm and 64% have concomitant aortoiliac aneurysms [39]

- Fifty percent have bilateral popliteal artery aneurysms [36, 39].

High incidence of thromboembolic events (74% complication rate over 5 years)

- Seventy-five percent patients present with symptoms that include claudication, embolization with ischemia, thrombosis, or swelling and pain from expansion and compressive symptoms [40].

Diagnosis

- High level of suspicion in patients with very easily palpated, wide popliteal pulse
- Ultrasound is highly sensitive and specific
- CTA for operative planning is useful
  - Conventional arteriography unnecessary unless acute limb ischemia present

Indications for repair:

- **Current recommendations for popliteal aneurysm repair include presence of symptoms, size of 1.5–2.0 cm with presence of thrombus, or all aneurysms >2 cm.**

Repair techniques: Open vs. endovascular depends on factors including patient comorbidities, runoff vessel patency, popliteal artery tortuosity, and length of vessel involvement.

- *Open repair:* **Posterior vs. medial approach**.
  - **Posterior** approach with aneurysm resection and interposition graft replacement. More commonly used currently vs. medial approach.
    Preferred in large aneurysms with tibial nerve and popliteal vein compression
    Benefit includes complete aneurysm decompression
  - Aneurysm exclusion with above-knee to below-knee bypass through **medial** approach

Medial approach preferred if aneurysmal degeneration extends into superficial femoral artery or infra-genicular arterial tree.

Historically was the preferred method but found to have collateral filling of aneurysm sac and subsequent expansion.

- Limb loss rate similar between both approaches
- Autogenous vein has better 5-year patency as compared to polytetrafluoroethylene (PTFE) grafts (94% vs. 85%) [41].

Thrombolytic therapy is indicated in patients with thromboembolic complications of popliteal artery aneurysms where there is no outflow vessel visualized on CT angiography or arteriography.

- Associated with improved graft patency and limb salvage rates after initial thrombolysis compared to early operative intervention alone [42, 43].
- *Endovascular* repair: Benefits include shorter operative time, decreased hospital length of stay, and less perioperative morbidity [40].
  - Ideal candidates:

    Multi-vessel runoff

    2 cm proximal and distal landing zones (1.5 cm minimum)
  - Relative contraindications:

    Extension of disease into superficial femoral artery or into tibial vessels

    Single-vessel runoff

    Large aneurysms causing compressive symptoms
  - Inferior patency with endovascular repair in the early post-operative period based on Vascular Quality Initiative from 2015 [44].

    Superior 1-year patency rates with open repair

- Outcomes:

    Directly related to status of runoff vessels [45].

    Five-year patency for asymptomatic lesions was 91%. Symptomatic lesions 5-year patency of 54%.

    Overall survival and rate of limb loss equivalent between open and endovascular repairs

    - Lower 1-year patency rates in endovascular repair, but 4-year cumulative primary patency rates were 86% for endovascular vs. 88% for open repair, respectively, when patients on dual antiplatelet therapy.
- *Infra-popliteal aneurysms:* Very rare and usually secondary to trauma or infection

    Symptoms can range from asymptomatic to claudication, to limb ischemia

    Diagnosed by ultrasound, CT angiography, or conventional arteriography.

    Repair of infra-popliteal artery aneurysms is indicated when aneurysmal segment is two times the size of normal adjacent artery or symptomatic aneurysms (pain, ischemia).

    - Can be treated by ligation or coil embolization if adequate collateral circulation.
        - In absence of collateral circulation, vein interposition or ligation with bypass is appropriate.
- *Femoral artery aneurysms:*

    Normal diameter per Society of Vascular Surgery of common femoral artery (CFA) is 7.8–11.2mm in men, and 7.8–8.5 mm in women

    - Common femoral artery aneurysms
        - **Type 1:** Involve the CFA down to the femoral bifurcation

            44–85% of cases
        - **Type 2:** CFA with extension into the profunda femoris

- Like other peripheral aneurysms, associated with atherosclerotic disease
  - Ninety-five percent of patients with a femoral artery aneurysm had a second aneurysm
  - Fifty-nine percent bilateral femoral aneurysms [39]

Thirty to 40% of patients with associated thromboembolic events in presence of femoral artery aneurysms

Rupture is rare (with exception of profundal femoris aneurysms)

Diagnosis made by palpation of femoral artery or angiography.

Indications for repair (Vascular Low-Frequency Disease Consortium) [46]:

- Symptomatic aneurysms of any size
- Aneurysms with intramural thrombus
- Aneurysms >3.5 cm (compared to prior recommendation of >2.5 cm)
- Age < 60
- Aneurysms showing growth on surveillance
- Change in baseline pulse exam indicating embolization

Treatment

- Resection of aneurysm with interposition graft
  - Prosthetic preferred due to the size of common femoral artery
- *Stent grafting for common femoral aneurysms is rarely, if ever, indicated.*
  - High rate of stent fracture and compression given hip motion
  - Complicates future femoral access and compromises profunda artery.

– *Subclavian and axillary artery aneurysms*

Account for 1% of all peripheral aneurysms [46].

Thoracic outlet syndrome responsible for majority of subclavian artery aneurysms (74%). Can be atherosclerotic in nature.

- Associated with aberrant subclavian anatomy
  - **Kommerell diverticulum**—Aneurysm-like widening at origin of aberrant subclavian artery
- Trauma accounts for majority of axillary artery aneurysms (54%)

Associated with distal embolization (68%). Thrombosis and rupture are rare.

Ninety percent of patients are usually symptomatic at time of diagnosis

- Digital cyanosis, shoulder pain, claudication, pulsatile mass, nerve/venous compression.
- **Horner syndrome**, stridor, hoarseness in subclavian artery aneurysms.

Indications for repair: Most aneurysmal axillary and subclavian arteries require treatment given highly symptomatic nature.

- Approach depends on size, cause, and location of aneurysm with status of distal circulation.
  - Aneurysm should be excluded with restoration of arterial continuity using interposition graft or bypass.
    - Cervical rib resection when present.
    - Thoracic outlet decompression (scalenectomy, first rib resection) if neurogenic thoracic outlet symptoms exist.
    - Supraclavicular approach is preferred for subclavian artery aneurysms. Median sternotomy may be needed for proximal control.
  - Endovascular approach in high-risk patients.
    - Scant long-term data
    - Can be useful with arteriovenous fistulae or pseudoaneurysms, but limited by short fixation zones and significant branch coverage.
    - Twenty-eight percent morbidity rate with stent graft use for subclavian and axillary aneurysms [47].

Eighty-nine and 99% primary and secondary patency rates reported [47].

- Axillary artery aneurysms can be treated through axillary approach, infra-clavicular approach, or combined supra-clavicular and infra-clavicular approach depending on anatomy.
  - Resection of axillary artery potentially hazardous given involvement of brachial plexus.
  - If brachial plexus compressive symptom present, resection with interposition bypass is required. If no compressive symptoms, proximal and distal ligation with bypass can be utilized which avoids risk of brachial plexus injury.

Questions and Answers

1. Which of the following is false regarding AAA?
   (a) Tobacco is the strongest associated risk factor for AAA development
   (b) Diabetes mellitus is a negative risk factor for the development of AAA
   (c) Saccular aneurysms are more prone to rupture than fusiform
   (d) There is survival benefit for early repair of AAA before 5.0 cm in men
   (e) Aneurysmal aortas have a decrease in both collagen and elastin
2. T/F: Endovascular repair for popliteal aneurysms has inferior patency rates at 1 year compared to open repair.
3. What is the most common type of endoleak after EVAR for AAA?
   (a) Type 1
   (b) Type 2
   (c) Type 3
   (d) Type 4
   (e) Type 5

Answer: 1 (d). There is no survival benefit to early AAA repair as evidenced in the UK Small Aneurysms Trial, though most progress onto requiring repair.

Answer: 2 True. Open repair has been associated with superior patency rates as compared to endovascular treatment of popliteal aneurysms.

Answer: 3 (b). Type 2 endoleak is the most common endoleak after EVAR and is secondary to retrograde flow from collateral vessels (i.e. lumbars) that continuously perfuse the aneurysm sac. These are often self-limiting but warrant treatment if surveillance CT shows increasing aortic aneurysm size.

References

1. Belardi P, Lucertini G. Regarding "peripheral aneurysms and arteriomegaly: is there a familial pattern?". J Vasc Surg. 1999;30(3):581.
2. Heron M. Deaths: leading causes for. Natl Vital Stat Rep. 2011;59:1–95.
3. Go A, Mozaffarian D. Heart disease and stroke statistics—2013 update | Circulation. 2013. Ahajournals.org. Accessed 20 Sept 2019.
4. Kent KC, Zwolak RM, Egorova NN, Riles TS, Manganaro A, Moskowitz AJ, et al. Analysis of risk factors for abdominal aortic aneurysm in a cohort of more than 3 million individuals. J Vasc Surg. 2010;52(3):539–48.
5. Wilson SE, Van Wagenen P, Passaro E Jr. Arterial infection. Curr Probl Surg. 1978;15:1–89.
6. Lederle FA. Prevalence and associations of abdominal aortic aneurysm detected through screening. Ann Intern Med. 1997;126(6):441.
7. Pleumeekers H, Hoes A, Does EVD, Urk HV, Hofman A, Jong PD, et al. Aneurysms of the abdominal aorta in older adults. Am J Epidemiol. 1995;142(12):1291–9.
8. Powell J, Sweeting M, Brown L. Systematic review and meta-analysis of growth rates of small abdominal aortic aneurysms. J Vasc Surg. 2011;54(6):1847.
9. Lazaris AM. Regarding "The Society for Vascular Surgery practice guidelines on the care of patients with an abdominal aortic aneurysm". J Vasc Surg. 2019;69(3):975.
10. Powell J. Final 12-year follow-up of surgery versus surveillance in the UK Small Aneurysm Trial. Br J Surg. 2007;94(6):702–8.
11. Lederle FA. The Aneurysm Detection and Management Study Screening Program (ADAM). Arch Intern Med. 2000;160(10):1425.

12. Deery SE, Lancaster RT, Baril DT, et al. Contemporary outcomes of complex abdominal aortic aneurysm repair. J Vasc Surg. 2016;63:1195–200.
13. Schmitto JD, Fatehpur S, Tezval H, Popov AF, Seipelt R, Schöndube FA, et al. Hypothermic renal protection using cold histidine–tryptophan–ketoglutarate solution perfusion in suprarenal aortic surgery. Ann Vasc Surg. 2008;22(4):520–4.
14. Crawford ES, et al. Thoracoabdominal aortic aneurysms: preoperative and intraoperative factors predicting immediate and long-term results of operations in 605 patients. J Vasc Surg. 1984;3:389–404.
15. Zwolak RM, Sidawy AN, Greenberg RK, Schermerhorn ML, Shackelton RJ, Siami FS. Lifeline registry of endovascular aneurysm repair: open repair surgical controls in clinical trials. J Vasc Surg. 2008;48(3):511–8.
16. Schermerhorn M, Omalley A, Javeri A. Endovascular versus open repair of abdominal aortic aneurysms in the Medicare population. J Vasc Surg. 2008;47(5):1120.
17. Björck M, Troëng T, Bergqvist D. Risk factors for intestinal ischaemia after aortoiliac surgery: a combined cohort and case-control study of 2824 operations. Eur J Vasc Endovasc Surg. 1997;13(6):531–9.
18. Johnston K. Ruptured abdominal aortic aneurysm: Six-year follow-up results of a multicenter prospective study. J Vasc Surg. 1994;19(5):888–900.
19. Harkin D, Dillon M, Blair P, Ellis P, Kee F. Endovascular Ruptured Abdominal Aortic Aneurysm Repair (EVRAR): a systematic review. J Vasc Surg. 2007;46(6):1309.
20. Mehta M. Endovascular aneurysm repair for ruptured abdominal aortic aneurysm: the Albany Vascular Group approach. J Vasc Surg. 2010;52(6):1706–12.
21. IMPROVE Trial Investigators. Comparative clinical effectiveness and cost effectiveness of endovascular strategy v open repair for ruptured abdominal aortic aneurysm: three year results of the IMPROVE randomised trial. BMJ. 2017;359:j4859.
22. Crawford E. Ruptured abdominal aortic aneurysm: an editorial. J Vasc Surg. 1991;13(2):348–50.
23. Marty-Ané C, Alric P, Picot M, Picard E, Colson P, Mary H. Ruptured abdominal aortic aneurysm: influence of intraoperative management on surgical outcome. J Vasc Surg. 1995;22(6):780–6.
24. Becquemin J-P, Majewski M, Fermani N, Marzelle J, Desgrandes P, Allaire E, et al. Colon ischemia following abdominal aortic aneurysm repair in the era of endovascular abdominal aortic repair. J Vasc Surg. 2008;47(2):258–63.
25. Peppelenbosch A, Windsant IV, Jacobs M, Tordoir J, Schurink G. Open repair for ruptured abdominal aortic aneurysm and the risk of spinal cord ischemia: review of the literature and risk-factor analysis. J Vasc Surg. 2010;52(5):1423.
26. Bown M, Nicholson M, Bell P, Sayers R. The systemic inflammatory response syndrome, organ failure, and mortality after abdominal aortic aneurysm repair. J Vasc Surg. 2003;37(3):600–6.

27. Levi N, Schroeder T. Isolated iliac artery aneurysms. Eur J Vasc Endovasc Surg. 1998;16(4):342–4.
28. Krupski WC, Selzman CH, Floridia R, Strecker PK, Nehler MR, Whitehill TA. Contemporary management of isolated iliac aneurysms. J Vasc Surg. 1998;28(1):1–13.
29. Tilson M, Toset A, Tyrie L. Chicken embryology of human aneurysm resistant arteries. Matrix Biol. 2006;25:134.
30. Bacharach JM, Slovut DP. State of the art: management of iliac artery aneurysmal disease. Catheter Cardiovasc Interv. 2008;71(5):708–14.
31. Ailawadi G, Eliason JL, Upchurch GR. Current concepts in the pathogenesis of abdominal aortic aneurysm. J Vasc Surg. 2003;38(3):584–8.
32. Sandhu RS, Pipinos II. Isolated iliac artery aneurysms. Semin Vasc Surg. 2005;18(4):209–15.
33. Dix F, Titi M, Al-Khaffaf H. The isolated internal iliac artery aneurysm—a review. Eur J Vasc Endovasc Surg. 2005;30(2):119–29.
34. Laine MT, Björck M, Beiles CB, Szeberin Z, Thomson I, Altreuther M, et al. Few internal iliac artery aneurysms rupture under 4 cm. J Vasc Surg. 2017;65(1):76–81.
35. Nachbur B, Inderbitzi R, Bär W. Isolated iliac aneurysms. Eur J Vasc Surg. 1991;5(4):375–81.
36. Clark ET, Mass DP, Bassiouny HS, Zarins CK, Gewertz BL. True aneurysmal disease in the hand and upper extremity. Ann Vasc Surg. 1991;5(3):276–81.
37. Flinn W, Bergan JJ. Aneurysms of secondary and tertiary branches of major arteries. New York: Grune & Stratton; 1982.
38. Diwan A, Sarkar R, Stanley JC, Zelenock GB, Wakefield TW. Incidence of femoral and popliteal artery aneurysms in patients with abdominal aortic aneurysms. J Vasc Surg. 2000;31(5):863–9.
39. Dent TL. Multiple arteriosclerotic arterial aneurysms. PubMed – NCBI [Internet]. 2019. http://ncbi.nlm.nih.gov. Accessed 1 Sept 2019.
40. Stumm MV, Teufelsbauer H, Reichenspurner H, Debus E. Two decades of endovascular repair of popliteal artery aneurysm—a meta-analysis. Eur J Vasc Endovasc Surg. 2015;50(3):351–9.
41. Golchehr B, Tielliu I, Verhoeven E, Möllenhoff C, Antonello M, Zeebregts C, et al. Clinical outcome of isolated popliteal artery aneurysms treated with a heparin-bonded stent graft. Eur J Vasc Endovasc Surg. 2016;52(1):99–104.
42. Varga ZA, Locke-Edmunds JC, Baird RN. A multicenter study of popliteal aneurysms. J Vasc Surg. 1994;20(2):171–7.
43. Ravn H, Björck M. Popliteal artery aneurysm with acute ischemia in 229 patients. Outcome after thrombolytic and surgical therapy. J Vasc Surg. 2007;45(6):1288.
44. Eslami MH, Rybin D, Doros G, Farber A. Open repair of asymptomatic popliteal artery aneurysm is associated with better outcomes than endovascular repair. J Vasc Surg. 2015;61(3):663–9.
45. Shortell CK, Deweese JA, Ouriel K, Green RM. Popliteal artery aneurysms: a 25-year surgical experience. J Vasc Surg. 1991;14(6):771–9.

46. Lawrence PF, Harlander-Locke MP, Oderich GS, Humphries MD, Landry GJ, Ballard JL, et al. The current management of isolated degenerative femoral artery aneurysms is too aggressive for their natural history. J Vasc Surg. 2014;59(2):343–9.
47. Mohan IV, Stephen MS. Peripheral arterial aneurysms: open or endovascular surgery? Prog Cardiovasc Dis. 2013;56(1):36–56.

12 Lower Extremity Occlusive Disease

Sheela T. Patel

Lower Extremity Occlusive Disease

- PAD refers to atherosclerosis involving the aorta, iliac, and lower extremity arteries
- Spectrum of disease
  - Asymptomatic
  - Intermittent claudication
  - Limb-threatening ischemia: rest pain, ulcer, gangrene
- Classification of severity of PAD
  - **Rutherford** [1]
    - 0 Asymptomatic
    - 1 Mild claudication
    - 2 Moderate claudication
    - 3 Severe claudication
    - 4 Ischemic rest pain
    - 5 Minor tissue loss
    - 6 Ulceration of gangrene
  - **Fontaine**
    - Stage I: asymptomatic

S. T. Patel (✉)
Department of Surgery, Loma Linda University, Loma Linda, CA, USA
e-mail: stpatel@llu.edu

A. Murga et al. (eds.), *The Vascular Surgery In-Training Examination Review (VSITE)*,
https://doi.org/10.1007/978-3-031-24121-5_12

Stage IIa: mild claudication
Stage IIb: moderate-severe claudication
Stage III: ischemic rest pain
Stage IV: ulceration or gangrene

- Risk factors
  - Smoking
  - Diabetes mellitus
  - Hypertension
  - Hyperlipidemia: elevated cholesterol, reduced HDL
  - Obesity
  - Family history of PAD
  - Chronic renal disease
  - Advanced age
- PAD screening (ABI testing) [2]
  - Age ≥ 65
  - Age 50–65 with risk factors for atherosclerosis or family history of PAD
  - Age < 50 with DM and an additional risk factor for atherosclerosis
  - Known atherosclerotic disease in another vascular bed
- Epidemiology
  - Twenty percent of those over 55 have PAD
  - Prevalence and severity elevated in African Americans and Hispanics
  - PAD is marker for significant systemic atherosclerosis
- History
  - Assessment of functional status, ambulation potential, frailty, living situation
  - Burden of comorbidities: prior history of stroke, myocardial infarction, interventions
- Physical examination
  - Pulse exam
  - Inspect for ulcerations, calluses, trophic skin changes (dry shiny skin), hair loss, nail hypertrophy, infection
  - Surgical incisions (prior bypass, previous vein harvest)

- Diagnosis
  - Noninvasive testing
    - ABI
      - Handheld Doppler probe placed over the dorsalis pedis or posterior tibial artery
      - Blood pressure cuff inflated at ankle; cuff deflated and pressure reading when the Doppler signal returns is recorded
      - Higher of 2 ankle systolic pressures divided by the higher of the brachial systolic pressures
      - 1.0–1.2 normal
      - ABI < 0.9, start to get claudication
      - ABI < 0.5, start to get rest pain
      - ABI < 0.4, ulcers
      - ABI < 0.3, gangrene
      - If medial wall calcification (diabetics), ABI may be noncompressible which can falsely elevated ABI
    - Exercise testing
      - Symptomatic patients with palpable distal pulses and normal resting ABI
      - ABIs measured after 5 min of walking on a treadmill
      - Drop in ABI indicates stenosis; unmask hemodynamically significant disease
    - Segmental limb pressures and pulse volume recordings (PVRs)
      - Cuffs placed at high-thigh, low-thigh, high-calf, and low-calf levels
      - Pressures measured at four levels; pressure decrease between cuff segments > 20 mmHg indicates obstruction
      - Magnitude and contour of pulse volumes at four levels
      - Provides localization of anatomic lesions
      - Normal PVR tracing with sharp upstroke, distinct pulse peak, rapid decline
      - With increasing arterial obstruction, PVR tracing becomes progressively flattened and prolonged

Toe pressures <20–30 mmHg are associated with advanced ischemia
  - May be more reliable in diabetic patients
  - Digital arteries less frequently affected by calcific disease

Transcutaneous oxygen measurement <20–30 torr indicates lack of perfusion

Duplex ultrasound
  - Assess anatomic location and degree of stenosis
  - PSV > 200 cm/s or systolic velocity ratio > 2.5 correlates to >50% stenosis

– CTA

Calcification can obscure true degree of stenosis and can be misleading in tibial arteries

Radiation exposure

Contrast nephropathy

– MRA

With renal insufficiency, gadolinium with increased risk of nephrogenic systemic fibrosis

Cannot use in patients with metallic implants

– Arteriography

Pull-back pressures across lesions using provocative vasodilators (papaverine 30–60 mg, nitroglycerine 100–200 μg can be used to unmask a stenosis

Include oblique views
  - Contralateral oblique projection shows iliac artery bifurcation
  - Ipsilateral oblique projection shows femoral artery bifurcation

CO_2 angiography to avoid contrast load; only useful for larger proximal arteries

Detailed runoff views, including magnified lateral views of the foot
  - May need to advance catheter selectively into SFA or popliteal artery to obtain adequate views of the infrapopliteal and pedal circulations

Ipsilateral antegrade approach only used if normal inflow

IVUS (intravascular ultrasound) provides transverse 360° image of lumen (useful for dissections, post angioplasty/stent)

TASC II (Trans-Atlantic Inter-Society Consensus) classification system used to gauge extent of angiographic disease in the aortoiliac, femoropopliteal, and infrapopliteal segments [8, 9]

- Types A–D
- Endovascular treatment for TASC type A lesions (focal, short lesions)
- Open surgical treatment for TASC type D lesions (long-segment occlusions, diffuse)
- Insufficient evidence for treatment for TASC type B and C lesions

Grading of Anatomic Severity of Disease in Global Anatomic Staging System (GLASS) developed to address endovascular treatment and target artery path [10]

- Plain XR
  - Osteomyelitis
- Echocardiogram
  - Rule out embolism from heart (acute ischemia)

- Preoperative evaluation
  - Cardiac risk
    - Forty percent of patients have coronary artery disease
    - Assume all CLTI patients have significant CAD
    - Postpone infrainguinal bypass to allow further cardiac workup if unstable angina, recent MI, poorly controlled CHF, critical aortic stenosis, symptomatic/untreated arrhythmia
  - Commitment to stop smoking
- Patterns of disease
  - Superficial femoral artery disease
    - Calf claudication
    - Older, DM, tobacco abuse

  - Aortoiliac disease
    - Associated with heavy tobacco use and hyperlipidemia
    - Young women smokers with premature disease: circumscribed occlusive lesions of midabdominal aorta
    - **Leriche's syndrome**
      - Bilateral thigh, hip, buttock claudication
      - Impotence: inadequate perfusion of internal pudendal arteries
      - Leg muscle atrophy
      - Absent femoral pulses
    - Rich collateral network develops; rarely cause of critical limb ischemia, except by embolization
- Intermittent claudication
  - Cramping pain with walking which is reproducible and abate with rest
    - SFA disease: calf claudication
    - Aortoiliac disease: buttock/hip/thigh claudication
  - Differential: degenerative hip disease, spinal stenosis (pseudoclaudication), disc herniation, venous occlusive disease, chronic compartment syndrome
    - Consider popliteal entrapment, cystic adventitial disease, thromboangiitis obliterans (Buerger disease), vasculitis (Takayasu disease, polyarteritis nodosa, Wegener granulomatosis) in young patient with leg pain
  - Initial treatment is nonoperative
    - Supervised structured walking program: 30–45 min, 3–5 days per week for a minimum of 12 weeks
    - Smoking cessation
    - Blood pressure management
    - Glucose control
    - ASA
    - Statin
    - **Pentoxifylline=Trental**
      - Reduces blood viscosity by improving red blood cell membrane flexibility and inhibits platelet aggregation

Cilostazol=Pletal
    - Phosphodiesterase III inhibitor with vasodilator and antiplatelet activity
    - May take up to 4 months to derive maximum benefit
  - 1–7% risk of limb loss at 5 years; clinical deterioration of limb in 25% [3–5]
  - Only 10% will require revascularization
  - Only offer revascularization in low-risk patient with significant disability; eschew elective revascularization in active smokers
- Chronic limb-threatening ischemia (CLTI)
  - **Tissue loss**: ulcer, gangrene
    Sensory neuropathy associated with DM may lead to neuropathic ulcers
    Dry gangrene: noninfected black eschar
    Wet gangrene: tissue maceration, pus
  - **Ischemic rest pain**
    Burning pain in toes or distal forefoot
    Dependent rubor and elevation pallor
    Awoken by pain at night and dangle foot down for relief
    ABI < 0.5
    Doppler ankle pressure <35 mmHg (nondiabetics) and <55 mmHg (diabetics)
  - At least two levels of disease (aortoiliac, femoropopliteal, tibial)
  - Chronic: progression of atherosclerosis
  - Acute: plaque rupture with thrombosis, embolism
  - If untreated, high risk for amputation
  - Staging to define amputation risk (Society for Vascular Surgery Lower Extremity Threatened Limb Classification System; **WIfI**) [6, 7]
    Stratifies limb risk by grading three critical factors
    - Applies to all patients with rest pain or tissue loss
    - **W**ound
      - Wounds classified from grade 0 to grade 3 based on size, depth, severity, anticipated difficulty achieving wound healing

- **I**schemia
  - Ischemia classified from grade 0 to grade 4 according to ABI, ankle systolic pressure, toe systolic pressure, transcutaneous oximetry
- **f**oot **I**nfection
  - Infection classified from grade 0 to grade 3 based on objective clinical observations
- Sixty-four combinations assigned to four stages of clinical severity expected to correlate with amputation risk at 1 year and wound healing outcomes
- WIfI stage 1 with low amputation risk; stage 3 and 4 more likely to require revascularization and increased risk for limb loss

  Predicts wound healing time

- Acute limb ischemia
  - Sudden onset of ischemia

    6Ps: pain, pallor, paresthesia, pulselessness, poikilothermia, paralysis

    Acute ischemia affects sensory nerves first; loss of sensation is one of earliest signs

    Muscle tenderness is sign of advanced ischemia
  - **Thrombotic occlusion**

    Progressive atherosclerotic narrowing allows time for collateral formation

    Bypass graft occlusion

    Severity of ischemia depends on whether the profunda femoris is patent
  - **Embolism** (heart-atrial fibrillation, myocardial infarction, left ventricle aneurysm, valvular disease; thoracic or abdominal aortic penetrating ulcer or aneurysm, popliteal aneurysm)

    Lodges at arterial branch points (aortic bifurcation-saddle embolus, common femoral artery bifurcation, brachial artery bifurcation)

    Pulses often present in contralateral limb

    Paradoxical embolism: clot from venous system (DVT) travels through patent foramen ovale into arterial system; acute ischemia in young patient with concomitant DVT

- Consider aortic dissection if patient hypertensive and chest or back pain; high index of suspicion
- Arm ischemia seldom limb threatening

    Intervention to prevent exercise-induced arm fatigue and pain

    Usually due to cardiac embolus

    May be caused by thoracic outlet syndrome and proximal subclavian artery aneurysm
- Categories

    I-Viable: not immediately threatened, intact capillary refill, no muscle weakness, no sensory loss, Doppler signals

    II-Threatened

    - IIa: Marginal-salvageable if prompt treatment, slow capillary refill, no muscle weakness, minimal sensory loss, ± Doppler signals
    - IIb: Immediate-salvageable with immediate revascularization, slow or absent capillary refill, mild-moderate muscle weakness, some sensory loss, no Doppler signals

    III-Irreversible: major tissue loss, amputation regardless of treatment, absent capillary refill, profound paralysis (rigor), profound sensory loss, no Doppler signals
- Treatment

    Timely intervention paramount, no collateralization

    - Irreversible nerve and muscle damage may occur within 6 h

    Systemic heparinization (5000–10,000 units IV, then drip to maintain PTT 60–90 s) to prevent secondary thrombosis and further deterioration; no direct thrombolytic effect

    Intravenous hydration, supplemental oxygen, intravenous analgesia

    EKG to rule out atrial fibrillation, MI

    Class IIb requires immediate OR or angiography with lysis or suction thrombectomy

    Class III treated with primary amputation

Thromboembolectomy with Fogarty balloon catheters for thromboemboli

- Femoral arteriotomy
  - Transverse arteriotomy if non-diseased artery
  - Longitudinal arteriotomy if diseased artery; patch angioplasty
- Over-the-wire embolectomy catheters may be used to direct catheter into tibial arteries
- Popliteal arteriotomy may be needed to clean out tibial arteries
  - Embolectomy catheter least effective in small distal tibial and pedal arteries
- Fogarty balloon catheters passed proximally and distally until forward and backbleeding established
- Send extracted thromboemboli for pathologic examination to rule out atrial myxoma

Bypass grafting if failed thrombectomy

Acute popliteal aneurysm occlusion may need thrombolytic therapy to open up outflow target artery

Thrombolysis

- Particularly effective for bypass graft occlusion
- Retrograde contralateral femoral approach usually preferred
- Pulse spray with subsequent drip therapy via lysis catheter
- Mechanical thrombectomy devices (AngioJet, Penumbra Indigo, EKOS)
  - Rapidly debulks thrombus and increases exposure of residual thrombus to thrombolytic
  - Hemolysis with hemoglobinuria (AngioJet)
- Heparin drip through sheath to prevent pericatheter thrombus
- Identify culprit lesion
- Contraindications to lysis
  - Active bleeding diathesis
  - Recent gastrointestinal bleeding (<10 days)

- Intracranial or spinal surgery
- Intracranial trauma within previous 3 months
- Recent cerebrovascular accident within 2 months
- Uncontrolled hypertension
- Intracranial tumors
- Recent eye surgery

Compartment syndrome

- After restoration of perfusion, edema and pressure develop within muscles which are enveloped in fixed fascial compartments (ischemia-reperfusion injury)
- Rhabdomyolysis
- Muscle necrosis can lead to hyperkalemia, myoglobinemia
- Myoglobinuria can lead to renal dysfunction
  - Aggressive hydration, maintain urine output > 100 ml/h
  - Alkanization of urine; add bicarbonate to fluids
- Less risk of compartment syndrome with thrombolysis; more gradual resolution of clot
- **High index of suspicion**
- Tense swollen compartment
- Pain elicited with **passive movement** and **out of proportion** to exam and swelling
- May be confirmed with **elevated intracompartment pressure** using arterial line manometer or Stryker system; use for equivocal cases, unconscious patients, pediatric patients
  - Normal compartment pressure < 10–12 mmHg
- Anterior compartment most susceptible; leg pain with sensory deficits on dorsum of foot and weakness of toe dorsiflexion (deep peroneal nerve); foot drop
- Treatment is fasciotomy to prevent limb loss and permanent disability
- Consider **prophylactic fasciotomy** for all cases of acute arterial ischemia in which revascularization delayed **>4–6 h** or combined arterial and venous pathologies

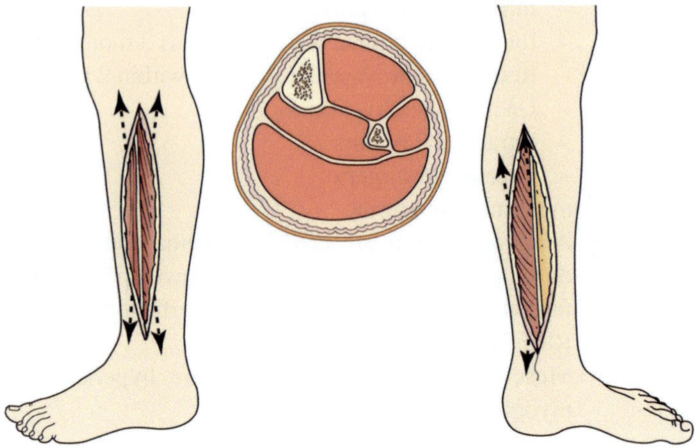

Fig. 12.1 Four compartment fasciotomy. (Taken from Rutherford's Vascular Surgery and Endovascular Therapy 9th Ed. Ch.102 P. 1349)

- Technique of lower leg fasciotomy (Refer to Fig. 12.1)
  - Four anatomic compartments: anterior, lateral, superficial posterior, deep posterior
  - Generous longitudinal incisions on lateral (decompress anterior and lateral compartments) and medial (decompress superficial posterior and deep posterior compartments) aspects of leg
  - Avoid injury to **superficial peroneal nerve** when performing lateral incision, particularly near fibular head as it descends along septum separating anterior and lateral compartments
  - Avoid injury to greater saphenous vein when performing medial incision
  - Deep posterior compartment decompressed by dividing soleus muscle from tibial border

- Thigh contains three compartments: anterior, posterior, medial
  - Single lateral incision can be used to decompress posterior and anterior compartments
  - Medial compartment rarely requires decompression
- If no culprit lesion found, hypercoagulable workup, rule out malignancy, consider HIT if patient on heparin and falling platelet count

- Atheromatous embolization
  - Also known as **cholesterol embolization** or **blue toe syndrome**
  - Microembolization of arteriosclerotic debris to terminal arteries in foot
  - Origin from heart, aneurysms, ulcerated plaques (shaggy aorta)
  - May occur spontaneously or may be precipitated by intraarterial manipulation of wires or catheters during angiography
  - High index of suspicion
  - Skin manifestations: bluish mottled painful spots over toes, livedo reticularis, splinter hemorrhages, petechiae
  - Palpable pedal pulses
  - Eosinophilia in up to 80% of cases
  - Controversial whether use of anticoagulation associated with higher incidence of atheroemboli; may prevent thrombus formation over unstable plaque thus allowing cholesterol crystals to embolize or may initiate intraplaque hemorrhage
  - Severe inflammatory reaction contributes to vascular obstruction
  - Eliminate embolic source with surgery or stenting; be cautious of manipulating lesion and causing recurrent embolization
  - Supportive treatment of end-organ damage; statins, aspirin may be helpful

- Chronic limb-threatening ischemia (CLTI)
  - Usually multilevel disease (aortoiliac, femoropopliteal, tibial)
  - Foot protection
    - Heel protection: soft gauze pad secured with gauze roll, no tape on skin
      - Elevate off bed or place in boots (Rooke boots)
    - Lambswool or gauze between toes
    - Lotion to prevent cracking
    - Bedsheets draped over footboard
    - Head of bed elevated 6 in. to improve foot perfusion by gravity
  - Local debridement and drainage of infected tissue
  - Revascularization is an essential component in relief of CLTI
- Treatment of aortoiliac disease
  - TransAtlantic Intersociety Consensus (TASC) II guidelines delineate which anatomic lesions are best served by endo vs. open surgical therapy
    - TASC A and B lesions (focal, short-segment lesions <3 to 10 cm, unilateral or bilateral) are best treated with endo
    - TASC D lesions (long segment occlusions and diffuse stenoses, particularly bilateral) are best treated with open surgery
    - TASC C with either technique
  - **Aortoiliac endarterectomy**
    - Occlusive disease limited to **distal aorta and common iliac arteries**
    - Contraindicated if aortic or iliac aneurysm, aortic occlusion to the level of the renal arteries, occlusive disease in the external iliac or femoral arteries\
  - PTA/stent
    - Balloon-expandable stents in CIA; better radial force for calcified lesions, more precise placement near aortic bifurcation

        - Kissing iliac balloons/stents to treat iliac lesions at aortic bifurcation; protect contralateral CIA from plaque dislodgement or embolization
        - Sheath has to be advanced beyond the lesion to avoid stent dislocation
      - Self-expandable stents in EIA; more flexible in tortuous areas
      - Covered stents (Viabahn, iCAST)
        - Restenosis develops at edges that are not covered by graft material
        - COBEST Trial: covered stent group with lower restenosis rate and greater freedom from stent occlusion vs. bare metal stent group [11]
- Aortofemoral bypass
  - Gold standard for severe symptomatic aortoiliac occlusive disease
  - Primary patency 85–95% at 5 years
  - Femoral arteries exposed first through bilateral longitudinal incisions
  - Aortic exposure
    - Transperitoneal approach
      - Transverse colon retracted cephalad
      - Small bowel shifted to patient's right side
      - Ligament of Treitz taken down and duodenum mobilized to right
    - Retroperitoneal approach
      - Hostile abdomen
      - Concurrent renal or mesenteric arterial disease requiring suprarenal exposure
      - Right lateral decubitus position on inflatable beanbag
      - Table retroflexed at waist
      - Hips rotated back towards left
      - Difficult to expose right renal and right iliac artery
      - Oblique incision from left lateral border of rectus abdominis to posterior axillary line; lateral third of 11th rib excised

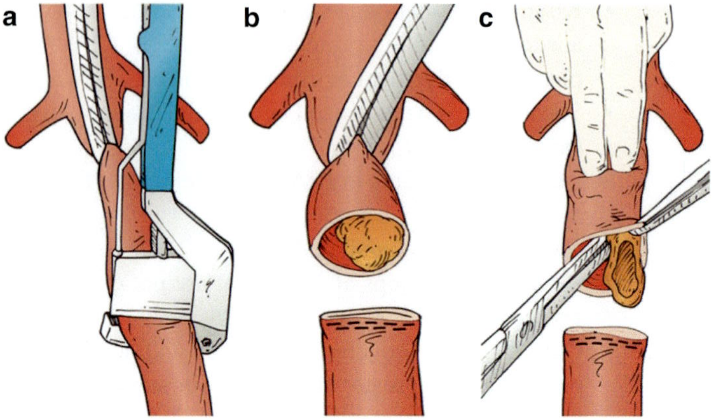

Fig. 12.2 End-to-End proximal anastomosis configuration for aortobifemoral reconstruction. (**a**–**c**) End-to-end aortic anastomosis and ligation of distal infrarenal aorta. (Taken from Rutherford's Vascular Surgery and Endovascular Therapy 9th ed. Ch. 106 P. 1406)

End-to-end proximal anastomosis (Refer to Fig. 12.2)

- Transection of aorta between clamps 1–2 in. below renal arteries; oversew or staple distal aorta
- More anatomic position-doesn't protrude anteriorly; better retroperitoneal coverage
- Exclusion of distal aorta and iliac arteries may reduce atheroembolism from clamping
- Complete thromboendarterectomy of infrarenal neck can be performed
- Suprarenal clamp may be needed to ensure thorough removal of all intraluminal debris from infrarenal aortic cuff
  - Retraction of left renal vein can facilitate adequate exposure of juxta-renal aorta; can divide left renal vein but preserve adrenal, lumbar, and gonadal branches
  - Concurrent clamping of renal arteries to prevent inadvertent emboli

  - Adjunctive mannitol and lasix can be used to trigger diuresis before aortic cross clamping
- Main body of graft shortened to minimize graft redundancy and allow limbs to straddle transected aortic stump

End-to-side proximal anastomosis (Refer to Fig. 12.3)

- Beveled anastomosis performed after longitudinal aortotomy
- Large IMA present; maintain flow for colonic perfusion
- EIA disease; preserves antegrade flow to hypogastric arteries and avoids pelvic ischemia

Distal anastomosis

- To the common femoral artery if widely patent profunda femoris and superficial femoral arteries
- Carry graft onto proximal SFA if orifice of SFA stenotic and profunda femoris artery normal
- Carry graft onto profunda femoris artery (profundaplasty) if SFA stenosis/occlusion
- To the profunda femoris artery if CFA and SFA occluded
  - Ligate lateral femoral circumflex vein crossing anteriorly over the proximal profunda femoris artery
  - Can use lateral approach with medial retraction of the sartorius to avoid scarred or infected groin

Bifurcated knitted Dacron prosthesis impregnated with collagen or gelatin

- Usually 16 × 8 mm for males; 12 × 6 mm for women

Iliac limbs tunneled into groins

- On the **left**, **beneath sigmoid mesentery and ureter** and lateral to the nerve plexus overlying terminal aorta

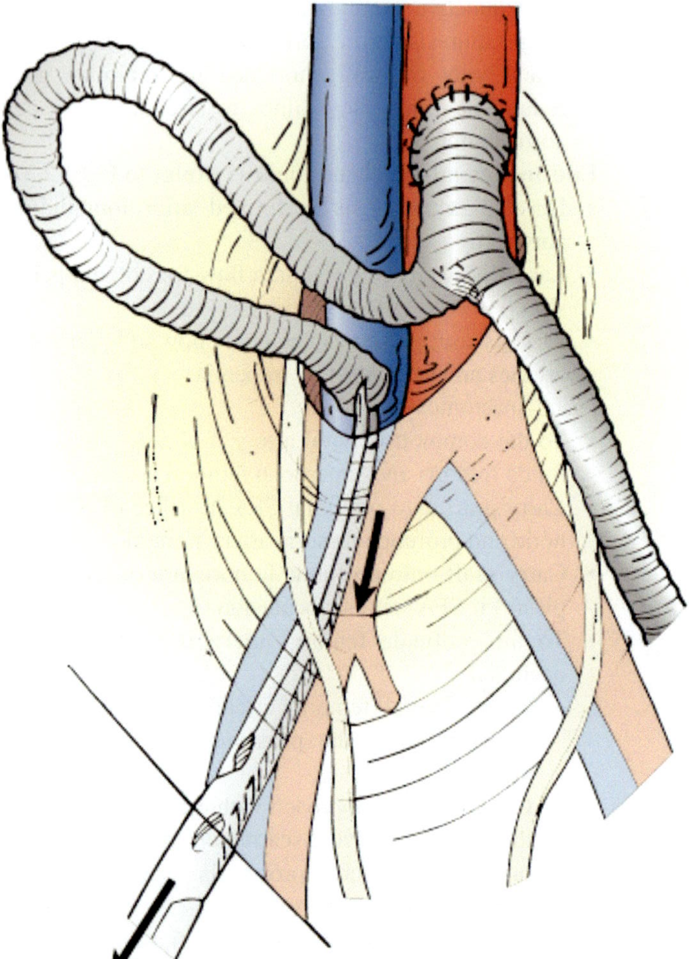

Fig. 12.3 Aortobifemoral graft limb tunneling. (Taken from Rutherfod's Vascular Surgery and Endovascular Therapy 9th ed. Ch. 106 P. 1407)

- On the **right**, along the course of the right iliac artery **beneath the ureter**
- Crossing vein normally present beneath the inguinal ligament must be ligated or avoided to prevent bleeding

Concomitant distal bypass if tissue loss

Revascularization of the IMA (bypass or reimplantation) if IMA large (>3.5–4 mm), if poor backbleeding, or if IMA pressure < 40 mmHg; poor collateralization from SMA

- Any bloody bowel movement within 48 h of aortic reconstruction should prompt sigmoidoscopy

Sexual dysfunction

- Impaired or absent penile erection
- Retrograde ejaculation
- Important to minimize dissection in the area of aortic bifurcation and left common iliac artery to avoid autonomic nerve plexus regulating erection and ejaculation

Gastrointestinal hemorrhage, especially hematemesis, in any patient with history of prosthetic aortic graft, must raise suspicion of aortoenteric fistula, usually years later

- Make sure retroperitoneum closed over the proximal anastomosis
- Herald bleed presages a large gastrointestinal bleed
- CTA: proximity of duodenum to graft with inflammation
- EGD to rule out other sources of bleeding, rarely may see graft material eroding into duodenum
- Treatment: extra-anatomic bypass (axillo-bifemoral bypass), graft resection with aortic stump oversew, bowel repair
  - In situ graft replacement for indolent infections (femoral vein graft: neo-aortoiliac system NAIS, rifampin-soaked dacron, cryopreserved allogenic aortic homograft)

- Extra-anatomic bypasses

  Less durable than aortobifemoral bypass; patency 50–75% at 5 years

  Iliac occlusion and normal contralateral iliac/axillary artery

  Hostile abdomen (previous surgery, radiation)

  Significant cardiopulmonary comorbidities

  Femoral-femoral bypass (Refer to Fig. 12.4)

  - Vertical groin incisions
  - Subcutaneous suprapubic tunnel with graft in C configuration anterior to deep fascia
  - 6 or 7 mm ringed Dacron or PTFE
  - Sixty to 80% 5-year patency

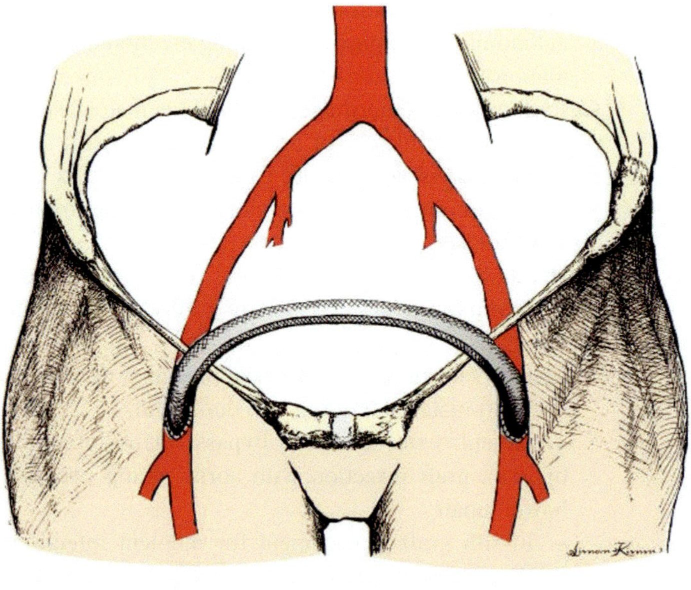

Fig. 12.4 Standard "inverted C" configuration of femorofemoral bypass. (Taken from Rutherford's Vascular Surgery and Endovascular Therapy 9th ed. Ch. 107 P. 1418)

Axillofemoral bypass (Refer to Fig. 12.5)

- Axillobifemoral graft with better patency than axillounifemoral graft
- First portion of axillary artery exposed via infraclavicular incision
- Split pectoralis major muscle
- Tunnel along midaxillary line anteriorly above the iliac crest and in front of inguinal ligament in subcutaneous plane
- Tunnel posterior to the pectoralis minor; may divide pectoralis minor
- 8 mm ringed Dacron or PTFE
- Place anastomosis as far medially as possible on the axillary artery
- Thirty to 85% 5-year patency

Obturator bypass (Refer to Fig. 12.6)

- Utilize if arterial infection in the femoral triangle, hostile groin
- Inflow: ipsilateral common or external iliac artery via oblique lower abdomen incision and retroperitoneal exposure
- Outflow: above knee popliteal or superficial femoral artery
- Graft tunneled through obturator foramen posterior to adductor longus
- Obturator foramen approached medial to external iliac vein and posterior to superior aspect of pubis ramus
- Incise obturator membrane anteromedially to avoid obturator nerve and artery
- Use autologous vein graft

– Thoracofemoral bypass

Descending thoracic aorta exposed through a 6th or 7th interspace incision

10 mm graft tunneled through diaphragm and down through retroperitoneal space to left groin

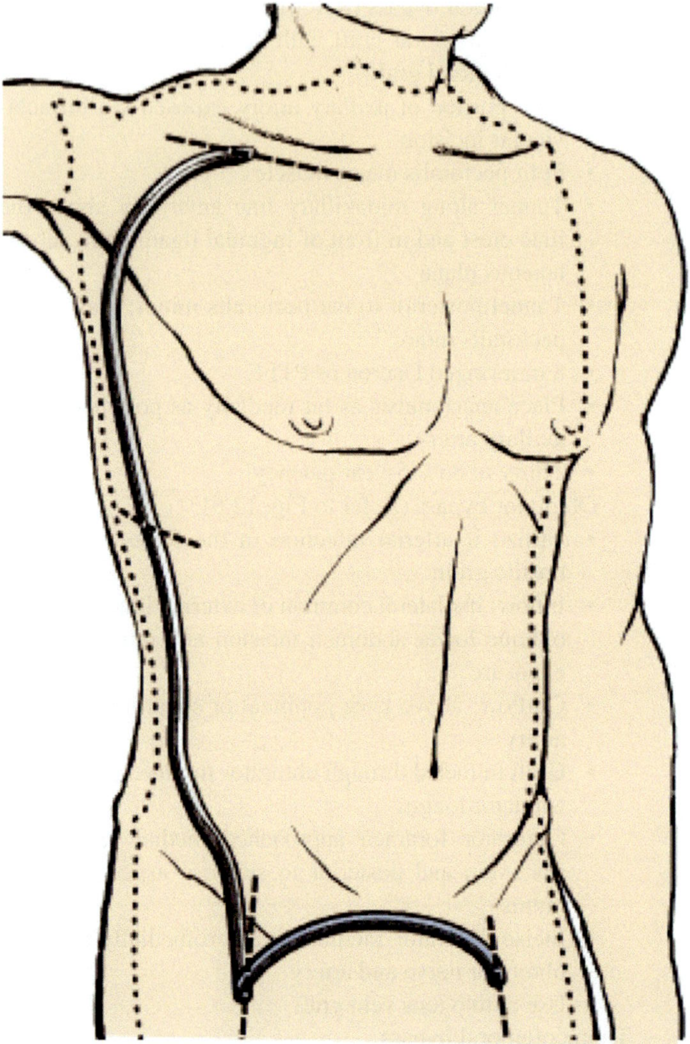

Fig. 12.5 Configuration of axillary femorofemoral bypass. (Taken from Rutherford's Vascular Surgery and Endovascular Therapy 9th ed. Ch. 107 P. 1420)

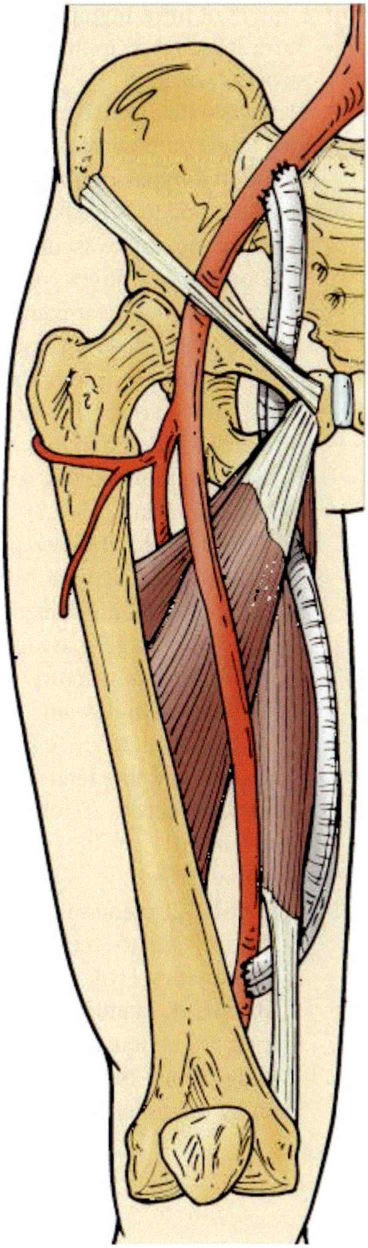

Fig. 12.6 Obturator bypass graft configuration. (Taken from Rutherford's Vascular Surgery and Endovascular Therapy 9th ed. Ch. 107 P. 1421)

- Treatment of infra-inguinal disease
  - Infra-inguinal revascularization less durable than aortoiliac revascularization
  - Patients with extensive foot gangrene, long occlusions, limited target outflow arteries, and good saphenous vein should be offered bypass over endovascular treatment to establish in-line blood flow to the foot
  - Caveats with endovascular treatment
    - Don't burn bridges; may have to bypass to more distal target if endo treatment fails [12]
    - Preserve collateral vessels (avoid covered stent)
    - Angiosome directed treatment; anatomic area that is fed by source artery (i.e., heel ulcer requires posterior tibial artery intervention to promote healing)
  - **BASIL (Bypass versus Angioplasty in Severe Ischemia of the Leg) trial**: [13–15]
    - Four hundred fifty-two patients randomized 1999–2004
    - Patients treated with bypass first had comparable outcomes to patients treated with balloon angioplasty first at 6 months; surgery associated with higher morbidity
    - After 2 years, surgery associated with reduced risk of amputation and death
    - If life expectancy exceeds 2 years, surgery is more appropriate first intervention
    - Bypass success after failed endovascular therapy is compromised
  - Ongoing trials
    - **BASIL-2**: randomized patients with infrapopliteal arterial disease to vein bypass first vs. best endovascular therapy first [16]
    - **BASIL-3**: randomize patients with femoropopliteal disease to balloon angioplasty ± bail out bare metal stent or drug coated balloon ± bail out bare metal stent or primary drug-eluting stent [17]

  BEST-CLI (Best Endovascular vs. Best Surgical Therapy in Patients with Critical Limb Ischemia)
  - Multicenter clinical trial to randomize 2100 pts with CLTI to either best open or best endovascular therapy [18]

- **Global Vascular Guidelines on CLTI**: decisions regarding revascularization based upon PLAN principles

  Patient risk estimation
  - Candidacy for limb salvage
  - Peri-procedural risk
  - Life expectancy

  Limb threat severity using the SVS Wound Ischemia Foot infection (WIfI) staging system

  ANatomic pattern of disease using the Global Anatomic Staging System (GLASS) [10]

- Goal of revascularization is to establish straight in-line flow from the hip to the foot
- Shorter bypasses are preferred because of improved patency; SFA or popliteal artery may provide inflow if no proximal arterial disease
- Conduits

  Preoperative duplex mapping
  - Patients scanned with light tourniquet in place and with limb dependent
  - At least 3 mm in diameter
  - Soft, compressible

  Type and quality of bypass conduit are most important determinants of infrainguinal bypass success

  Autogenous greater saphenous vein best, especially for below knee popliteal and tibial reconstructions

  Use contralateral greater saphenous vein if limb asymptomatic and ABI > 0.6

  Arm vein: cephalic or basilic veins, may need to be spliced to secure adequate length, more fragile-careful with distention

Lesser saphenous vein; short, useful for posterior approaches to popliteal artery

Femoropopliteal deep vein: short, larger caliber

Vein preparation

- Cannulate with 3 mm olive or Marks tip needle
- Gently distend with chilled autologous blood (50 cc) to which 1000 units of heparin and 60 mg papaverine added

Prosthetic: dacron, PTFE (6 mm), PTFE bonded with heparin (Propaten), Distaflo (6 mm, minicuff used for tibial anastomoses)

Cryopreserved vein

- Results have been disappointing
- Expensive
- Useful in setting of gross infection

Vein configuration: reversed, in situ, nonreversed

- No difference in patency
- Valvulotome (Mills, LeMaitre) used for in situ and non-reversed veins; may be better size match

Vein adjuncts at distal anastomosis when prosthetic used: Taylor patch, Linton patch, Miller cuff, St. Mary's boot (Refer to Fig. 12.7)

- May improve compliance mismatch at anastomosis

Composite sequential bypass: proximal component PTFE, distal component vein

For endarterectomy patch angioplasty: PTFE or Dacron patch, bovine pericardial patch, endarterectomized segment of native occluded SFA, vein

Isolated popliteal artery: patent popliteal artery segment at least 5 cm long but with only geniculate collaterals and no major distal tibial or peroneal runoff artery in direct continuity with foot

- Blind popliteal artery bypass may be useful for claudication, rest pain

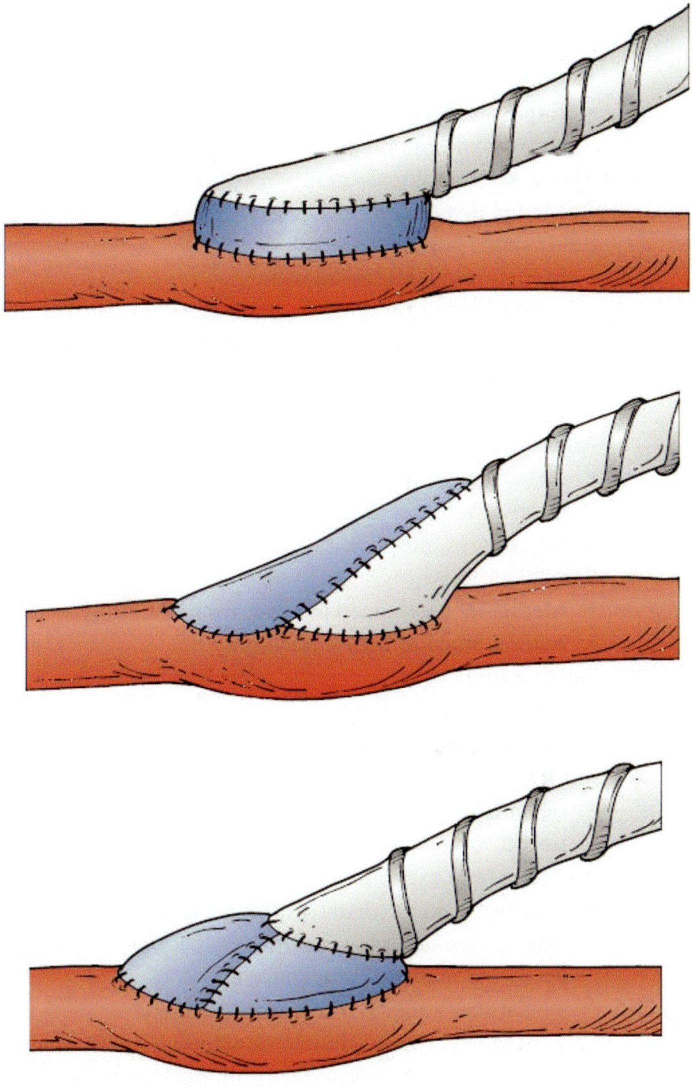

Fig. 12.7 Vein adjuncts at distal anastomosis when prosthetic used: Taylor patch, Linton patch, Miller cuff, St. Mary's boot. (Taken from Rutherford's Vascular Surgery and Endovascular Therapy 9th ed. Ch. 109 P. 1447)

- Surgical exposure

    Common femoral artery

    - Longitudinal groin incision
    - Exposure of common femoral, profunda femoris, and superficial femoral arteries

    Above-knee popliteal artery

    - Medial distal thigh incision

    Below-knee popliteal artery

    - Medial proximal leg incision
    - Medial head of gastrocnemius retracted inferiorly

    Tibioperoneal trunk, proximal posterior tibial artery

    - Medial knee incision
    - Detach soleus muscle from tibial border

    Anterior tibial artery

    - Anterolateral leg incision between tibia and fibula
    - Groove between anterior tibialis and extensor digitorum longus muscles

    Peroneal artery

    - Medial incision, deep to posterior tibial artery
    - Lateral incision with fibulectomy

    Pedal arteries

    - Dorsalis pedis artery
    - Lateral and plantar arteries off the posterior tibial artery
    - Inframalleolar target artery maximizes forefoot perfusion

    Avoiding redo exposure [19]

    - Can use mid or distal profunda femoris artery for inflow via lateral approach; incision placed in upper thigh lateral to sartorius muscle
        - Sartorius and SFA retracted medially
        - Raphe between adductor longus and vastus medialis incised to expose the profunda femoris artery
    - Lateral approach to popliteal artery
        - Above-knee

            Lateral incision between the iliotibial tract and biceps femoris muscle

            Avoid common peroneal nerve

    - Below-knee
        - Identify peroneal nerve as it courses around neck of fibula
        - Excise 6–10 cm of fibula
- Tunneling
    - Large-caliber hollow-bore metal tunneller with removable obturator
    - For below knee popliteal artery, anatomic tunnel between two heads of the gastrocnemius
    - Tunnel bypasses subcutaneously to avoid scarring and render graft surveillance and revision easier
    - Bypasses to the anterior tibial artery can be tunneled through the interosseous membrane or a lateral subcutaneous plane
- Femoropopliteal bypass
    - Best conduit is autogenous saphenous vein; 80% primary patency over 5 years
    - Vein superior to all prosthetic materials, even in the above-knee position
    - Dacron, PTFE acceptable for above knee popliteal anastomosis
- Femorotibial bypass
    - Primary patency of vein superior to PTFE for infrapopliteal bypass (49% vs. 12% at 4 years)
    - Anterior and posterior tibial arteries preferred because in direct continuity with pedal arch; peroneal artery if only patent artery
- Intraoperative assessment
    - Distal pulse palpation and Doppler flow assessment with and without manual compression of the graft
    - Completion arteriography
    - Intraoperative duplex scanning
    - Angioscopy-arm vein conduit, adequacy of valve lysis
- Duplex surveillance of vein bypass grafts to maintain patency [20–22]
    - Increased peak systolic velocity across stenotic area (PSV > 300 cm/s) or velocity ratio > 3.5–4.0

    Decrease in peak systolic flow velocity < 45 cm/s in the graft beyond area of stenosis
    0.15 fall in ABI
    Surveillance of prosthetic grafts not as convincing as whether it improves outcomes; occlusion causes loss of outflow [23, 24]
- Early graft thrombosis
    Technical error at anastomosis
    Embolus
    Inadequate runoff to maintain graft flow
    Graft kinking
    Poor vein conduit
    External compression
    Hypercoagulable state
    Explore distal anastomosis first, gentle distal thrombectomy
    If reversed vein, both proximal and distal anastomoses require exploration
- Late graft thrombosis usually due to myointimal hyperplasia (<2 years) or atherosclerotic progression; usually need new bypass
- Percutaneous endovascular intervention
    Best results for short focal lesions
    Preferred in high-risk patients with shorter life expectancies
    Situational perfusion enhancement: transient boost in arterial perfusion could be sufficient to accomplish healing of ulcer; short-term durability of endovascular procedure may be inconsequential
    Direct angiosome targeted revascularization may provide better outcomes for ulcer healing
    Tibial disease challenging and less durable
    Most common mode of failure: restenosis due to intimal hyperplasia
    Outcomes dependent on
    - Indication for the procedure
    - Lesion characteristics

- Runoff status
- Comorbidities
- Technical factors: dissection, persistent stenosis

Approaches

- Contralateral femoral artery using up-and-over approach
- Ipsilateral femoral artery using antegrade approach
  - Cannot evaluate inflow aortoiliac arteries
  - Better guidewire and catheter control in infrapopliteal intervention
- Left brachial artery if extensive bilateral iliofemoral arterial disease

Always obtain oblique projections of the iliacs, femorals, and lateral views of the foot

PTA

- Plain old balloon angioplasty (POBA): intraluminal
- Subintimal angioplasty
  - Wire used to intentionally create a subintimal dissection plane just proximal to an occlusion
  - Reentry into true lumen
- Drug-coated balloons (paclitaxel) may decrease myointimal hyperplasia
  - Bard Lutonix balloon catheter [25]
  - IN.PACT Admiral balloon catheter [26]
- Cutting balloons for infrainguinal bypass graft stenoses
  - Blades mounted on balloon which score the lesion
- Treatment considered successful if residual stenosis <30% or if no pressure gradient

Stenting

- For femoropopliteal disease, use self-expandable stents
- For covered stents, avoid coverage of significant collaterals (Gore Viabahn)
- Supera stent: interwoven nitinol helical stent; more radial force and crush resistance compared to standard self-expanding nitinol stents [27]

- Balloon-expandable drug-eluting coronary stents (Taxus, Cypher)
- Paclitaxel-eluting Zilver self-expanding nitinol stents [28]
- Avoid stent placement in infrainguinal vein grafts

Atherectomy: excisional, orbital, laser

- **Excisio**nal: SilverHawk, TurboHawk
- Orbital: Diamondback 360
- Laser: TurboElite excimer laser
- Plaque debulking
- Excisional atherectomy catheters remove and collect atheroma
- Ablative devices fragment atheroma into small particles (orbital, laser)

Reentry devices

- Facilitate crossing chronic total occlusion by subintimal approach
- Outback reentry catheter: external marker to help orient retractable needle to pierce intima and gain access into true lumen using fluoroscopy
- Pioneer catheter: uses IVUS technology to guide reentry needle toward true lumen

Devices specifically designed for crossing a chronic total occlusion (CTO)

- Plaque microdissection (Frontrunner XP CTO Catheter)
- Bidirectional catheter spinning (CrossBoss CTO Catheter)
- Catheter tip deflection capability with spiral wedges (Wildcat Catheter)

Embolic protection devices

- Primary amputation if significant comorbidities, dementia, non-ambulatory, extensive nonsalvageable tissue loss, inadequate plantar skin

- Diabetic foot
  - Foot disorders (ulcer, infection, gangrene) are the leading cause of hospitalization in patients with diabetes
  - Amputations are preceded by foot ulcer in more than 85% of cases [29]
  - Among patients who have undergone a major amputation, up to 40% will undergo amputation of the contralateral limb within 3 years
  - Pathogenesis: neuropathy, infection, ischemia
  - Peripheral neuropathy: mixture of sensory, motor, autonomic involvement
  - Loss of normal protective sensation: apply pressure on selected dorsal and plantar areas of the foot with deformable Semmes-Weinstein monofilament (10 g)
  - Intrinsic muscle weakness of foot leads to digital contractures and equinus deformity
  - Autonomic neuropathy leads to dry feet, anhidrosis, noncompliant skin, hyperkeratosis, fissures, cracking
  - Infection often subtle and often tracks deep
  - Mal perforans ulcer: plantar ulcer at the metatarsal heads in diabetic patients with neuropathy
    - Treatment with ray amputation when underlying osteomyelitis
  - Patients with foot ulcer and systemic signs of infection should be assumed to have a foot infection
  - Diagnosis
    - Plain XR with multiple views of the foot
      - Gas in soft tissue may indicated deep tissue infection
      - Bony deformities
    - MRI, bone biopsy to rule out osteomyelitis
  - Treatment
    - Topical wound agents
    - IV antibiotics

Hyperbaric oxygen therapy (HBOT)

- May stimulate cellular proliferation and angiogenesis

Offloading

- Proper fitting shoes
- Orthotic inserts to distribute weight evenly
- Total contact casting
- Irremovable cast walkers

Surgical debridement

- Infection manifested by swelling, erythema, pain, fever, malodorous drainage, gangrene
  - Usually polymicrobial
- Scalpel, curette; make generous longitudinal incisions to drain
- Negative pressure wound therapy
- Aim for moist pink granulation bed

Osteomyelitis suspected when deep or extensive ulceration

- Probes to bone
- MRI may be helpful in assessing extent
- Bone biopsy to assess antibiotic susceptibility
- 6–8 weeks of antibiotics

Revascularization if ischemia

- Infrapopliteal disease and incomplete pedal arch common
- Plain XRs can demonstrate arterial calcification and suitability of open bypass

Amputation

- Determination of level of amputation: clinical judgment, segmental arterial pressures, Doppler waveforms, toe pressures, transcutaneous oxygen pressures
- Work of walking increases dramatically as level of amputation becomes more proximal
- Ray amputation: removal of toe and metatarsal head

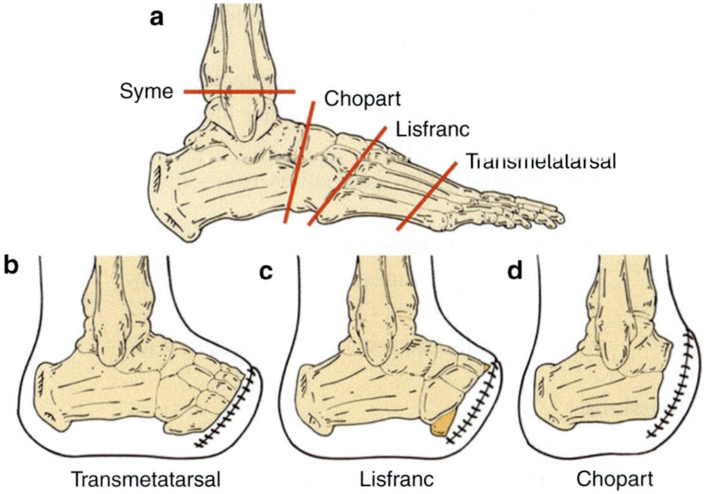

Fig. 12.8 Levels of foot amputations. (**a**) Levels of amputations. (**b**) Transmetatarsal. (**c**) Lisfranc. (**d**) Chopart. (Taken from Rutherford's Vascular Surgery and Endovascular Therapy 9th ed. Ch. 112 P. 1501)

- Forefoot amputations preserve length but ambulation may be difficult (Fig. 12.8)
  - Transmetatarsal amputation (TMA)
  - **Lisfranc** (tarsometatarsal joint) amputation
  - **Chopart** (midtarsal joint) amputation
  - **Syme** (tibial-talar joint) amputation
- Below-knee amputation
  - Long posterior flap
  - For severe foot infections, guillotine transtibial amputation just proximal to ankle followed by formal revision to BKA
- Above-knee amputation
  - Nonambulatory, elderly, nursing-home patient with knee contractures and extensive heel gangrene should be considered for primary AKA
  - Fish-mouth incision

    - Heel ulcers challenging; calcanectomy
  - Charcot neuroarthropathy
    Severe destruction of pedal architecture
    Mid-foot collapse leads to plantar ulcer
    Chronic, progressive
    Erythematous, hot, edematous foot—not an infectious process
    Rocker bottom deformity is late sign of disease
    Treatment: early immobilization, offloading
    - Total contact cast (TCC)
    - Treat until inflammation becomes quiescent

Questions

1. A patient presents to the emergency department with new onset of bilateral thigh, hip and buttock pain that has worsen over the last couple of months. On physical exam you notice absent femoral pulses bilateral. What is the most likely diagnosis?
   (a) Treves-Stewart Syndrome
   (b) Leriche's Syndrome
   (c) Barlow Syndrome
   (d) Behcets Syndrome
   (e) Mirizzi Syndrome
2. Of the following 6Ps which is not associated with acute limb ischemia?
   (a) Pain
   (b) Pallor
   (c) Paresthesia
   (d) Pulselessness
   (e) Panuveitis
   (f) Paralysis

Answers: 1 (b), 2 (e)

References

1. Rutherford RB, Baker JD, Ernst C, et al. Suggested standards for reports dealing with lower extremity ischemia: revised version. J Vasc Surg. 1997;26:517–38.
2. Gerhard-Herman MD, Gornik HL, Barrett C, et al. 2016 AHA/ACC guideline on the management of patients with lower extremity peripheral artery disease: executive summary: a report of the American College of Cardiology/American Heart Association Task Force on Clinical Practice Guidelines. J Am Coll Cardiol. 2017;69(11):1465–508.
3. O'Riordan DS, O'Donnell JA. Realistic expectations for the patient with intermittent claudication. Br J Surg. 1991;78:861–3.
4. Cox GS, Hertzer NR, Young JR, et al. Non-operative treatment of superficial femoral artery disease: long term follow-up. J Vasc Surg. 1993;17:172–81.
5. Muluk SC, Muluk VS, Kelley ME, et al. Outcome events in patients with claudication: a 15 year study in 2777 patients. J Vasc Surg. 2001;33:251–7.
6. Mills JL Sr, Conte MS, Armstrong DG, et al. The Society for Vascular Surgery Lower Extremity Threatened Limb Classification System: risk stratification based on wound, ischemia, and foot infection (WIfI). J Vasc Surg. 2014;59(1):220–34.
7. Mills JL. The application of the Society for Vascular Surgery Wound, Ischemia, and foot Infection (WIfI) classification to stratify amputation risk. J Vasc Surg. 2017;65(3):591–3.
8. Norgren L, et al. Inter-society consensus for the management of peripheral arterial disease (TASC II). J Vasc Surg. 2007;45(suppl S):S5–S67.
9. Dormandy JA, et al. Management of peripheral arterial disease (PAD). TASC Working Group. Trans Atlantic Inter-Society Consensus (TASC). J Vasc Surg. 2000;31:S1–S296.
10. Conte MS, Bradbury AW, Kolh P, et al. Global vascular guidelines on the management of chronic limb-threatening ischemia. J Vasc Surg. 2019;69(6S):3S–125S.
11. Mwipatayi BP, Sharma S, Daneshmand A, et al. Durability of the balloon-expandable covered versus bare-metal stents in the Covered versus Balloon Expandable Stent Trial (COBEST) for the treatment of aortoiliac occlusive disease. J Vasc Surg. 2016;64:83–94.
12. Nolan BW. Prior failed ipsilateral percutaneous endovascular intervention in patients with critical limb ischemia predicts poor outcome after lower extremity bypass. J Vasc Surg. 2011;54:730–6.
13. Bradbury AW, BASIL Trial Participants. Bypass versus angioplasty in severe ischemia of the leg (BASIL): multicenter, randomized controlled trial. Lancet. 2005;366:1925–34.

14. Bradbury, et al. Bypass versus Angioplasty in Severe Ischemia of the Leg (BASIL) trial: analysis of amputation free and overall survival by treatment received. J Vasc Surg. 2010;51(5 Suppl):18S–31S.
15. Bradbury AW, Adam DJ, Bell J, et al. Bypass versus Angioplasty in Severe Ischemia of the leg (BASIL) trial: a survival prediction model to facilitate clinical decision making. J Vasc Surg. 2010;51(5 Suppl):52S–68S.
16. Popplewell MA, et al. Bypass versus angioplasty in severe ischemia of the leg – 2 (BASIL-2) trial: study protocol for a randomized controlled trial. Trials. 2016;17(1):11.
17. Hunt BD, Popplewell MA, Davies H, et al. on Behalf of the BASIL-3 Collaborative Group. Balloon versus Stenting in severe Ischemia of the Leg – 3 (BASIL-3): study protocol for a randomized controlled trial. Trials. 2017;18:224.
18. Menard MT, Farber A. The BEST-CLI Trial: a multidisciplinary effort to assess whether surgical or endovascular therapy is better for patients with CLI. Semin Vasc Surg. 2014;27:82–4.
19. Veith FJ, Cayne NS. Unusual surgical exposures to avoid scarred or infected standard access routes to the common femoral, deep femoral, and popliteal arteries. J Vasc Surg. 2016;64:1160–8.
20. Visser K, Idu MM, Buth J, et al. Duplex scan surveillance during the first year after infrainguinal autogenous vein bypass grafting surgery: cost and clinical outcomes compared with other surveillance programs. J Vasc Surg. 2001;33:123–30.
21. Mills JL, et al. The importance of routine surveillance of distal bypass grafts with duplex scanning: a study of 379 reversed vein grafts. J Vasc Surg. 1990;12:379–86.
22. Wixon CL, Mills JL, Westerband A, et al. An economic appraisal of lower extremity bypass graft maintenance. J Vasc Surg. 2000;32:1–12.
23. Lalak NJ, et al. Duplex scan surveillance of infrainguinal prosthetic bypass grafts. J Vasc Surg. 1994;20:637–41.
24. Dunlop P, et al. The effect of a surveillance programme on the patency of synthetic infrainguinal bypass grafts. Eur J Vasc Endovasc Surg. 1996;11:441–5.
25. Rosenfield K, Jaff MR, White CJ, et al. LEVANT 2 Investigators. Trial of paclitaxel-coated balloon for femoropopliteal artery disease. N Engl J Med. 2015;373(2):145–53.
26. Laird JR, Schneider PA, Tepe G, et al. IN.PACT SFA Trial Investigators. Durability of treatment effect using a drug-coated balloon for femoropopliteal lesions: 24-month results of IN.PACT SFA. J Am Coll Cardiol. 2015;66(21):2329–38.
27. Garcia L, Jaff MR, Metzger C, et al. SUPERB Trial Investigators. Wire-interwoven nitinol stent outcome in the superficial femoral and proximal popliteal arteries: twelve-month results of the SUPERB trial. Circ Cardiovasc Interv. 2015;8(5):e000937.

28. Dake MD, Ansel GM, Jaff MR, et al. Durable clinical effectiveness with paclitaxel-eluting stents in the femoropopliteal artery: 5-year results of the Zilver PTX randomized trial. Circulation. 2016;133(15):1472–83.
29. Levin ME. Management of the diabetic foot: preventing amputation. South Med J. 2002;95:10–20.

Mesenteric Arterial Disease 13

Rahul Kar and Allen Murga

Anatomy, Normal Arterial and Venous Anatomy: Collateral Circulation

Celiac Artery

– Arises at level of L1, bordered by the median arcuate ligament (MAL) at aortic hiatus superiorly and superior border of pancreas inferiorly
– 3 branches:[1] left gastric, splenic, common hepatic arteries.

SMA

– Inferior to celiac trunk, origin is crossed by neck of pancreas and splenic vein. Comes off superior to uncinate process and 3rd portion of duodenum

[1] Multiple variations exist (Most common-common hepatic arises from SMA or directly from abdominal aorta).

R. Kar · A. Murga (✉)
Department of Vascular Surgery, Loma Linda University, Loma Linda, CA, USA
e-mail: Rkar@llu.edu; amurga@llu.edu

A. Murga et al. (eds.), *The Vascular Surgery In-Training Examination Review (VSITE)*,
https://doi.org/10.1007/978-3-031-24121-5_13

- SMV runs parallel and usually along its right border
- 1st Branch: usually inferior pancreaticoduodenal artery—supplies collateral circulation with celiac via gastroduodenal and superior pancreaticoduodenal
- 2nd Branch: middle colic artery—arises at inferior border of pancreas.

IMA

- 3–4 cm above aortic bifurcation and just left of midline at level of L3.
- Main trunk divides into sigmoidal branches and left colic artery.
- Collateral circulation: ascending left colic artery forms inferior marginal artery of Drummond (major collateral arcade between SMA and IMA)
- Meandering mesenteric artery (of Moskowitz) known as "arc of Riolan": runs centrally medial to mesenteric border of colon and through middle mesenteric arcade near inferior mesenteric vein. Sigmoidal branches lead to left and right superior rectal arteries: collateralize with hypogastric arteries in pelvis.

Diagnosis and Management of Mesenteric Disease

Clinical Presentation/History

Acute mesenteric ischemia (AMI): associated with sudden abdominal pain and often rapid clinical deterioration.

- Pain out of proportion to physical examination.
- Guarding and rebound tenderness early in disease course
- Peritonitis with diffuse pain at later stages with signs of intestinal ischemia

Nonocclusive mesenteric ischemia (NOMI) or mesenteric venous thrombosis (MVT): slower more insidious course. Associated with critical illness, hospitalization, often on pressors.

- Abdominal pain and distension with nausea/vomiting, and bloody stools.

Chronic mesenteric ischemia (CMI): associated with postprandial pain and progressive weight loss.

- Dull/crampy pain located in epigastric region 15–45 min after meals, severity varies according to size and type of meal.
- "Food fear" and decreased oral intake.
- Frequently in elderly women (70% of patients).
- Physical exam: nonspecific, undernourished and cachetic, abdominal bruit may be heard, guarding and rebound tenderness often absent.

Imaging

Duplex US-color Doppler to assess flow velocities and resistance index in splanchnic arterial beds [1].

- SMA: PSV ≥295 cm/s associated with 50% stenosis,
  - PSV ≥400 cm/s associated with ≥70% stenosis
- Celiac: PSV ≥240 cm/s associated with 50% stenosis
  - PSV ≥320 cm/s associated with ≥70% stenosis.
- Celiac or SMA with stent:
  - PSV ≥445 cm/s associated with ≥70% stenosis in SMA
  - PSV ≥289 cm/s associated with ≥70% stenosis in celiac.

CTA: 93% sensitivity and 96% specificity for detecting AMI.

- Ease and speed of performance and ability to simultaneously image mesenteric arteries, veins, and visceral organs.

  - CT findings in AMI—bowel wall thickening, dilation, attenuation.
  - Pneumatosis intestinalis, portal venous gas, mesenteric edema, and ascites can be seen on CT as well associated with AMI.
  - Venous engorgement, "target sign" in SMV with thrombus in center of the lumen can be seen in patients with MVT.

Magnetic Resonance Angiography (MRA): longer to perform than CTA but avoids radiation.

- Poor visualization of the IMA, peripheral splanchnic vessels, calcified plaque, previously placed stents vs. CTA.

Conventional angiography: "gold standard."

- AP and lateral views of the visceral aorta, and selective catheterization of the celiac, SMA, IMA provides most accurate localization of lesions
- Allows for therapeutic options: balloon angioplasty, stenting, thrombolysis, and percutaneous thrombus extraction.

Management

Medical treatment: usually not effective alone in patients with symptomatic mesenteric ischemia.

- High intensity statins recommended
- Aggressive fluid resuscitation with restoration of urine output, correction of electrolyte abnormalities and acidosis should be done/started before operation.
- Patients with chronic mesenteric ischemia who are malnourished should receive TPN or enteral nutrition.
- Broad spectrum IV antibiotics recommended in patients with AMI
- After stent placement—300 mg clopidogrel load followed by 1–3 months of 75 mg daily and maintained on aspirin and high dose statin indefinitely.

Endovascular treatment: Balloon angioplasty and stenting in CMI, generally accepted as primary therapy now.

Surgical treatment—laparotomy with visceral revascularization.

- Bowel should be reassessed after vascular reconstruction and reperfusion.
- Intraoperative angiography can be done to assess mesenteric flow.
- Second look laparotomy in 24 h recommended to reassess bowel viability.

Acute Mesenteric Ischemia (AMI)

Embolus—arterial emboli are the most common cause of AMI (40–50% of cases) [2].

- Source is frequently an intracardiac mural thrombus (from afib, MI, cardiomyopathy, structural heart defects, cardiac tumors).
- Other sources: septic embolic from endocarditis, mural thrombus from proximal aneurysm in abdominal or thoracic aorta, atheromatous plaque.
- SMA is most common source for emboli in aorta—usually lodges several cm from origin, distal to middle colic artery.

Thrombosis—second most common cause of AMI (20–35% of cases).

- Preexisting plaque is most common.
- Hypercoagulability syndromes can predispose to thrombosis as well.
- Affected segment is usually at the origin at the level of the aorta.
- Mortality for AMI patients higher with mesenteric thrombosis vs. emboli.

NOMI—due to impaired perfusion in the absence of thromboembolic disease. Five to 15% of cases.

- Can be due to a low-flow state which is made worse by presence of atherosclerotic disease.
- Most commonly occurs secondary to cardiac disease (e.g. sever CHF patients undergoing cardiac surgery, afib causing reduced left ventricular function).
- Risk factors: older age, hypovolemia, systemic vasoconstrictors, vasoactive drugs (e.g. Digoxin, alpha-adrenergic agents, beta-blocking agents, cocaine), aortic insufficiency, cardiopulmonary bypass, abdominal compartment syndrome, liver failure, patients on hemodialysis (incidence 40× higher).

Treatment selective mesenteric angiography and catheter based infusion of intra-arterial vasodilators (papaverine and prostaglandin E1 [PGE1]) as well as angioplasty and stenting if needed.

- Intravenous PGE1 infusion has been shown to treat vasospasm associated with NOMI as well.
- Low doses of intra-arterial iloprost (inhibitor of platelet aggregation with fibrinolytic activity) have shown significant vasodilatory effect on mesenteric blood flow.

Mesenteric Venous Thrombosis and Portal Vein Thrombosis 5–15% of cases, involvement usually limited to superior mesenteric vein but can also involve IMV, splenic vein, and portal veins [3].

- Primary (idiopathic).
- Secondary—when underlying disease process is present
  - 3 main categories: direct injury (surgery, trauma), local venous stasis/congestion (due to increased intraabdominal pressure, hypersplenism, CHF, obesity), thrombophilia (protein C/S deficiency, antithrombin 3 deficiency, factor V leidin, OCP use, polycythemia vera, HIT, antiphospholipid syndrome, CMV infection)

- *Treatment*: prompt initiation of systemic anticoagulation (improves survival and reduces risk of recurrence).
  - Abdominal exploration with laparotomy if peritonitis/ severe gastrointestinal bleeding/or intestinal stricture.
  - Lifelong anticoagulation with vitamin K antagonists recommended.

Chronic Mesenteric Ischemia

Most common cause: atherosclerosis.

- Hx of smoking, HTN, HLD, and atherosclerotic disease in other areas common. Can also be associated with vasculitis and inflammatory conditions (e.g. lupus, Buerger disease, radiation arteritis)

Medical treatment: high intensity statins and risk factor modification.

Surgical treatment: Revascularization is indicated in all patients with symptoms of CMI.

- Goal is to relieve symptoms, restore normal weight and prevent bowel infarction.
- Primary endovascular stenting is first choice in treatment in >80% of patients
- SMA is the primary target for revascularization.
  - Ideal lesion for endovascular treatment: short, focal stenosis or occlusion with minimal to moderate calcification or thrombus.
  - Celiac lesions have high rates of restenosis with angioplasty and stenting.
- Open revascularization: type of open reconstruction based on patient's anatomy and risk assessment.
  - 2-vessel reconstructions (CA and SMA) with a bifurcated polyester graft from supraceliac aorta accounts for >80% of mesenteric reconstructions [4].

- Antegrade mesenteric bypass: bypass from distal thoracic or supraceliac aorta (often spared from disease) via transperitoneal upper midline or bilateral subcostal incision [4].

Key Steps

– Supraceliac aorta exposed after division of diaphragmatic crura.
– systemic heparinization and clamp using two aortic clamps or a Satinsky clamp
– Aortotomy and proximal anastomosis with graft to aorta
– Graft is gently beveled and right graft limb anastomosed end-to-end to the celiac axis or hepatic artery
– Left limb of graft is tunneled behind pancreas and end-to-side anastomosis done with SMA.

Retrograde mesenteric bypass: inflow from infrarenal aorta/prior infrarenal aortic grafts/or the iliac arteries.

- Usually only reconstruct one artery (SMA) in retrograde bypasses.
  – Common iliac artery is most commonly used as source of inflow (avoids aortic cross clamp).
  – Large 8 or 10 mm graft should be used and prefer "C" shaped graft when iliac is used as inflow.
  – Either right or left iliac may be used, but right iliac usually lays better when used for inflow.

Retrograde Open Mesenteric Stenting (ROMS) [2]—hybrid approach done via midline laparotomy to expose SMA.

– Used in selected patients with AMI due to in situ thrombosis when there is an indication for laparotomy, or if severe aortic/iliac calcifications and there is no good inflow source for bypass.

SMA Dissection

- SMA is most commonly affected mesenteric artery where spontaneous dissection occurs (followed by celiac). Still rare with 0.06% incidence [5]. Typically older men in 50s-60s. Can be caused by connective tissue diseases (Marfans, Ehlers Danlos syndrome, Loeys-Dietz syndrome), but also associated with obesity, tobacco use, atherosclerosis, alcohol abuse, obesity, heavy weight lifting, pregnancy
- Usually originates 1–3 cm from SMA origin (where SMA transitions from a fixed retropancreatic position to a mobile mesenteric root).
- Symptomatic vs. Asymptomatic presentation

Symptomatic: abdominal pain 90% of cases [5] (severe, tearing, mid-epigastric area, occasional radiation to back) or abdominal pain out of proportion to exam (suggestive of mesenteric ischemia)

Diagnosis CTA (gold standard) and contrast enhanced CT, less commonly (Duplex Ultrasound, MRI)

Sakamoto Classification based on CT [5–7]:

Type 1: patent false lumen with both entry and reentry tears
Type 2: a “cul de sac” shaped false lumen without reentry
Type 3: thrombosed false lumen with ulcer defect
Type 4: completely thrombosed false lumen without ulcer

Type 1—can be treated conservatively with anticoagulation and medical management

Type 2—follow closely for signs of ischemia, if present treat endo vs. open

Type 3—high likelihood of requiring intervention either endo or open

Type 4—do not require any intervention

Management

Asymptomatic—medical management with anticoagulation/antiplatelet agents

Symptomatic—initial Tx: bowel rest and fluid resuscitation, anticoagulation

If patients fail to improve or signs of ischemia-

Surgery: (if hemorrhage or concern for bowel necrosis)

Visceral bypass (aortavisceral bypass, extraanatomic bypass (gastroepiploic or hepatic artery to SMA bypass), intimectomy/fenestration combined with vein patch, or autogenous graft with saphenous vein

Endovascular

- SMA stent via transfemoral or transbrachial access
- Self-expanding nitinol bare metal stent preferred (or covered stent graft if aneurysmal degeneration present)
- Recommended lifelong antiplatelet
- CTA or duplex surveillance at 1 month, every 6 months for first year, then annual surveillance

Splanchnic Artery Aneurysm

Incidence/Etiology

Dilation of enlargement of artery to 1.5–2× normal diameter. 1/3 of patients will have associated aortic, renal, iliac, lower extremity, or cerebral artery aneurysm. Overall incidence 0.1–2%. Etiology: atherosclerosis, medial degeneration, collagen vascular disease.

- Risk factors: multiparity, portal hypertension, inflammatory conditions (associated with splanchnic pseudoaneurysms).

- Genetic disease and connective tissue disorders have also been implicated.

Surgical Treatment

Open Repair

Ligation of proximal and distal branches without reconstruction in cases of frank rupture and hemodynamic collapse during elective cases if there is adequate collateralization

Celiac and hepatic artery can be ligated if there is collateralization from gastroduodenal and pancreaticoduodenal arteries and portal vein is patent

Endovascular Therapy

Associated with shorter hospital stay, lower cost, faster recovery

- Treatment: coil and glue embolization, injection of particles or gelfoam, placement of covered stents or flow diverting stents, injection of ethyl alcohol or thrombin.

Splenic artery aneurysms Most common (60%), females:males 4:1 [8]. Most are saccular and located in the mid or distal splenic artery and its bifurcations. Risk factors: multiparity, fibromuscular dysplasia, portal hypertension, blunt trauma, infection, pancreatitis.

Lower rupture risk in patients who are not pregnant (>50% rupture during pregnancy)

"Double rupture" phenomenon—occurs after initial tamponade in lesser sac followed by free rupture into retroperitoneum

Treatment: Any patient with symptoms should undergo intervention, women who are pregnant or are of childbearing age should undergo treatment as well. If there is a pseudoaneurysm it should be treated as well. Otherwise treatment indicated if >2 cm in size.

Open surgery: complete resection with splenectomy, proximal and distal ligation of the aneurysm, or ligation with arterial reconstruction.

- Splenectomy is not always needed due to collaterals from short gastritis (unless ligation is done at splenic hilum).

Endovascular: coil or glue embolization associated with 96% technical success

- Post-embolization syndrome (fever, abdominal pain, nausea/vomiting) can occur after embolization but usually resolves.
- Covered stent repair limited to proximal lesions (limited ability to get adequate wire support due to tortuosity)

Hepatic artery aneurysms Second most common (20%) [6]. Most hepatic aneurysms found in extrahepatic vasculature (75–80%) and most commonly in the common hepatic artery, right hepatic artery is second most common. Male to Female ratio 3:2. No association with pregnancy with incidence or rupture risk. Percutaneous and endoscopic interventions have led to increased rise of hepatic artery aneurysms.

Treat any symptomatic aneurysm, pseudoaneurysm, and aneurysms >2 cm.

Open surgery: Via right subcostal or midline laparotomy, can use intraoperative ultrasound to identify aneurysm.

- Common HAA can be ligated or endovascular embolization if GDA is patent. HAA distal to GDA can be treated by arterial reconstruction after ligation.
- Aneurysms within the liver can be treated with resection, ligation, or embolization.
- Should not do hepatic artery ligation in presence of cirrhosis. If Right hepatic artery is ligated or embolized must do a cholecystectomy.

SMA aneurysms 6% of cases, slight male predominance. Almost exclusively occur in the first 5 cm of the artery [6].

Etiology—commonly infection, mycotic etiology accounts for 60% of SMA aneurysms. Other causes: atherosclerosis, connective tissue disease, pancreatitis with trauma.

Presentation: Nonrutured cases likely to cause colicky pain, intestinal angina, weight loss—in 70–90% of patients. High association with rupture as well compared to other splanchnic aneurysms (38–50%).

Treatment: recommend observation of small (<2.5 cm) aneurysms.

- All pseudoaneurysms and those with a mycotic etiology should be repaired.
- Treatment operations: surgical aneurysmectomy, arterial reconstruction, simple ligation (in rare cases).
- If mycotic or inflammatory in etiology then do NOT use PTFE or Dacron bypass grafts.
- Open approach via midline or retroperitoneal, proximal dissection may extend underneath renal vein and if necessary, the adrenal vein may be ligated.
- Must confirm presence of a replaced or aberrant right hepatic branch.
- Endovascular management can be done with either coil embolization or stent grafts.

Celiac artery aneurysms: 4% of splanchnic aneurysms [6]

Etiology—infectious, atherosclerosis, medial degeneration, median arcuate ligament syndrome implicated in formation of some celiac aneurysms.

Presentation—rupture rates of 10–20%, history of colicky abdominal pain, or intestinal angina. Acute abdominal pain and hemorrhagic shock in cases of rupture.

Treatment: recommend repair for aneurysms >2.5 cm.

Surgical options: ligation with or without reconstruction, aneurysmectomy, aneurysmorrhaphy.

- Arterial reconstruction depends on collaterals.
- Endovascular options include coil or glue embolization, percutaneous thrombin or ethanol injection, stent graft placement.

Rare splanchnic aneurysms (gastric/gastroepiploic, pancreaticoduodenal and gastroduodenal, IMA, jejunal/ileal/colic artery aneurysms)

Gastric Artery and Gastroepiploic Artery Aneurysms

- 4% of all splanchnic aneurysms, usually due to atherosclerosis, trauma, infection [6]. Usually along left or right gastric artery.
- 90% are ruptured on initial presentation. Any GAA or GEAA discovered before rupture should be treated.
- Open surgical aneurysmectomy or exclusion. Simultaneous revasculariation usually not required.
- If endovascular: must embolize both distal and proximal (aneurysm may recruit a new vascular supply in a retrograde manner if proximal embolization is done without distal embolization).

Pancreaticoduodenal/Gastroduodenal Aneurysms Extremely rare, ~2% of all splanchnic aneurysms [6].

- Usually associated with pancreatic pathology, celiac occlusion or stenosis, or abdominal trauma or iatrogenic injury.
- Male to female ratio 4:1.
- *Presentation*: vague epigastric abdominal pain, may radiate to back, gi bleeding, hypotension, emesis, diarrhea, jaundice.
- GI or biliary tract is site of rupture in 65% of cases.
- No correlation between size and rupture risk.
- Treat regardless of size.

- Endovascular management is ideal—coil embolization techniques.
- Open repair with ligation may require partial pancreatectomy or pancreaticoduodenectomy.

IMA/Jejunal/Colic Artery Aneurysms extremely rare, usually small <1 cm.

- Usually symptomatic and often ruptured on presentation.
- Recommend treatment for any lesion seen, most ruptured are <1 cm.
- Open surgical treatment by aneurysmectomy, or ligation.
- Endovascular treatment by coil embolization.

Celiac Artery Compression Syndrome (aka Median Arcuate Ligament Syndrome [MALS]) anatomic and clinical illness resulting from extrinsic compression of the celiac axis.

Presentation postprandial and exercise induced abdominal pain, nausea, vomiting, weight loss, "food fear." Female:Male 3:1, nausea/vomiting, unintentional weight loss, exercise induced pain, second-sixth decade of life, autonomic dysfunction, fibromyalgia.

- Median arcuate ligament comes from diaphragmatic crura from L1 to 4 which projects cephalad to join the anterior longitudinal ligament of the spine overlying the celiac axis.
- Composed of the edge of crura that crosses the aorta at the level of the celiac artery. Splays over the aorta and laterally to the suspensory ligament and fourth portion of the duodenum.
- In most cases: the ligament does not encroach the celiac artery and causes no compression. 10–24% may have no symptoms.
- Underlying pathophysiology unknown, possible hypothesis is that compression of the celiac plexus nerve fibers may lead to pan and alter gastric myoelectrical activity/impair motility.

- CTA/MRA to evaluate structural elements of celiac artery, median arcuate ligament and viscera.
- Abdominal duplex ultrasound.
- Normally distance between celiac artery and median arcuate ligament increases during inspiration and decreases with expiration. PSV >200cm/s, no flow, or retrograde common hepatic arterial flow during inspiration or expiration consistent with 70% stenosis of celiac artery. Elevated PSV with expiration which normalize or decrease with inspiration and standing suggestive of MALS.

Angiography—asymmetric focal narrowing of proximal celiac axis with poststenotic dilation; narrowing increases with expiration. Increased collaterals in celiac distribution means significant stenosis.

Gastric Tonometry: blood gases and PCO_2 measured during peak exercise and recovery after 10 min bicycle test.

- Positive result: gastric arterial PCO_2 gradient >0.8 after exercise, increase in gastric PCO_2; arterial lactate levels <8 mmol/L.

Management: open or laparoscopic release of the median arcuate ligament. Percutaneous celiac ganglion block perioperatively can be done as a diagnostic and potentially therapeutic test.

- Endovascular therapy with percutaneous transluminal angioplasty (PTA) or stenting alone is NOT recommended (does not address the issue of extrinsic compression by the ligament).

Middle aortic syndrome developmental aortic narrowing from coarctations in the aorta.

- Can be distinguished based on the most cephalad extent of the involved portion (suprarenal 69%, suprarenal-infrarenal 23%, infrarenal 8%) [3]

Etiology overfusion of the two dorsal aortas during 4th week of gestation.

Most frequent genetic diseases in utero associated with abdominal aortic coarctations: neurofibromatosis-1 (NF1), and tuberous sclerosis; maternal rubella during 1st trimester.

- Nondevelopmental coarctation has been associated with umbilical artery catheterization during neonatal period.

Clinical symptoms hypertension from suprarenal or intrarenal aortic narrowing (often refractory to medication), rarely—lower extremity fatigue with exercise/or claudication, postprandial intestinal angina (6%) [3].

Evaluation CTA/MRA, Renal Doppler US (often used first line to assess renin mediated hypertension caused by aortic or renal artery disease), catheter based angiography

Medical management antihypertensive drugs (ACE inhibitors, ARBs), combined alpha and beta blockers (labetalol), beta-blockers, central alpha agonists (clonidine), diuretics, calcium channel blockers, peripheral alpha antagonists, vasodilators.

Surgical Treatment

Isolated abdominal aortic coarctations: patch aortoplasty.

- If segment of aorta is too narrow or with disease affecting the renal or splanchnic arteries:
  - Thoracoabdominal bypass with ePTFE.
  - Grafts positioned behind the left kidney with a gentle curve to the distal aorta.
  - Oversize grafts to recognize aortic growth in children. 8–12 mm grafts in young children, 12–16 mm grafts for early adolescents, 14–20 mm grafts in late adolescents and adults.

Questions

1. A 62-year-old female presents to the clinic with complaint of post prandial abdominal pain for the last 3 months associated with 5 lb of weight loss. A US mesenteric duplex was done showing a PSV of 200 cm/s in the celiac artery and 410 cm/s in the SMA; the IMA was unable to be visualized. Which of the following is consistent with the above clinical picture?
   (a) Mild-moderate SMA stenosis <70%
   (b) High grade SMA stenosis >70%
   (c) High grade celiac artery stenosis >70%
   (d) Aortoiliac occlusive disease
2. A 30-year-old female is found to have an incidental 3.2 cm splenic artery aneurysm on CT trauma "pan scan" after an MVC. She is afebrile, hemodynamically stable, denies any abdominal pain. What is the optimal management of her splenic artery aneurysm?
   (a) Admission for urgent operative resection and splenectomy
   (b) US surveillance in 1 month
   (c) US surveillance in 1 year
   (d) Elective splenic artery embolization
3. A 66-year-old female presents to the ED with complaint of post-prandial abdominal pain for 6 months, 10 lb weight loss, as well as abdominal pain during her spin classes causing her to need to stop. Her history is notable for DM2 and Fibromyalgia. Which are these would you expect to see on diagnostic imaging?
   (a) Angiography showing occlusion of the proximal SMA without flow seen in distal SMA
   (b) Angiography showing widely patent Celiac with moderate ostial stenosis of SMA <70%
   (c) US Mesenteric duplex showing celiac artery PSV >230 cm/s during expiration with normalizes with inspiration
   (d) US Mesenteric duplex showing elevated SMA velocities during inspiration >225 cm/s which normalizes with expiration

4. A 57-year-old male with chronic mesenteric ischemia and 20 lb weight loss over the past 5 months presents to your clinic. His PMH is notable for DM2, HTN, HLD, and CKD stage 4. On CTA there is circumferential calcification of the abdominal aorta, mild stenosis of the celiac origin, occlusion of the proximal SMA with retrograde filling distally, occlusion of the IMA, common iliac arteries are patent without significant disease, patent right EIA without significant disease, and circumferential calcification of the left EIA. What is the best operative plan?
   (a) Medical management
   (b) Retrograde SMA bypass with inflow from R CIA
   (c) Hybrid approach with Retrograde SMA stent placement
   (d) Antegrade bypass to SMA
5. A 40-year-old male with PMH notable for HTN, HLD, A-Fib, ESRD on HD, and PAD presents to the ED with acute abdominal pain starting 2 h ago. On abdominal exam he is diffusely tender throughout with light palpation. He is afebrile but his BP is 90/50 and HR is 110 s. Labs show WBC 11; Hgb 9.0; Lactate 6; SCr 1.4. What is your next best step in management.
   (a) Urgent mesenteric arterial duplex
   (b) NPO/NGT placement and Serial Abdominal Exams
   (c) IVF resuscitation and IV antibiotics with noncontrast CT abdomen/pelvis
   (d) IVF resuscitation/heparin drip/IV antibiotics with stat CTA abdomen/pelvis

Answers: 1 (b), 2 (d) 3 (c) 4 (b) 5 (d)

References

1. Lo RC, Schermerhorn ML. In: Cronenwett JL, et al., editors. Rutherford's vascular surgery. Philadelphia: Saunders/Elsevier; 2010. p. 1728–33.
2. Wyers MC, Martin MC. In: Cronenwett JL, et al., editors. Rutherford's vascular surgery. Philadelphia: Saunders/Elsevier; 2010. p. 1754–70.
3. Biteman BR, Brody F. In: Cronenwett JL, et al., editors. Rutherford's vascular surgery. Philadelphia: Saunders/Elsevier; 2010. p. 1780–6.

4. Oderich GS, Riberio M. In: Cronenwett JL, et al., editors. Rutherford's vascular surgery. Philadelphia: Saunders/Elsevier; 2010. p. 1735–52.
5. Dougherty MJ, Troutman DA. In: Cronenwett JL, et al., editors. Rutherford's vascular surgery. Philadelphia: Saunders/Elsevier; 2010. p. 1771–8.
6. Acosta S, Bjorck M. In: Cronenwett JL, et al., editors. Rutherford's vascular surgery. Philadelphia: Saunders/Elsevier; 2010. p. 1787–92.
7. Sakamoto I, Ogawa Y, Sueyoshi E, et al. Imaging appearances and management of isolated spontaneous dissection of the superior mesenteric artery. Eur J Radiol. 2007;64:103–10. Rutherford's p. 1773.
8. Kwong JM, et al. In: Cronenwett JL, et al., editors. Rutherford's vascular surgery. Philadelphia: Saunders/Elsevier; 2010. p. 1109–20.

14 Renal Artery

Christopher B. Khoury and Allen Murga

Anatomy of Renal Vasculature

- Renal arteries arise from aorta at the **level between L1 and L2**
- Both renal arteries give off a branch to the adrenal gland superiorly, then divide into 4–5 branches near the renal hilum
- **Renal hilum anterior to posterior**—renal vein, renal artery, and renal pelvis
- Right renal artery passes behind the IVC
- **Accessory renal arteries** present in **30%**, arise from aorta between SMA and common iliac arteries.
- Horseshoe kidneys ↑ chance of multiple accessory arteries
- **Renal veins—left renal vein** receives the **left adrenal** and **left gonadal veins** prior to crossing aorta and draining into the IVC**. Right adrenal** and **right gonadal veins** drain directly into **IVC**

C. B. Khoury
Department of Surgery, Loma Linda University, Loma Linda, CA, USA
e-mail: ckhoury@llu.edu

A. Murga (✉)
Department of Vascular Surgery, Loma Linda University,
Loma Linda, CA, USA
e-mail: amurga@llu.edu

A. Murga et al. (eds.), *The Vascular Surgery In-Training Examination Review (VSITE)*,
https://doi.org/10.1007/978-3-031-24121-5_14

- Both renal veins may receive a lumbar vein
- Left renal vein landmark for locating renal arteries. Left renal artery is found posterior and cephalad to the vein, while the right renal artery is found posterior and caudally once the IVC is retracted medially

Diagnosis and Management of Renal Disease

Renal Artery Aneurysm

- Incidence: occurs less than 1% of the population
- Bilateral in 10%
- Peak incidence age 40–60 years
- Less than 3% rupture
- Rupture associated with 10% mortality in men and nonpregnant females
- Rupture in pregnancy has mortality of 55% and fetal death rate of 85%

Diagnosis

- Presentation:
  - Majority asymptomatic and found incidentally
  - Risk of rupture: pain, distension, syncope
  - May be associated with severe HTN and hematuria
- Imaging:
  - CTA preferred
  - MRA when CT contraindicated

Management

- Medical
  - Antiplatelet therapy with aspirin
  - Annual surveillance until stable for 2 years then imaging q2-3 years

- Intervention
  - Consider if size >3 cm, symptomatic, pregnant/women of childbearing age regardless of size, refractory HTN with renal artery stenosis, false aneurysms, acute dissections causing aneurysms
  - Endovascular
    - Embolization for distal and parenchymal aneurysms
    - Stent graft exclusion for main artery aneurysms
  - Open
    - Aneurysmorrhaphy with primary or patch repair vs. autologous bypass

Renovascular Hypertension

- >90% of patients referred for renal artery stenting have atherosclerotic lesions
- Renovascular hypertension secondary to renal artery occlusive disease is the most common form of surgically correctable hypertension [1]
- Occlusive lesions are divided into three main categories: Renal artery atherosclerosis, congenital stenosis, and fibromuscular dysplasia.
- **Pathophysiology**
  - A stenosis causing an 80% reduction in renal artery cross-sectional area (the so-called critical stenosis) induces a pressure gradient sufficient to cause increased renin release from the kidney. Renin and its effects on angiotensin and aldosterone account for the elevated blood pressure of renovascular hypertension (see Fig. 14.1a and b)
  - **Critical renal artery stenosis** causes a **pressure gradient of 10–15 mmHg** across the lesion, stimulating **renin** release from juxtaglomerular cells of afferent arteriole
  - **Renin-**enzyme, hydrolyzes angiotensinogen (liver) → angiotensin I (Ang I) in plasma
    - Renin cleared by the liver

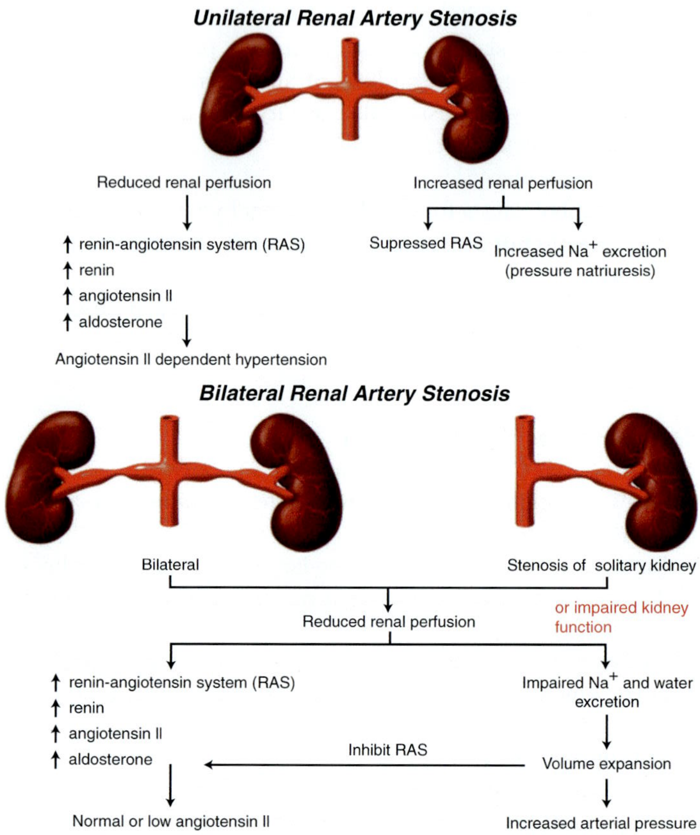

Fig. 14.1 Renal artery stenosis. (Reproduced with permission from Syndromes of Renovascular Hypertension)

- Renin release ↑ by:
  - ↑ stretch of baroreceptors (juxtaglomerular apparatus)
  - Changes in renal interstitial volume and pressure
  - ↑ pressure in afferent renal arterioles
- **Angiotensin I → Angiotensin II (Ang II)** catalyzed by **angiotensin-converting enzyme (ACE)** in pulmonary endothelium.

- **Ang II**—primary driver of renovascular hypertension, short half-life (~4 min)
- Ang II has four effects:
  - ↑ aldosterone secretion (zona glomerulosa)
  - ↑ thirst
  - ↑ renal conservation of H_2O and Na
  - ↑ vasoconstriction of arteriolar smooth muscle
- **Renal: systemic renin index (RSRI)**—[individual renal renin activity (renal vein)—peripheral renin activity (plasma)]/systemic renin activity (plasma)
- **RSRI >0.48—**↑ renin secretion, **RSRI <0.24—**↓renin secretion [2].

Renal Artery Stenosis [3] (See Fig. 14.2a and b)

- **Diagnosis**
  - Presentation
    - Severe HTN **refractory** to medical management
    - Acute rise in serum creatinine following the initiation of ACE/ARB, which may resolve after withdrawal of the medication

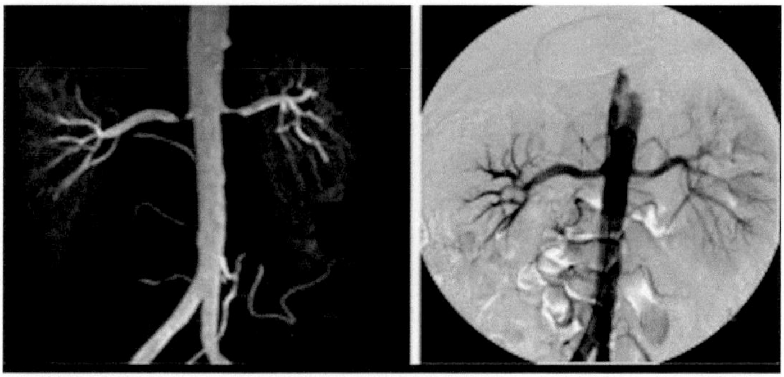

Fig. 14.2 Angiogram showing renal artery stenosis. (Reproduced with permission from Syndromes of Renovascular Hypertension)

Recurrent episodes of **hypertensive crisis, flash pulmonary edema, or congestive heart failure** requiring hospitalization

Progressive **reduction in GFR** without evidence of an alternative cause of renal disease

Abdominal bruits, edema (due to heart failure), or diminished pulses in extremities (due to atherosclerotic peripheral arterial disease)

- Imaging

  Renal Duplex US (screening)

  CTA and MRA vs. DSA (gold standard)

- **Management**
  - Nonoperative Management

    Risk factor modification (smoking cessation, diet, exercise, strict diabetes control)

    Patients should receive antiplatelet and statin therapy regardless of baseline lipid levels, unless contraindicated

    Aggressive management of HTN

    - Systolic BP of <140 mmHg and diastolic BP <90 mmHg
    - <130/80 for patients with concomitant diabetes or renal insufficiency
    - Typically requires multiple classes of antihypertensive
      - 1st line: ACE/ARB, thiazides, CCBs, beta-blockers
  - Endovascular Management

    Renal artery angioplasty and stenting

    Indications: severe hypertension refractory to max medical therapy, decline in renal function, and decreased renal perfusion from the lesion

    Contraindications: anatomic limitations such as stenosis of terminal main renal artery, branches of main renal artery, and lesions in multiple small renal arteries
  - Open Management

    Open renal artery revascularization (aortorenal bypass, renal artery thromboendarterectomy, hepatorenal bypass, and splenorenal bypass).

Indications: multiple small renal arteries or early primary branching of the main renal artery, need for aortic reconstruction near the renal arteries for other indications (i.e. aneurysm repair or severe aortoiliac occlusive disease), or failure of endovascular intervention.

Open bypass preferred in pediatric population

Ischemic Nephropathy

Causes of acute renal ischemia include renal artery thrombosis, embolism, trauma, aortic or renal artery dissection, iatrogenic injury, and renal vein thrombosis

Diagnosis

- Symptoms and signs of acute renal ischemia include abdominal or back pain, dyspnea, nausea, vomiting, hematuria, anuria, and acute hypertension
- Imaging:
  - CTA

    More sensitive than ultrasound and less time consuming than magnetic resonance angiography (MRA), with a reported sensitivity of 80%
  - MRA

    Reliability similar to that of CTA; its distinct advantages for evaluating renal segmental arteries and parenchymal disease make it a potentially valuable technique when contrast imaging is contraindicated due to renal dysfunction.

    Compared with CTA and/or ultrasound, rapid access to MRI is often relatively limited within emergency department and hospital environments, where acute renal ischemia is commonly evaluated.
  - US

    Does not require contrast or radiation exposure

Less sensitive than CTA for renal ischemia

Renal infarcts typically appear as wedge-shaped, hypoechoic lesions with absent blood flow on duplex ultrasound

- **Renal Artery Embolism**
  - Risk factors include atrial fibrillation, ischemic heart disease, cardiomyopathy, previous arterial thromboembolism, mitral or aortic valve disease, cardiac tumor, atherosclerotic aortic plaque, and paradoxical embolism in the setting of a patent foramen ovale.
  - Incidence among hospitalized patients of 0.007%
  - Treatment

    Heparin anticoagulation once suspected

    Evaluation for embolic source

    Revascularization considered in patients with acute ischemia and potentially salvageable renal function, especially in the setting of bilateral embolism.

    - Catheter-directed thrombolysis
    - Aspiration thrombectomy, angioplasty, and stenting may also be utilized as adjuncts to thrombolysis in the setting of embolic renal artery occlusion
    - Open embolectomy
      - Infrequently utilized for acute embolism because it is relatively invasive and time consuming compared with endovascular treatment

    Anticoagulation alone can be used for definitive management in patients with unilateral embolism and limited potential for renal salvage

- **Renal Artery Thrombosis**
  - Nonembolic renal artery thrombosis may result from a variety of both renal and extrarenal disease processes, including atherosclerotic renal artery stenosis, distal aortic occlusion from aneurysmal or atherosclerotic disease with proximal thrombus propagation, aortic or renal artery dissection, renal artery aneurysm, fibromuscular dysplasia, arteritis (e.g. Takayasu), stent thrombosis, hypercoagulable state, or

trauma. Iatrogenic thrombosis may also result from renal artery coverage or injury during endovascular procedures.
  - Treatment
    - Systemic anticoagulation
    - Management of intravascular volume status
    - Endovascular treatment
      - Angioplasty and stenting, thrombolysis, mechanical catheter thrombectomy, and aspiration thrombectomy
        - Frequently used in combination depending on etiology
    - Open Surgery
      - Renal artery thrombectomy, bypass, and/or endarterectomy
      - Reserved for situation in which renal salvage is substantial, or endovascular treatment failure, extensive thrombus burden
- **Renovascular Trauma**
  - Incidence of <1% in blunt abdominal trauma
  - 75% of patients also have an abdominal solid organ injury involving the kidney, liver, or spleen
  - 17% have multiple abdominal vascular injuries (most commonly to the renal vein or inferior vena cava)
  - Treatment
    - Factors associated consideration for revascularization include bilateral injury or injury to solitary functioning kidney
    - Observation with interval imaging, endovascular intervention, open revascularization, or nephrectomy
    - **Unilateral dissection or occlusion** after blunt trauma **should not be treated surgically**.
    - Revascularization has ↓ **chance of success with >4 h warm ischemia time** but most surgeons will attempt salvage revascularization up to **20–24 h** after **bilateral renal injury**
    - Limited success of endovascular treatment since ↓ or no heparin use due to concomitant injuries → ↑risk of

thrombus formation (at access or interventional sites) and wire/catheter manipulation of the injured vessel can result in overt hemorrhage and decompensation of an otherwise stable patient

Only 50% of those who underwent endovascular intervention had renal function salvage (with significant rates of re-occlusion)

- **Renal Vein Thrombosis**
  - Less than one case per million annually
  - Risk factors include malignancy, nephrotic syndrome, inherited thrombophilia, local surgery or inflammation, oral contraceptive use, pregnancy, and infection.
  - Iatrogenic renal vein thrombosis may also occur with vena cava filter or central venous catheter.
  - Treatment

    Anticoagulation at time of diagnosis

    Incidence of recurrent renal vein thrombosis is 1% per patient year of follow-up

    Thrombectomy or thrombolysis—reserved for failure or complication of oral anticoagulation (such as thrombus propagation or pulmonary embolism), bilateral thrombosis or thrombosis of a solitary kidney, associated caval thrombosis, acute renal failure, or persistent severe symptoms (most commonly flank pain)

    Nephrectomy has a limited role but may be the treatment of choice in the setting of postinfarction hemorrhage.

Renal Fibromuscular Dysplasia

- FMD is nonatheromatous, noninflammatory, proliferative process that primarily affects the **media** in long, unbranched, medium-sized arteries, including the renal artery [4].
- 5–10% of renovascular HTN secondary to FMD
- 90% female predominance

Diagnosis

- Duplex US, MRA, and CTA unreliable in excluding FMD
- **DSA** is gold standard for detection of FMD
  - Multifocal disease, which appears as a "**string of beads**" that are numerous and larger than the diameter of the vessel
  - Focal FMD, which reveals a concentric, smooth, band-like focal stenosis or a tubular stenosis

Management

- Medical management—aggressive antihypertensive treatment
- Endovascular management
  - Treatment considered in patient with uncontrolled HTN, impaired renal function, or ischemic nephropathy
  - **Percutaneous transluminal renal angioplasty** ***without stenting*** is treatment of choice
- Open management
  - Include aortorenal bypass with vein or prosthetic grafts or kidney autotransplantation
  - Reserved for patients with large aneurysm, especially at a branch site, thrombosis, or dissection that cannot be corrected endovascularly. Also, repeated failed endovascular tx.

Diagnostic Studies to Detect Functionally Significant Stenosis

Anatomic diagnostic criteria: stenosis >70%, post stenotic dilatation, presence of collateral circulation, kidney length of ≥7 cm, reduced kidney size (length decrease >1 cm or length discrepancy of at least 1–1.5 cm between kidneys) [5]

- **CTA**
  - Benefits—94% sensitivity, 93% specificity, 99% negative predictive value
  - Risks—nephrotoxic contrast, radiation exposure
- **MRA—**vascular structures enhance in **T1 phase** with gadolinium
  - Benefits—no radiation or nephrotoxic contrast
  - Risks—if GFR <30 mL/min, gadolinium based contrast agents may cause nephrogenic systemic fibrosis.
- **Digital subtraction angiography (DSA)—gold standard** for diagnosis and treatment [6]
  - Benefits—Hemodynamic assessment (direct pressure measurement) + catheter-based interventions (balloon and stent angioplasty).
  - Risks—nephrotoxic contrast and radiation exposure
  - Generally reserved for patient undergoing planned renal artery reconstruction.
- **Duplex US—**Normal renal flow: monophasic, low resistance with constant forward flow throughout the cardiac cycle
  - Benefits—non-invasive, no radiation or contrast exposure
  - Risks—inadequate imaging based on location/body habitus, technician dependent
  - Technique—fasting state, scan in B mode and color flow modes, low frequency (2.25–3.0 MHz) to achieve adequate depth
  - Interpretation—severity of stenosis measured by **peak systolic velocity (PSV)** at the SMA/aorta compared to the renal arteries
  - Normal renal PSV <180 cm/s. Normal aortic PSV 50–100 cm/s
  - **Renal PSV >200 cm/s** indicates **>60% stenosis**
  - **Renal-to-Aortic Ratio (RAR) ≥3.5 is used to identify a >60% stenosis** (with a normal aortic PSV)
  - **Renal Resistive Index ([PSV − EDV]/[PSV])** quantifies renal parenchymal resistance to flow. RRI upper limit of normal is 0.80. High RRI values (i.e. >0.80) are associated with clinical failure of renal revascularization procedures.

Endovascular Renal Aneurysm Repair

- Degenerative renal artery aneurysms have been treated with transcatheter embolization with detachable platinum coils that occlude the aneurysms but maintain renal flow [7]
- Alternatively, using liquid embolization, stenting, stent grafts, and ethylene vinyl alcohol copolymer has been used.
- Endovascular stent graft exclusion—ideal for main renal artery aneurysms not involving branch vessels.

Renal Artery Aneurysm Repair [8]

Key Steps

- If emergent/rupture—supraceliac aorta control may be required.
  - In unstable patients—nephrectomy is often required
- Renal artery exposure
  - Left—descending colon, pancreas, and spleen are reflected medially, dividing the splenorenal and splenophrenic ligaments.
  - Right—right medial visceral rotation, right colon mobilized medially from the cecum to hepatic flexure → Kocher maneuver. IVC and right renal vein identified. →Mobilization of the right renal vein exposing posterior right renal artery.
  - The renal vein is mobilized for retraction as the renal artery lies beneath it along the cephalad border.
- After heparinization, proximal and distal control are obtained with vascular clamps. The saccular aneurysm is resected with primary repair or patch angioplasty.

Renal Artery Bypass: Aortorenal, Splenorenal, Hepatorenal [9]

Key Steps

- Exposure of the supraceliac aorta, the infrarenal aorta, and the pararenal aorta.
  - Midline laparotomy incision, the posterior peritoneum overlying the aorta is opened, and the ligament of Treitz is divided to mobilize the duodenum to the patient's right.
  - Extension of the peritoneal incision in a caudal direction will expose the entire infrarenal aorta to the level of the aortic bifurcation.
  - The supraceliac aorta is exposed by dividing the left triangular ligament of the liver, incising the gastrohepatic ligament, retracting the esophagus and stomach laterally, and dividing the median arcuate ligament and the peritoneum overlying the aorta.
  - The peritoneum along the **left** renal vein is incised and followed along the inferior border of the pancreas, which facilitates its retraction for exposure of the left renal hilum where the artery lies posterior to the vein.
  - Exposure of the **right** renal artery is achieved through mobilization of the duodenum and hepatic flexure of the colon medially, where the artery lies posterior to the right renal vein.
- **Aortorenal/iliorenal bypass** [10]
  - The infrarenal aorta is controlled proximally and distally, and the patient is systemically heparinized.
  - For iliorenal bypasses, the exposure is continued distally from the aorta onto the iliac vessels. Avoid ureters!
  - The aorta is clamped, and an aortotomy is made using an aortic punch device.
  - Proximal and distal anastomosis performed using conduit of choice

- **Hepatorenal bypass** for right renal artery reconstruction [11].
  - Distal exposure of the right renal artery is obtained by mobilizing the ascending colon and duodenum medially. This is followed by retraction of the right renal vein.
  - The hepatic artery is exposed by incising the lesser omentum. The artery is identified to the left of the common bile duct.
  - Control of the common hepatic, gastroduodenal, and proper hepatic arteries is obtained.
  - Systemically heparinize, and the proximal anastomosis is performed in end-to-side fashion with the heel oriented to the right.
  - The graft is tunneled behind the duodenum, the right renal artery is divided, the conduit is spatulated, and the distal anastomosis is performed in an end-to-end fashion.
- **Splenorenal bypass** for left renal artery reconstruction.
  - The splenic artery is exposed by developing an avascular plane at the inferior border of the pancreas in the retropancreatic space and identifying the artery at the superior border of the pancreas.
  - An avascular plane is developed at the inferior border of the pancreas as the peritoneum is incised, leading to the left renal hilum where the left renal artery lies posterior to the left renal vein.
  - Systemic heparinization is performed, and the splenic artery is clamped and divided distally, mobilized, and directed inferiorly toward the left renal artery.
  - The left renal artery is divided, and both the splenic and renal artery ends are spatulated to perform an end-to-end anastomosis.

    If not enough length of splenic artery, a saphenous vein conduit may be used as an alternative.

Questions

1. A 35-year-old female without smoking history, presents to the emergency room in hypertensive crisis. She has been progressively placed four antihypertensive medications without improvement and has recent hospitalization for congestive heart failure and flash pulmonary edema. Duplex US shows peak systolic velocity of 250 mm/s in mid-right renal artery. Once medically optimized, what is the best treatment for this patient?
   (a) Right renal artery angioplasty with stent placement
   (b) Right renal artery angioplasty without stent placement
   (c) Hepatorenal bypass
   (d) Thromboendarterectomy of right renal artery
2. A 65-year-old male with history of smoking, uncontrolled hypertension on three antihypertensive medications and diabetes is found to have unilateral right renal artery stenosis. He is deemed an appropriate surgical candidate. Due to heavily calcified infrarenal aorta, you plan to perform a hepatorenal bypass. What is true regarding exposure of the hepatic artery?
   (a) Left medial visceral rotation
   (b) Dividing median arcuate ligament
   (c) Kocher maneuver
   (d) Identifying the hepatoduodenal ligament and incising lesser omentum
3. A 50-year-old male with history of smoking, stroke and peripheral artery disease, presents for consultation regarding uncontrolled hypertension. He states he has been on four medications without improvement in his blood pressure. What is the gold standard for diagnosis of this patient's disease?
   (a) Duplex US
   (b) DSA (Digital subtraction angiography)
   (c) CTA
   (d) MRA
   (e) Serum markers

Answer: 1 (b). Young female without atherosclerotic risk factors and >60% renal artery stenosis is consistent with FMD.

Answer: 2 (d)

Answer: 3 (b)

References

1. Rickey A, Corriere M. Renovascular hypertension. SCORE. 2021 [cited 2022 May 7]. Available from: surgicalcore.org.
2. Herrmann SM, Textor SC. Syndromes of renovascular hypertension. In: Singh A, Agarwal R, editors. Core concepts in hypertension in kidney disease. Berlin: Springer; 2016.
3. Iannuzzi J. Atherosclerotic renal artery disease. SCORE. 2021 [cited 2022 Jun 7]. Available from: surgicalcore.org.
4. Endicott K, Toursavadkohi S. Nonatherosclerotic renal artery disease. SCORE. 2021 [cited 2022 Apr 28]. Available from: https://www.surgicalcore.org.
5. Sidawy A, Perler B. Rutherford's vascular surgery and endovascular therapy. 9th ed. Amsterdam: Elsevier; 2018.
6. Mulholland MW, Lillemoe KD, Doherty GM, Maier RV, Simeone DM, Upchurch GR Jr. Greenfield's surgery. 5th ed. Philadelphia: Lippincott Williams & Wilkins; 2010.
7. Maldonado T, Lee V. Renal artery aneurysm. SCORE. 2021 [cited 2022 May 7]. Available from: surgicalcore.org.
8. Nedeau A. Renal artery aneurysm repair—open and endovascular. SCORE. 2021 [cited 2022 Jun 7]. Available from: surgicalcore.org.
9. Maijub J, Fajardo A. Renal artery bypass—aortorenal, splenorenal, hepatorenal. SCORE. 2021 [cited 2022 Jun 7]. Available from: surgicalcore.org.
10. Hoballah JJ. Bilateral aortorenal bypass. In: Hoballah JJ, Scott-Conner CEH, editors. Operative dictations in general and vascular surgery. Berlin: Springer; 2011.
11. Hoballah JJ. Hepatorenal artery bypass. In: Hoballah JJ, Scott-Conner CEH, editors. Operative dictations in general and vascular surgery. Berlin: Springer; 2011.

15 Thoracic Aortic Disease

Sheela Patel and Sandeep Jhajj

- Aneurysms:
- Introduction
  - Normal thoracic aorta is divided into four parts
    - Aortic root
    - Ascending aorta
    - Aortic arch
    - Descending thoracic aorta
  - Most common thoracic aneurysm occurs in ascending aorta
  - Thoracic aneurysms less frequent than abdominal aortic aneurysms (AAA)
- Definition
  - Dilatation at least 1.5 times its normal value
  - Diameter is strongest predictor of rupture
  - Saccular: eccentric dilatation of aorta; mycotic
  - Fusiform: chronic uniform dilatation involving whole circumference of aorta

S. Patel (✉) · S. Jhajj
Department of Surgery, Loma Linda University, Loma Linda, CA, USA
e-mail: stpatel@llu.edu; SJhajj@llu.edu

A. Murga et al. (eds.), *The Vascular Surgery In-Training Examination Review (VSITE)*,
https://doi.org/10.1007/978-3-031-24121-5_15

- Pathology
  - Medial degeneration (80%)
  - Aortic dissection (20%)
  - Frank atherosclerosis rare
  - Robust inflammatory component in media and adventitia (atherosclerosis affects intima)
  - Patients with TAAA secondary to dissection are younger and more extensive than from degeneration
  - Other acute aortic syndromes: intramural hematoma, penetrating aortic ulcer
  - Connective tissue disorders (Marfan syndrome, Ehlers-Danlos syndrome, Loeys-Dietz syndrome)
  - Vasculitis (giant cell arteritis, Takayasu arteritis, Behcet disease)
  - Infection: saccular, mycotic (bacterial)
  - Traumatic: dissection, pseudoaneurysm
  - Coarctation
    - Disparate upper and lower extremity pulses
    - Can cause heart failure, refractory hypertension, diminished pulses
    - Coarctation in thoracoabdominal aorta can be treated by patch aortoplasty or thoracoabdominal bypass
    - Stenting for descending thoracic aortic lesions
  - Aberrant right subclavian artery (see Fig. 15.1)
    - Right subclavian artery takes course posterior to the esophagus
    - Dysphagia lusoria
    - Kommerell diverticulum: artery becomes aneurysmal
    - Can be treated endovascular, open or hybrid
- Epidemiology
  - Average age: 65 years old
  - Equal gender distribution
  - More than 20% of patients have first-degree relative affected by aneurysm disease
  - 20–30% will also have AAA
  - 19th leading cause of death in the US [1]

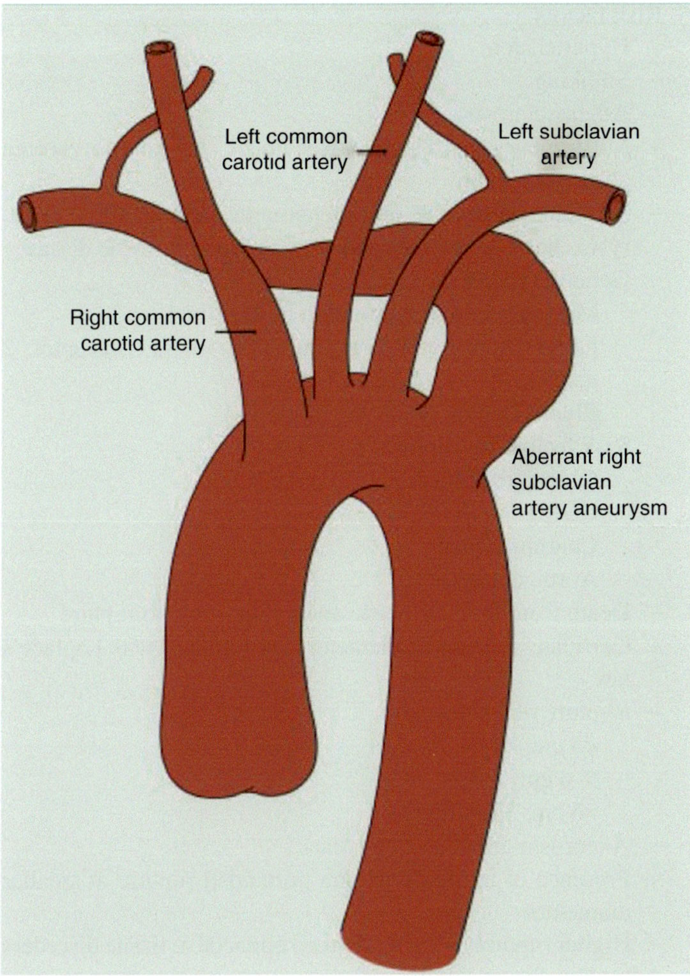

Fig. 15.1 Right aberrant subclavian artery. (Taken from Rutherford's Vascular Surgery and Endovascular Therapy 10th Ed. Ch. 86)

- Risk factors
  - Hypertension
  - Smoking
  - Atherosclerosis
  - Most aneurysms degenerative; up to 20% due to chronic aortic dissection
  - Familial; up to 20% of patients with thoracic aortic aneurysms have 1st degree relative with thoracic aortic disease
  - Genetic syndromes
    - Marfan syndrome: mutation in fibrillin-1
    - Loeys-Dietz syndrome: mutation in TFG-receptor 2 gene
    - Ehlers-Danlos syndrome (Type IV)
  - Risk factors for rupture
    - Older age
    - COPD
    - Continued pain
    - Aortic diameter
  - Death from thoracic aortic aneurysm is due to rupture
  - Correlates with aortic diameter in accordance with Laplace's law
  - Rupture risk at 5 years
    - <5 cm: <1%
    - 5–6 cm: 3–8%
    - >6 cm: 35–60% [2]
  - Aneurysm growth >1 cm/year
  - Presence of aortic dissection portended rupture at smaller diameters
  - Higher rupture risk with defined connective tissue disorders
- Anatomic classification
  - Based on extent of aortic involvement
  - Classification for descending thoracic aortic aneurysms
    - A: from distal origin of left SCA to 6th intercostal space
    - B: from T6 to T12
    - C: Entire descending thoracic aorta from left SCA to T12

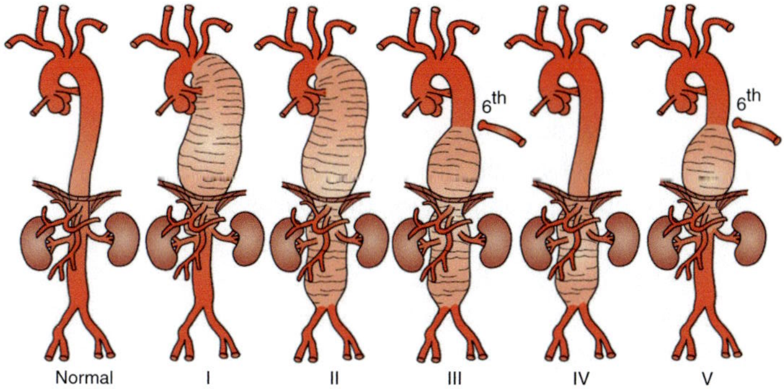

Fig. 15.2 Crawford classification for thoracoabdominal aortic aneurysms. (Taken from Rutherford's Vascular Surgery and Endovascular Therapy 10th Ed. Ch. 78)

- Crawford classification for thoracoabdominal aortic aneurysms (TAAA) (see Fig. 15.2)
  - Type I: distal to left subclavian artery to renal arteries; 25%
  - Type II: distal to left subclavian artery to aortic bifurcation; 30%
  - Type III: from sixth intercostal space to aortic bifurcation; <25%
  - Type IV: entire abdominal aorta from diaphragm to aortic bifurcation
  - Type V: below the sixth intercostal space to just above the renal arteries

- Clinical findings
  - Most are asymptomatic
  - Vague pain in chest, back, flank, abdomen (sudden expansion)
  - Sharp pain (rupture or impending rupture)
  - Differential: angina, aortic dissection, degenerative spine disease

  - Compressive symptoms
    - Hoarseness: stretching or compression of the left recurrent laryngeal nerve
    - Tracheal deviation
    - Persistent cough
    - Dysphagia: compression of esophagus
    - Hemoptysis or hematemesis: erosion of TAAA into bronchi or esophagus
  - Paraplegia: aortic dissection, embolization with occlusion of intercostal arteries
  - Blue toe syndrome: distal embolization
  - Most patients with symptoms have diameter >5 cm
- Imaging
  - Computed tomography
  - CXR
    - Widened mediastinum
    - Enlargement of the aortic knob
    - Tracheal deviation
    - Left main stem bronchus displacement
  - Transesophageal echocardiography (TEE)
    - Ascending and descending aorta can be visualized
    - Useful for acute aortic dissection
    - Heart function
  - Intravascular ultrasound (IVUS)
    - Imaging of aortic wall
    - Useful for aortic dissection
    - Requires intraarterial access
- Medical therapy
  - Stringent blood pressure control (beta blocker, ACE-I, or ARB)
    - Goal 140/90 in patients without DM; 130/80 in patients with DM or CRI
  - Cessation of smoking
  - Lipid profile optimization with statins
- Selection of treatment
  - Physiologic reserve

  - Anatomy
  - Size criteria
    - For most patients, threshold of >6 cm used
    - Positive family history or presence of connective tissue disorder might serve to lower threshold for repair
  - Saccular morphology
  - Rapid expansion (≥5 mm in 6 months, >1 cm/year)
  - Symptomatic aneurysms
  - Traumatic pseudoaneurysm
- Preoperative evaluation
  - Cardiac disease is the leading cause of mortality after open TAAA repair
  - Evaluation of coronary arteries and heart valves
  - If patient needs CABG prior to TAAA repair, avoid use of left internal mammary artery; important collateral to the spinal cord
  - Pulmonary function tests if COPD
- Treatment options
  - Despite lack of randomized trial data comparing it with open surgical repair, TEVAR has become the preferred treatment [3]
  - TEVAR has been used for mycotic aneurysms as definitive management or as bridge to stabilize to eventual open operation
  - For both open and endovascular repair, paraplegia is a devastating complication
  - Minimize paraplegia risk
    - Controlled hypothermia
    - Spinal fluid drainage
    - Optimized mean arterial pressure
    - Staging of repair of extensive aneurysms
  - Considerations for open repair
    - If connective tissue disorder, use less traumatic vascular clamps, use hypothermic circulatory arrest to avoid clamping, aortic wall reinforcement with felt pledgets or strips

Perfusion techniques for open repair

- Simple cross-clamp "clamp-and-sew" (Crawford technique) with adjuncts
  - Regional spinal cord hypothermia using epidural catheter with infusion of cold saline
  - Spinal fluid drainage
  - Steroids
  - Endorphin receptor antagonists
  - More left heart strain and HTN from proximal aortic clamping
- Assisted circulation; distal aortic perfusion with sequential clamping
  - Left atrial to femoral artery bypass (partial heart bypass) utilizing a Bio-Medicus pump
  - Left inferior pulmonary vein cannulated with catheter tip directed towards left atrium
  - Outflow via a 8- or 10-mm Dacron graft placed end-to side on left common femoral artery; retrograde perfusion of the pelvic and visceral arteries during proximal repair
  - Roller pumps provided perfusion via visceral cannulas
  - Visceral perfusate is cold blood
  - Renal perfusate is cold crystalloid solution (4 °C lactated Ringer's with mannitol and methylprednisolone) via separate roller pump
  - Bypass flow rate adjustable so proximal and distal arterial perfusion pressures can be maintained; offload heart, reduce cardiac strain with very proximal aortic clamping
  - Utilize if patient cannot tolerate one lung anesthesia
  - Utilize if patient cannot tolerate cardiac strain of proximal clamping

    Moderate passive hypothermia
- Hypothermic circulatory arrest

    - No place to proximally clamp aorta, some acute dissection cases
    - Long cooling and rewarming times
    - Total heparinization; more bleeding
    - Requires complete cardiopulmonary bypass with arterial perfusion catheters in femoral artery or ascending aorta
    - Venous return through femoral vein cannula which usually extends to right atrium and superior vena cava
    - Left ventricle sump drain to prevent cardiac dilatation
    - Cool to 16–18 °C; extreme systemic hypothermia provides excellent organ protection from ischemia of aortic occlusion
    - Circulation arrested during proximal anastomosis
  - Passive distal aortic perfusion with selective perfusion of mesenteric arteries
    - No pump devices; passive bypass circuit
    - Gott shunt
    - Axillofemoral artery bypass
    - Aortoiliac bypass
    - Renal artery perfusion with 4 °C renal preservation solution
- Anesthesia
  - Arterial lines
  - General endotracheal anesthesia
    Double lumen ventilation if extensive proximal aortic replacement
  - TEE
  - Neuromonitoring leads to motor-evoked (MEPs) and somatosensory evoked potentials (SSEPs)
    MEPs involve stimulating brain with electrical currents and monitoring the resulting signals in peripheral muscles

  - Lumbar spine drain
    - Drain spinal fluid to improve spinal cord flow during aortic occlusion
    - CSF pressure kept at 10 mmHg or less
  - Avoid arterial dilators (nitroprusside, hydralazine); can steal spinal cord blood flow
  - Methylprednisolone (30 mg/kg) after induction; stabilizes neuronal cell membranes
  - Naloxone (1 mg/kg/h) infused during and after procedure; reduces release of excitatory neurotransmitters
  - Mannitol given before and during aortic occlusion and after renal perfusion (12.5 g)
  - Moderate systemic hypothermia (31–34 °C) used to prolong spinal cord and organ ischemic tolerance
  - Keep MAP >90 mmHg to maximize collateral perfusion of the spinal cord
- Patient positioning
  - For thoracoabdominal incision
    - Right lateral decubitus position with left side up
    - Shoulders positioned perpendicular to table
    - Pelvis tilted posteriorly so left femoral vessels can be accessed for aortofemoral bypass, arterial line, or cannulation if left heart bypass
    - Extreme pelvic tilting to expose right groin
    - Beanbag to secure positioning
- Surgical exposure
  - Aneurysm confined to descending thoracic aorta: thoracotomy in 4th, 5th, 6th, 7th intercostal space
  - Crawford type III, IV: 8th or 9th intercostal space
  - Crawford type I, II: 5th or 6th intercostal space
    - Incision begins posterior to tip of scapula and proceeds medially along T6
    - Incision extended inferiorly at midline towards umbilicus
    - Latissimus dorsi divided and serratus anterior muscle mobilized
    - Cut costochondral junction

    - 6th rib resected or cut posteriorly and left in place
    - Diaphragm incised through aortic hiatus using circumferential or radial incision; allows complete exposure of descending thoracic and abdominal aorta
    - Retroperitoneal plane developed with spleen, colon, left kidney mobilized medially to right of abdominal aorta (left medial visceral rotation)
    - SMA can be exposed more completely by dissecting anterior to kidney
    - Left iliac artery easily exposed
    - Right iliac artery exposure may require dividing the IMA at origin to mobilize distal aorta
    - Avoid ureters; ureteral stents can be placed prior to surgery in redo surgery or inflammatory aortas
  - Aneurysms at the arch level usually require fifth intercostal space incision
    - Dissection begins at pulmonary hilum with opening of pericardium to expose left inferior pulmonary vein and ligamentum arteriosum divided
    - Avoid phrenic nerve and vagus nerve (recurrent laryngeal nerve)
      - RLN injury: vocal cord dysfunction, hoarseness
      - Phrenic nerve injury: diaphragm dysfunction
    - If large mediastinal or arch hematoma, pericardium opened to access the proximal arch for aortic control
- Open aneurysm repair (aortic arch aneurysm)
  - Requires sternotomy
  - Extracorporeal circulatory support
  - Often with deep hypothermic circulatory arrest
  - Hemiarch or total arch replacement
  - With concomitant descending thoracic aortic involvement, "elephant trunk" technique can be used where a second intervention addresses the descending thoracic aorta component via left thoracotomy or endovascular stent graft deployment

- Open aneurysm repair (descending thoracic aortic aneurysm)
  - Left thoracotomy
  - Aortic clamping
  - Inlay grafting
- Open aneurysm repair (TAAA)
  - Initial clamping

    Heparin flush (1000 units/L)

    Partial left heart bypass with centrifugal pump most commonly used

    If complete heart bypass used, total systemic heparinization (400 units/kg)

    MAP kept >100 while aorta clamped
  - Proximal anastomosis

    Segmental clamp applied to proximal descending thoracic aorta and mid thoracic aorta

    Aorta is divided completely and separated from underlying esophagus

    Collagen or gelatin-impregnated woven Dacron graft

    Felt strips or pledgets may be used to reinforce anastomosis

    After completing proximal anastomosis, patient put in Trendelenburg and test anastomosis and clamped moved distally

    Upper intercostal arteries ligated

    Lower thoracic arteries temporarily occluded with balloon catheters

    May have to re-implant intercostals between T8 and L2

    Graft passed through aortic hiatus

    Distal clamp moved to infrarenal aorta
  - Visceral-renal reattachment (Fig. 15.3)

    With left heart bypass, retrograde perfusion of renal and mesenteric vessels as the proximal anastomosis is fashioned and distal aortic clamp proximal to the visceral vessels

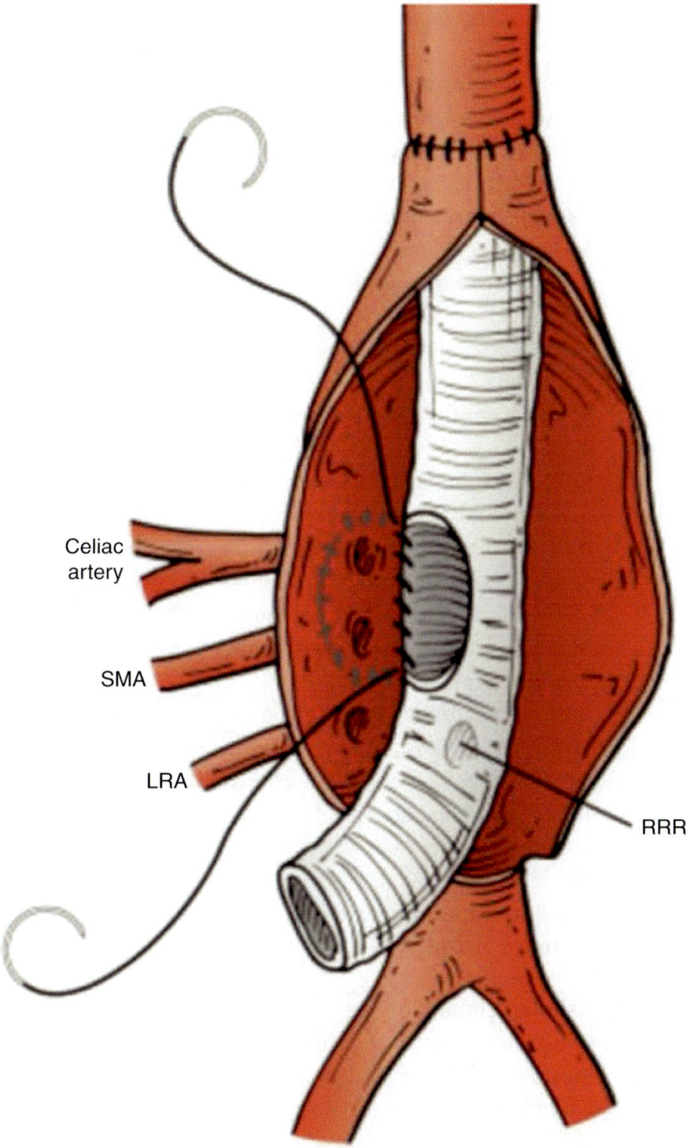

Fig. 15.3 Visceral-renal reattachment. (Taken from Rutherford's Vascular Surgery and Endovascular Therapy 10th Ed. Ch. 79)

When clamp moved to infrarenal aorta, viscera perfused via balloon tipped catheters with cold blood (34 °C) from centrifugal pump

Each kidney cooled with 300–400 cc cold (4 °C) renal perfusion solution (12.5 g mannitol, 1000 units heparin/L lactated Ringers)

Patient's core temperature 33 °C

Visceral-renal reattachment done with Carrel patch directly to aortic graft using inclusion technique (see Fig. 15.3)

Keep Carrel patch as small as possible to avoid patch aneurysms

- Patch configuration determined by spacing of the vessels
- Usually celiac, SMA, right renal artery in 1 patch
  Left renal artery attached separately

Individual bypass grafts (Coselli branched graft)

- Usually in patients with connective tissue disorders (Marfan) to avoid patch aneurysms

May require endarterectomy of renal or visceral arteries if calcified plaque

Intravenous Indigo Carmine given to document when urine produced after renal reperfusion

  – Distal anastomosis performed after pulsatile flow restored to viscera and renal arteries
  – Distal aortic perfusion cannulas removed once T reaches 36 °C
  – Diaphragm reapproximated
  – Chest tubes placed
- Neuroprotection
  – Spinal cord circulation

    Great radicular artery (from artery of Adamkiewicz) most important; at T8-L2

    Collaterals from intercostal, lumbar, subclavian, hypogastric arteries

- Risk factors associated with spinal cord ischemia
    - Aneurysm extent
    - Location: aneurysm affecting lumbar region have less robust collateralization
    - Perioperative hypotension
    - Embolization from aortic atheromatous lesions
- Intraoperative hypothermia (34 °C)
- Deliberate hypertension (MAP 90–100 mmHg)
- Distal aortic perfusion
- CSF drainage
    - Maximum of 15 cc of CSF drained each hour to prevent intracranial hemorrhage

• Endovascular treatment
- CTA for preoperative planning
    - Postprocessing 3D software (M2S, Vitrea, Aquarius) with centerline measurements
    - Include aortic arch, chest, abdomen, pelvis
    - Assess tortuosity
    - Status of vertebral arteries
    - Assessment of pelvic perfusion and spinal cord circulation; prior aortic repair, long aortic segment coverage
    - Aortic length measurements
        - Natural tortuosity of aorta and natural tendency of endograft to sit against the greater curvature usually results in underestimation of length for graft coverage
- Landing zones for thoracic aorta interventions (Ishimaru zones) (see Fig. 15.4)
    - Proximal edge of TEVAR device in relation to branch vessels
    - Zone 0: proximal to the innominate artery
    - Zone 1: proximal to left common carotid artery
    - Zone 2: proximal to origin of left subclavian artery
    - Zone 3: proximal descending thoracic aorta (<2 cm from left SCA)
    - Zone 4: 2 cm distal to SCA extending to proximal half descending thoracic aorta (T6 vertebral body)

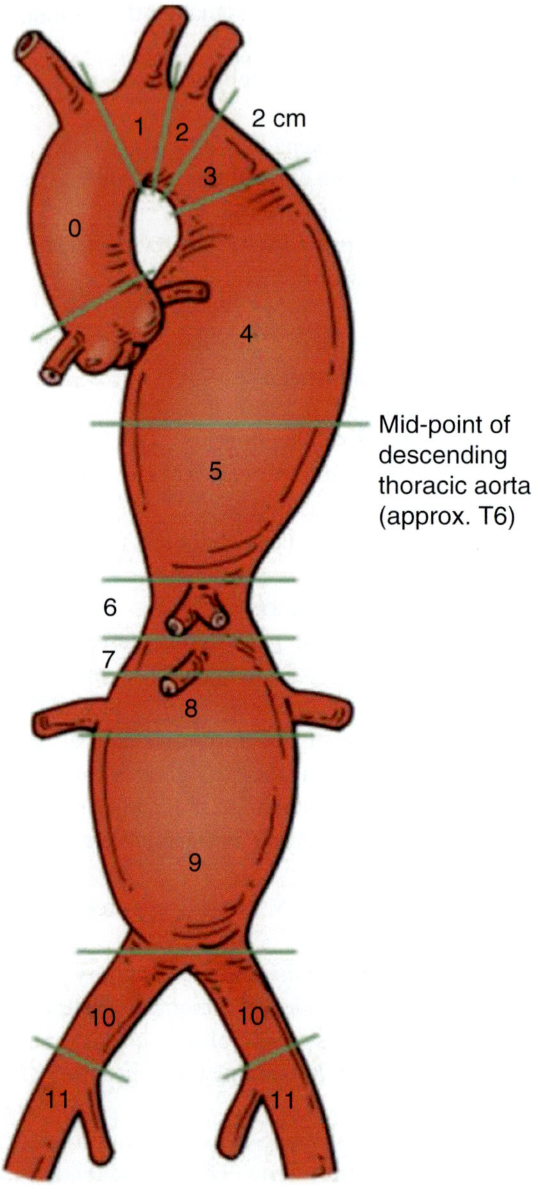

Fig. 15.4 Thoracic aorta landing zones. (Taken from Rutherford's Vascular Surgery and Endovascular Therapy 10th Ed. Ch. 80)

Zone 5: distal half descending thoracic aorta to celiac artery

Zone 6: celiac artery to top of SMA

Zone 7: SMA to suprarenal aorta

Zone 8: perirenal aorta

Zone 9: infrarenal aorta

Zone 10: common iliac arteries

Zone 11: external iliac arteries

Ideal landing zones in 3 and 4

- Anatomic criteria

  Suitable landing zones (≥20 mm) proximal and distal to allow adequate seal

  - Longer seal zone may be preferable in angulations

  Landing zone in straight segment of aorta which is cylindrical with parallel walls and without significant mural thrombus or calcification

  - Longitudinal stiffness of device can limit device apposition to inner curve (bird beaking)

  Largest FDA-approved thoracic stent graft is 46 mm diameter which is appropriate to treat a 41–42 mm aortic neck

  When multiple stent grafts are used, minimum of 3 cm of overlap

  10–20% oversizing at proximal landing zone; if oversize too much, retrograde aortic dissection, bird beaking, stent-graft collapse, accelerated aneurysm degeneration

  - Undersized grafts lead to migration and endoleaks

  With proximal landing zone in previous Dacron graft, longer length (4–5 cm) and more aggressive oversizing

  Coverage of left subclavian artery (zone 2)

  - Left SCA important for perfusion of spinal cord and brain via left vertebral artery
  - Coverage generally well tolerated because of rich collateral network; in unstable patients, coverage of left subclavian artery may be reasonable

- SVS guidelines recommend preserving left SCA flow due to risk of brainstem stroke and spinal cord and arm ischemia in elective situations (grade 2, level C evidence) [4]
- Mandatory left subclavian artery revascularization
  - Dominant left vertebral artery
  - Left internal mammary to coronary artery bypass
  - Presence of left arm hemodialysis access
  - Aberrant right subclavian artery
  - Hypoplastic or absent right vertebral artery
  - Termination of left vertebral artery into posterior inferior cerebellar artery
  - Occluded internal iliac arteries
  - Anomalous origin of left vertebral artery from arch
  - Consider left SCA revascularization if extensive aortic coverage, previous infrarenal aortic replacement
- Operations to revascularize left SCA
  - Left supraclavicular incision
  - Preserve left vertebral artery flow
  - Left CCA to left SCA bypass (see Fig. 15.5)

    Combine with ligation or embolization of the left subclavian artery proximal to the vertebral artery origin from ipsilateral brachial artery; avoids type II endoleak
  - Left SCA to left CCA transposition

    Preservation of posteriorly located vertebral artery can be difficult

    Cannot perform if left internal mammary artery has been used for coronary bypass graft
- Endovascular options to revascularize left SCA
  - In situ fenestration using back end of wire, laser

Debranching of arch vessels (zone 0–2)

- Hybrid procedures with in situ fenestration
- Extra-anatomic bypasses

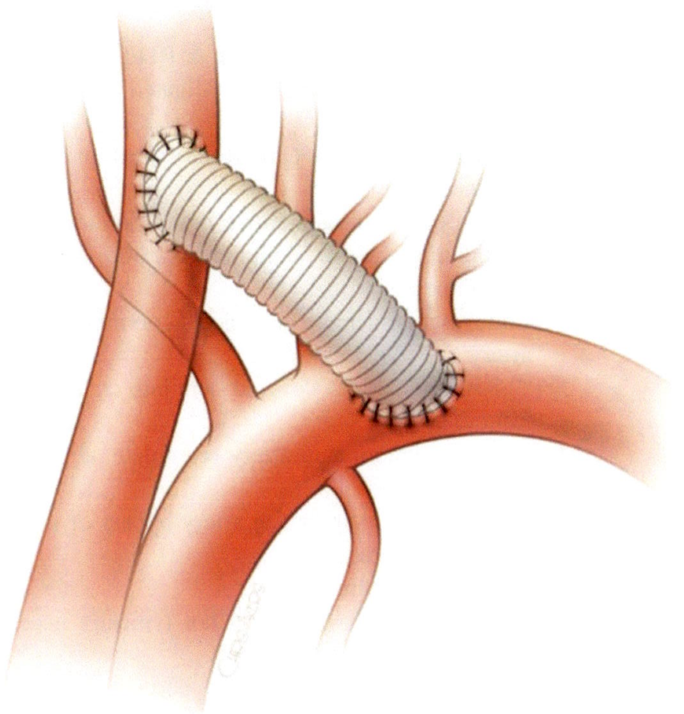

Fig. 15.5 Carotid subclavian bypass. (Taken from Rutherford's Vascular Surgery and Endovascular Therapy 10th Ed. Ch. 101)

- Endovascular debranching with chimney techniques
  Open aortic debranching
- Coverage of left carotid artery (partial arch debranching)
  - Extra-anatomic carotid-carotid bypass
    - Bilateral common carotid exposures through oblique neck incisions anterior to the sternocleidomastoid muscle
    - Retropharyngeal or subcutaneous tunnel with gentle downward curve

        Tunnel behind the manubrium with subcutaneous tunnel
    - Ringed 6- or 8-mm Dacron or PTFE graft
    - Left common carotid artery ligated proximal to the anastomosis
    - Avoid bilateral recurrent laryngeal or vagus nerve injury
    - Don't need intraoperative brain monitoring or shunting when common carotid arteries clamped
  - Endovascular debranching of left common carotid artery
    Retrograde CCA covered stent into arch (chimney)
- Coverage of innominate artery (complete arch debranching)
  - Left carotid to subclavian artery bypass or transposition done first
  - Median sternotomy
  - Cardiopulmonary bypass is not typically necessary
  - Side biting clamp on ascending aorta
  - Bifurcated Dacron graft or larger tube graft (8–12 mm) with side arm (6–8 mm) anastomosed to right innominate and left common carotid arteries end-to-end
  - 10 mm Dacron graft onto the hood of the ascending aortic graft can serve as conduit for antegrade deployment of stent graft; stent may not be long enough to reach ascending aorta from the groin
- Frozen elephant trunk
  - Aneurysm involves ascending aorta; no proximal landing zone for stent graft
  - Hypothermic cardiac arrest required "frozen"
  - Ascending aorta replaced with Dacron graft

  - Bypass taken off this graft to innominate and left carotid arteries
  - Arch opened
  - Modified Dacron graft with stent attached distally constrained in sheath and deployed into a distal landing zone in the descending thoracic aorta
  - Proximal end of modified graft sewn to ascending aortic graft

Coverage of celiac artery

- Intentional celiac coverage safe in presence of prominent SMA-celiac collaterals via gastroduodenal and pancreaticoduodenal arcades
- Preoperative angiography through SMA with temporary balloon occlusion of celiac artery
- Favorable angiographic features
  - Prominent gastroduodenal artery arcade
  - Replaced right hepatic artery
  - Preexisting celiac stenosis
  - Well-developed SMA
- If cannot sacrifice celiac artery
  - Parallel graft (downward periscope graft in celiac artery, snorkel, chimney, sandwich)
  - Custom-made stent graft with distal scallop or fenestration/branch
  - Open celiac debranching prior to TEVAR (end-to-end celiac artery anastomosis, end to side hepatic artery bypass)

Appropriately sized arterial access to deliver stent-graft

- Femoral artery should be $\geq$7 mm; thoracic stent device delivery systems large (22–24F)
- Iliac conduit may be required in 15%
  - 10 mm Dacron graft anastomosed end to side to common or external iliac artery through retroperitoneal incision in lower quadrant

This conduit can be accessed through same incision or be brought out through incision in lower abdomen or groin

Insert sheath through graft wall rather than open end more stable

At end of procedure, conduit can be ligated or converted to iliofemoral bypass

- Internal endoconduit: "crack and pave"

  10 or 13 mm covered self-expandable stent deployed across diseased iliac segment and aggressively inflated; controlled vessel rupture

  Usually loss of patency of internal iliac artery

  Allows for 22–24 F sheath placement

- Direct aortic access

Increased risk for spinal cord ischemia with longer aortic coverage

- Other endovascular options

  Debranching

  - Open surgical bypass to an aortic branch artery from a location proximal or distal to the intended placement of aortic endograft

  Scallop

  - U-shaped openings cut out at ends of endograft which allows filling of aortic branch
  - Vary in width and depth

  Parallel-stent grafting

  - Snorkel
  - Chimney: antegrade flow into branch
  - Periscope: retrograde flow into branch
  - Sandwich graft

  Fenestrations

  - Presence of opening in endograft fabric allows perfusion of aortic branch vessel
  - Circular or elliptical holes reinforced with nitinol ring
    Vary in diameter in both major and minor axis

      - Balloon-expandable stent-grafts placed through fenestration into target vessel; aortic end is flared with larger balloon

    Branches

      - Most often directed in caudal direction, but occasionally directed cranially
      - Branches may reside within (internal), exterior (external), or both (internal-external) to the aortic graft
      - Self-expandable stent-grafts required to bridge the branch to target artery
        - Self-expandable stent graft used to better accommodate long distances, tortuosity

- Commercially available devices

    Gore conformable thoracic aortic graft device

      - C-TAG device: ePTFE reinforced with nitinol self-expanding stent
      - Short open bare metal stents on proximal aspect
      - Deploys from middle of graft outward; prevents windsock effect

    Medtronic Valiant Captivia Device

      - Woven polyester graft attached to sinusoidal nitinol springs
      - Bare metal proximal FreeFlo configuration

    Cook Zenith Alpha

      - Woven polyester with external nitinol stents
      - Active fixation

    Bolton Relay

      - Woven polyester sewn to self-expanding nitinol stents
      - Transport delivery system consists of outer sheath and flexible secondary sheath
      - Active fixation with bare stents

- Investigational devices for TAAA

    Seal lengths 2–4 cm sought; proximal landing zone in healthy segment of thoracic aorta

    May need brachial or axillary access to cannulate visceral arteries

- When multiple sheaths required, 10- to 12-mm axillary conduit can be used

Physician modified endografts (PMEGs)

- Physician deploys standard endograft on back table and creates modifications by hand to accommodate branch vessels specific to patient's anatomy
- Modified graft re-sheathed for insertion and deployment in patient

Off-the-shelf designs

- p-Branch device (Cook): incorporates fenestrations for the SMA and bilateral renal arteries and scallop for the celiac artery
  - Renal fenestrations created within a pocket of redundant fabric which can "pivot" and thereby allow selection of renal artery and extension with stent-graft into renal artery
  - t-Branch device (Cook): 4 downward facing external cuffs
  - Thoracoabdominal Multibranch Endoprosthesis—TAMBE (Gore): 2 downgoing internal branches for celiac artery and SMA, 2 internal renal branches (antegrade or retrograde)

Investigational devices for aortic arch

- Designed for deployment in zones 0, 1, 2
- Avoidance of hypothermic circulatory arrest
- Partial or complete debranching of aortic arch
- Unique challenges
  - Greater vessel flow and pulsation
  - Tortuosity and angulation of arch
  - Proximity of aortic valve and coronary arteries
- Pre-cannulated side branches to facilitate device alignment and flexible bridging stents
- TEVAR endograft with single side-branch can be used to revascularize left subclavian artery without need for carotid-subclavian bypass or transposition

TEVAR for blunt traumatic aortic injury

    - TEVAR has become primary modality for repair of blunt traumatic aortic injury to descending thoracic aorta
- Operative technique
    - GETA to allow respiratory control and more precise imaging
    - Femoral artery accessed open or percutaneously
    - Aortogram in left anterior oblique projection
    - For celiac artery visualization, lateral projection ideal
    - Steady antegrade pressure on wire to keep device positioned against outer aortic curvature
    - Device tracking difficulties
        - Buddy wire
        - Long sheath
        - Distal graft deployment first
        - Brachial-femoral through-and-through guidewire (body floss); can use right brachial artery for improved tracking through arch
        - Temporary reduction of MAP decreases windsock effect; some used adenosine-induced cardiac asystole or rapid cardiac pacing
    - Avoid aggressive proximal ballooning to avoid retrograde type A aortic dissection
    - Care should be exercise during sheath removal to avoid iatrogenic iliac injury (iliac on a stick); maintain stiff wire access so if iliac rupture occurs, can repair with covered stent graft
- Hybrid endovascular repair for TAAA
    - Relocate visceral aortic branches with an open bypass procedure from distal inflow sites (CIA, infrarenal aorta; retrograde debranching bypass graft) followed by exclusion of TAAA with TEVAR
        - Avoids thoracotomy
        - Avoids division of diaphragm and aortic clamping
        - Reduces visceral ischemia time

- Trifurcated Dacron or standard bifurcated Dacron grafts used with 6- or 7-mm limbs sewn
  - 2 limbs used to bypass the right and left renal arteries with end-to-end distal anastomosis
  - Left renal artery exposed by mobilizing left renal vein; ligate inferior mesenteric, gonadal, adrenal veins
  - Right renal artery identified posterior to vena cava
  - 3rd limb used for the SMA end to side

    Mesocolon elevated

    Middle colic artery identified and followed proximally to SMA
  - Jump graft taken off SMA graft to celiac artery through transverse mesocolon and tunneled anterior to the pancreas (right iliac artery donor) or posterior to pancreas (left iliac artery donor)
  - Celiac artery exposed by entering lesser sac through gastro-hepatic ligament

    Dense celiac plexus divided

    Graft anastomosis end to side to hepatic or splenic artery; retrogastric route
- Visceral grafts routed in "lazy C" fashion
- Proximal end of recipient vessels ligated to prevent type II endoleak
- Grafts covered with omental flap to minimize graft-enteric erosion

– Neuroprotection

  Increased risk with long-segment aortic coverage and antecedent or concomitant abdominal aortic graft

  CSF drainage

  - Use selectively in patients at increased risk for spinal cord ischemia
  - Maintained for 48–72 h while CSF pressure $\leq$10 cm H_2O
  - Use third-generation cephalosporin; better CSF penetrance

        - Needs ICU admission
        - Hemorrhagic complications associated with catheter placement (intracranial hemorrhage with rapid drainage, epidural hematoma)
        - Postdural puncture headache; treat with bed rest, hydration, caffeine
        - Most common complication: CSF leak with spinal headache; treat with hydration and blood patch
        - Meningitis risk if prolonged catheter insertion

      Maintain MAP >90 mmHg to increase spinal cord collateral flow

      Ischemic preconditioning by staged repair

      Selective segmental artery coil embolization (MISACE)

        - Enhance collateralization before TEVAR

      Perfusion branch: creation of side branch intentionally left open to the aneurysm sac, creating a large endoleak that is used to perfuse critical intercostal vessels

        - Side branch is then closed using embolization at later time

- Stent-grafting in patients with connective tissue disorders not recommended
  - Unknown impact of persistent radial forces of stent graft in abnormal and weak aorta
  - Use as bail-out procedure or bridge to definitive open repair
  - Higher risk of retrograde aortic dissection
- Delayed paralysis after TAAA surgery
  - COPS protocol
  - CSF drainage

    Keep in place for 7 days

    Patient flat

    15 cc CSF drained each hour
  - Oxygen delivery

    Supplemental oxygen

    Treat anemia (keep Hb >12)

    Cardiac index >2.5 L/min

  - Patient status
    - MAP >90 mmHg
    - Increase spinal cord perfusion pressure
  - Undertake these maneuvers immediately
- Endoleak
  - Type I: inadequate apposition, degeneration of landing zone; treat with balloon inflation or additional stent graft
  - Type II: intercostal arteries, surveillance
  - Type III: inadequate overlap, interposition stent graft
- CTA surveillance at 1 month, then at 6 months, then yearly
  - Include delayed imaging to detect subtle endoleaks
- Aortic dissection
  - Introduction
    - Acute aortic dissection is most common catastrophic event affecting aorta
    - In chronic phase, aneurysmal degeneration and rupture of outer wall of false lumen
    - Death due to acute dissection of ascending thoracic aorta usually due to aortic rupture into pericardium (tamponade), acute aortic regurgitation, coronary ostia compromise
    - Death due to acute dissection of descending thoracic aorta due to end organ compromise due to acute obstruction of visceral or extremity arteries
    - Treatment is primary blood pressure control
  - Acute aortic syndromes
    - Aortic dissection
    - Intramural hematoma
      - Clotted blood in intramural space without obvious intimal tear
      - Regarded as precursor to dissection
    - Penetrating aortic ulcers
      - Focal ulceration of atherosclerotic plaque into media
      - May be associated with hematoma within aortic wall

- Classification

  Aortic dissections classified according to anatomic location of entry tear and the time between onset of symptoms and patient presentation [5–8]

  Acute: within first 2 weeks
  - 74% of patients who die from aortic dissections do so in the first 14 days

  Subacute: 2 weeks to 90 days
  - Dissection flap remains pliable
  - Best time to consider performing elective TEVAR coverage of proximal entry tear

  Chronic: after 90 days
  - Flap becomes stiff and fibrotic
  - Harder to remodel aorta

  Anatomic
  - Based on location of intimal tear and extent of aorta involved in dissection
  - Origin of entry tear is key predictor of early outcomes
  - Debakey classification (see Fig. 15.6)
    - Delineates both the origin of entry tear and extent of descending aortic dissection
    - Type I: dissection originates in ascending aorta, extends through aortic arch, and continues into descending aorta and/or abdominal aorta for varying distance
    - Type II: Dissection originates in and is confined to ascending aorta
    - Type IIIa: Dissection originates in descending aorta and is limited to descending
    - Type IIIb: Dissection involves descending and variable extent of abdominal aorta
  - Stanford classification for aortic dissection (see Fig. 15.6)
    - Most widely used

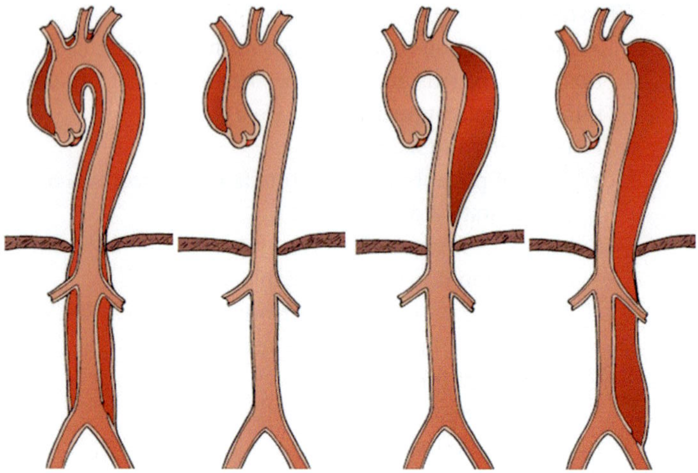

Fig. 15.6 Classification of aortic dissections. (Taken from Rutherford's Vascular Surgery and Endovascular Therapy 10th Ed. Ch. 83)

- Delineates according to origin of entry tear alone
- A: dissection originates in ascending aorta and arch; Debakey I and II; immediate surgery
- B: dissection originates in the descending thoracic aorta at or near ligamentum arteriosum and left subclavian artery; Debakey type IIIa, IIIb; medical management

Severity

- Complicated
  - Impending or frank rupture
  - Malperfusion
  - Persistent pain
  - Refractory hypertension
- Uncomplicated

- Epidemiology

  Men more frequently affected

  Type A peaks between 50 and 60 years

  Type B peaks between 60 and 70 years
  50% of patients with aortic dissection die before hospital admission
  Location of entry tear [9]
  - Ascending aorta 65%
  - Arch 10%
  - Descending aorta 20%
  - Abdominal aorta 5%

  Mortality associated with acute type A aortic dissection [10]
  - 30% first 24 h
  - 50% by 48 h
  - 90% at 1 year

  Early mortality for patients with acute uncomplicated type B aortic dissection: 10–12%
  Mortality of patients with acute complicated type B dissection: 25–50%
- Risk factors
  Hypertension
  Aortic wall structural abnormalities
  - Bicuspid aortic valve associated with ascending aortic dissections
  - Coarctation of the aorta
  - Chromosomal abnormalities: Turner, Noonan syndromes
    Marfan syndrome
    - Accounts for 50% cases of acute aortic dissection in patients <40 years
  - Ehlers-Danlos syndrome

  Pregnancy
  - Preeclampsia with hypertension
  - Pregnant women with Marfan syndrome at high risk
    - Presence of dilated aortic root (>4 cm) is best predictor of dissection in pregnant patient with Marfan syndrome

    - Most common site of dissection is the ascending aorta involving the sinuses of Valsalva or sinotubular junction (type A dissections in older patients more likely to originate higher in ascending aorta)

  Drug abuse: Cocaine and methamphetamines

- Pathogenesis

  Intimal tear followed by blood surging either antegrade or retrograde

  2 new channels referred to as true and false lumens (double-barreled aorta)

  Fenestrations between the 2 channels connect true and false lumens and usually occur at origin of branch vessels

  Compression of true lumen can result in malperfusion of the viscera or the limbs or rupture of false lumen

  In the descending aorta, the intimal tear typically originates within a few centimeters of the left SCA

    - Usually distal false lumen on the left posterolateral aspect of aorta
    - Celiac, SMA, right renal arteries typically emanate from true lumen
    - Left renal artery arises from false lumen

  Malperfusion occurs secondary to aortic branch compromise (see Fig. 15.7)

    - Dynamic obstruction: septum may intermittently prolapse into vessel ostium during cardiac cycle and the compressed true lumen flow is inadequate to perfuse branch vessel ostia which remains anatomically intact
      - Most common mechanism of branch compromise
    - Static obstruction: dissecting process extends into branch vessel; thrombosis beyond compromised ostia may further worsen perfusion
      - Usually requires stent graft into branch

- Clinical presentation

  Great masquerader

  Sudden tearing or stabbing pain in back, abdomen, chest

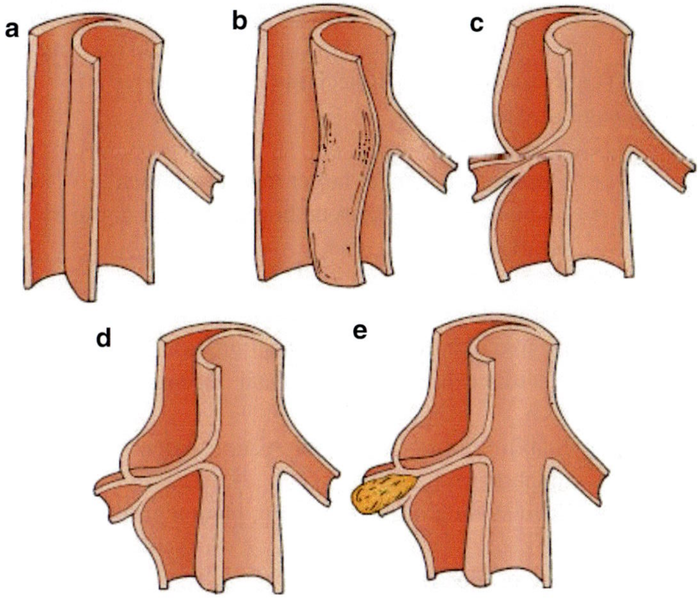

Fig. 15.7 Mechanism of aortic branches obstruction in acute aortic dissections. (Taken from Rutherford's Vascular Surgery and Endovascular Therapy 10th Ed. Ch. 83)

- Anterior in type A dissections
- Posterior in type B dissections; may be migratory

If abdominal pain, need to rule out mesenteric vascular compromise

Hypertension

Hypotension may be result of aortic valve disruption or cardiac tamponade

Spinal cord ischemia: interruption of intercostal vessels

Direct compression of nerves

- Hoarseness (recurrent laryngeal nerve)
- Horner syndrome (compression of sympathetic ganglion)

  Pulse deficit with or without extremity ischemia in a patient with severe chest or back pain should raise suspicion of acute aortic dissection

- Diagnostic evaluation

  CTA

  - False lumen usually larger than true lumen
  - Inability to assess ascending aorta and aortic valve clearly

  TEE

  - Delineate dissection flap in ascending aorta
  - Degree of aortic valvular regurgitation
  - Anatomic blind spot in distal ascending aorta and arch
  - Inability to document dissection extension beyond diaphragm

  CXR: widening of mediastinum, pleural effusions (type B)

- Treatment of type B dissection

  Prompt control of blood pressure in the ICU

  - Beta-blocker (esmolol) and vasodilator (nipride); beta-blocker first, then vasodilator
  - Aim for SBP 100–120 mmHg or MAP 60–70 and pulse 60–80

  If patient has hypotension, rule out tamponade

  Early recognition of malperfusion syndromes

  Treatment of malperfusion

  - Stent graft coverage of proximal entry tear to expand true lumen and restore flow to visceral arteries
    - If residual static branch vessel occlusion, secondary stent placement
    - PETTICOAT (Provisional Extension to Induce Complete Attachment) technique: composite TEVAR plus uncovered infra-diaphragmatic aortic stent; Zenith dissection endovascular stent [11]
  - Percutaneous fenestration (see Fig. 15.8)

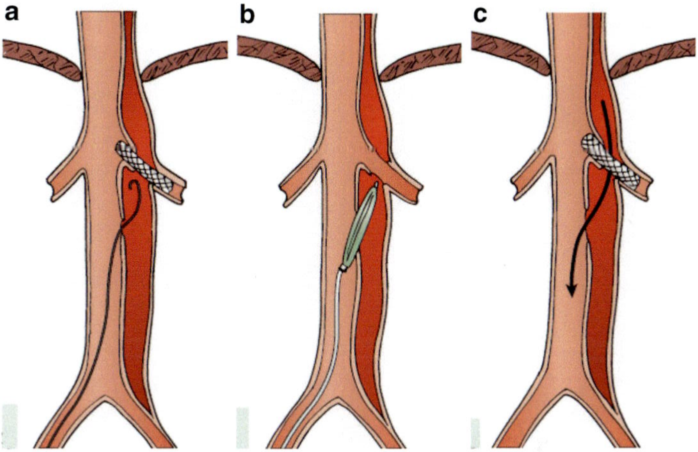

Fig. 15.8 Endovascular fenestration. (Taken from Rutherford's Vascular Surgery and Endovascular Therapy 10th Ed. Ch. 83)

  - Percutaneous catheterization of true and false lumens
  - Fenestration identified and selected with the aid of IVUS
  - If no natural fenestration identified, needle can be used to create fenestration close to compromised branch
  - Stiff wire advanced from true to false lumen
  - Angioplasty balloon (12–15 mm diameter × 2–4 cm length) used to create fenestration tear
  - Stent can be placed across fenestration
- Open surgical treatment (see Fig. 15.9)
  - Thoracoabdominal exposure through left 8th or 9th intercostal space
  - Supra-celiac clamping
  - Wide resection of dissected septum
  - May need to extend septectomy into visceral segment

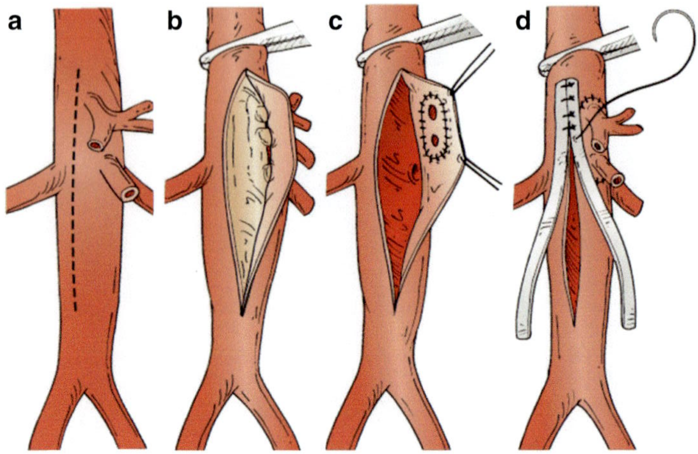

Fig. 15.9 Technique of surgical abdominal aortic fenestration. (Taken from Rutherford's Vascular Surgery and Endovascular Therapy 10th Ed. Ch. 83)

  - May need circumferential suture of vessel intima to aortic wall at ostia
  - Clamp moved to infrarenal aorta
  - Tube graft reconstruction of infrarenal aorta; Teflon strips to enhance anastomotic integrity
- Stent graft of uncomplicated type B dissection

  Stent-graft coverage of aortic entry tear in subacute phase helps to induce false lumen thrombosis and potentially reduce risk of late aneurysm degeneration (aortic remodeling)

  Factors associated with chronic aneurysm development after dissection

  - Poorly controlled hypertension
  - Maximal aortic diameter ≥4 cm in the acute phase
  - False lumen diameter over 22 mm
  - Continued patency of false lumen
  - Proximal entry tear ≥10 mm
  - Entry tear located on lesser curve

- Partially thrombosed false lumen where outflow fenestrations have thrombosed but proximal flow persists
- Elliptical true lumen combined with saccular false lumen

ADSORB trial [12]

- Prospective randomized trial
- Compared stent grafting to medical therapy for uncomplicated acute (<14 days) type B aortic dissection
- 61 patients randomized
- Incomplete false lumen thrombosis in 43% stent graft group vs. 97% of the medical group at 1 year
- True lumen increased in stent graft group; unchanged in the medical group

INSTEAD trial [13]

- Prospective randomized multicenter trial
- Compared stent grafting to medical therapy for treatment of subacute and chronic uncomplicated type B aortic dissection (>14 days)
- 140 patients randomized
- No difference in survival between 2 cohorts at 2 years
- 5-year survival superior in TEVAR cohort
- Following TEVAR, 90% of patients demonstrated aortic remodeling with complete false lumen thrombosis in thoracic aorta compared with 22% in optimal medial therapy group

Technique

- True lumen access from brachial or femoral approach and confirmed with IVUS
- Seal zone should be in at least 2 cm of normal aorta proximal to the entry tear
- IVUS used to assess true lumen expansion and flap mobility
- Don't balloon proximal seal zone in acute dissections so as to prevent retrograde dissection and rupture

Surveillance

- Patients will need CTA at 1 month, 6 months and 1 year in the first year, yearly after that

Question

1. TEVAR is not acceptable treatment for which of the following presentation:
   (a) Type B dissection not controlled pain despite anti-hypertensive
   (b) Connective tissue disorder
   (c) Descending thoracic aortic aneurysm
   (d) Thoracoabdominal aneurysm
2. What type of Ehler-Danlos syndrome is associated with vascular disease?
   (a) Type 1
   (b) Type 2
   (c) Type 3
   (d) Type 4
3. Which phase is aortic dissection recommended?
   (a) Hyperacute phase
   (b) Acute phase
   (c) Subacute phase
   (d) Chronic phase

Answer: 1 (b), 2 (d), 3 (c)

References

1. National Center for Injury Prevention and Control. WISQARS Leading causes of Death Report.; 2014.
2. Clouse WD, Hallett JW Jr, Schaff HV, et al. Improved prognosis of thoracic aortic aneurysms: a population-based study. JAMA. 1998;280:1926–9.
3. Abraha I, Romagnoli C, Montedori A, et al. Thoracic stent graft versus surgery for thoracic aneurysm (review). Cochrane Database Syst Rev. 2016.

4. Matsumura JS, Rizvi AZ. Left subclavian artery revascularization: Society for Vascular Surgery Practice Guidelines. J Vasc Surg. 2010;52(Suppl):65–9.
5. Estrera AL, Miller CC III, Safi HJ, et al. Outcomes of medical management of acute type B aortic dissection. Circulation. 2006;114(1 Suppl):I384–9.
6. Nienaber CA, Eagle KA. Aortic dissection: new frontiers in diagnosis and management: part I: from etiology to diagnostic strategies. Circulation. 2003;108(5):628–35.
7. Trimarchi S, Nienaber C, Rampoldi V, et al. Role and results of surgery in acute type B aortic dissection: insights from the International Registry of Acute Aortic Dissection (IRAD). Circulation. 2006;114(1 Suppl):I357–67.
8. Lombardi JV, Cambria RP, Nienaber CA, et al. Prospective multicenter clinical trial (STABLE) on the endovascular treatment of complicated type B aortic dissection using a composite device design. J Vasc Surg. 2012;55(3):629–40.
9. Hirst AE Jr, Johns VJ Jr, Kime SW Jr, et al. Dissecting aneurysm of the aorta: a review of 505 cases. Medicine (Baltimore). 1958;37(3):217–79.
10. Hagan PG, Nienaber CA, Isselbacher EM, et al. The International Registry of Acute Aortic Dissection (IRAD): new insights into an old disease. JAMA. 2000;283(7):897–903.
11. Lombardi JV, Cambria RP, Nienbaber CA, et al. Aortic remodeling after endovascular treatment of complicated type B aortic dissection with the use of a composite device design. J Vasc Surg. 2014;59:1544–54.
12. Brunwall J, Kasprzak P, Verhoeven E, et al. Endovascular repair of acute uncomplicated aortic type B dissection promotes aortic remodelling: 1 year results of the ADSORB trial. Eur J Vasc Endovasc Surg. 2014;48(3):285–91.
13. Nienaber CA, Kische S, Rousseau H, et al. Endovascular repair of type B aortic dissection: long-term results of the randomized investigation of stent grafts in aortic dissection trial. Circ Cardiovasc Interv. 2013;6(4):407–17.

16 Venous Disease

Morvarid Tavassoli, Shauna Trinh,
Cameron Hand, and Christian Bianchi

Anatomy (Fig. 16.1)

Lower Extremity

Superficial system
- Above muscular fascia, drains subcutaneous tissue [1, 2].
- Primary vein: great saphenous vein (GSV), isolated by saphenous fascia within saphenous compartment [1, 2].
- Tributaries connect via communicating veins [1, 2].

M. Tavassoli (✉) · S. Trinh
Department of General Surgery, Riverside University Health System, Moreno Valley, CA, USA
e-mail: m.tavassoli@ruhealth.org

C. Hand
Department of Family Medicine, Pomona Valley Hospital Medical Center, Pomona, CA, USA
e-mail: cameron.hand@pvhmc.org

C. Bianchi
Department of Vascular Surgery, Loma Linda University Medical Center, Loma Linda Veteran Affairs Medical Center, Riverside University Health System, Loma Linda, CA, USA
e-mail: Cbianchi@llu.edu

A. Murga et al. (eds.), *The Vascular Surgery In-Training Examination Review (VSITE)*,
https://doi.org/10.1007/978-3-031-24121-5_16

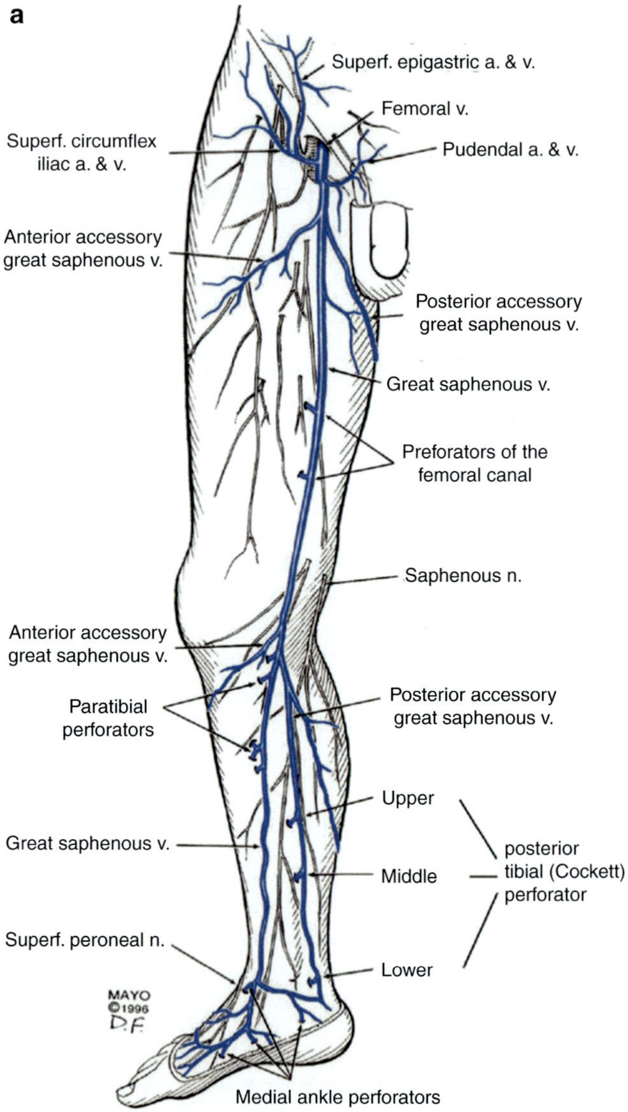

Fig. 16.1 Venous anatomy of lower extremity deep system (**a**), superficial and perforator systems (**b**). (From Meissner M, Moneta G, Burnand K, Gloviczki P, Lohr J, Lurie F et al. The hemodynamics and diagnosis of venous disease. J Vasc Surg. 2007;46(6):S4-S24. With permission from Elsevier)

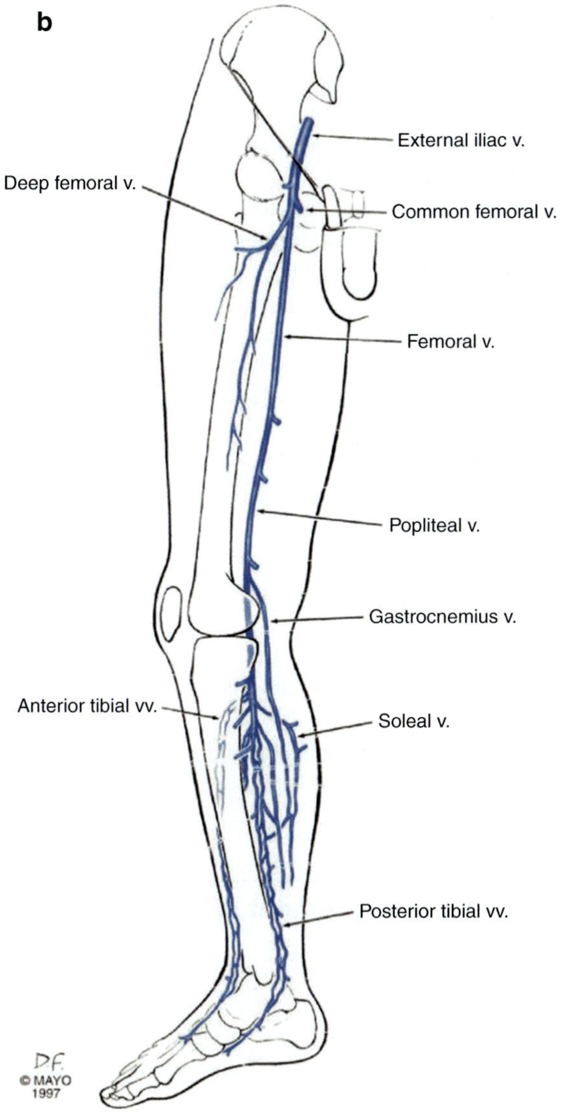

Fig. 16.1 (continued)

Deep system

- Underneath muscular fascia, drains deeper tissues and muscles [1, 2].
- Primary vein: femoral vein.
- Veins are paired below the calf. Popliteal or femoral veins occasionally paired [1, 2].
- Superficial system drains into deep system at confluence of the superficial inguinal veins (formerly saphenofemoral junction) in medial thigh [1, 2].

Perforator system

- Pierce fascia and connect deep and superficial systems either directly via deep axial veins or indirectly via muscle tributaries at 6 cm intervals [1, 2].
- Bicuspid valves prevent backflow and ensure unidirectional circulation from superficial to deep system [1, 2].

Upper Extremity

- Contains fewer valves [3].
- Superficial system primary veins: cephalic, basilic, and median antibrachial [3].
- Deep system primary veins: brachial and axillary veins [3].
- Confluence of brachial and basilic veins forms the origin of the axillary vein [3].

Diagnosis and Management of Venous Disease

Clinical Tests of Function

- Physical exam: skin changes, edema, varicosities. Cough impulse, Brodie-Trendelenburg, and Perthes tests check for reflux [4].
- Ankle-brachial index to evaluate for concomitant arterial disease, especially in presence of ulcers. If significant disease

presents, compression therapy may be contraindicated [4].

- Doppler scan, 97% sensitive, 73% specific for reflux [1, 4].
- Duplex ultrasound (US) is the gold standard for checking reflux and patency in all 3 venous systems—noninvasive, inexpensive, and reproducible. Reflux >1 s in deep system or > 0.5 s in superficial/perforator system is diagnostic of chronic venous insufficiency.
- Magnetic resonance venography or computed tomography provides cross-sectional imaging and better delineates the deep system. Adjunct studies for unequivocal US findings [1, 4].
- Air plethysmography: cuffs inflated around an extremity, then blood volume displaced is measured at rest and after exercise. Calf volume changes are used to calculate venous filling index. This is an indirect measurement of reflux, patency, and calf muscle pump dysfunction. Limitations: cannot visualize or localize reflux [1, 4].
- Photoplethysmography: intensity of LED reflection over the medial ankle at rest and with activity used as indirect measurement of RBC count to extrapolate venous refill and reflux [1, 4].

Invasive Tests

- Ascending or descending direct contrast venography: best for hemodynamic function and localization of individual dysfunctional valves. Limitations: invasive, risk of contrast reaction, technical limitations. Less frequently used modality since US [1, 4].
- Ambulatory venous pressure measures pressure and filling period at rest and with activity via needle pressure transducer. Consistently high pressure > 30 mmHg and rapid refill <20 s during activity indicate retrograde reflux [1, 4].

Chronic Venous Insufficiency (CVI)

- Caused by valvular incompetence, venous obstruction, or calf muscle pump dysfunction [1, 5].

- Valve insufficiency can affect all venous systems and may be primarily from weakened valves or secondary due to an injury, i.e. trauma, DVT [1, 5].
- Reflux results in subsequent venous hypertension, flow stasis, and venous expansion [1, 5].
- Immune response [1, 5].
  - Endothelial cells activate leukocytes, macromolecule, and iron extravasation. Increased TGF-b and PDGF production.
  - Chronic inflammation leads to altered collagen and increased matrix metalloproteinases accumulation.
- Risk factors: age, female, prolonged standing or sitting, obesity, smoking, prior lower extremity trauma, hormonal changes, hereditary conditions, venous thrombosis, non-thrombotic venous obstruction (May-Thurner syndrome), arteriovenous shunt, or malformation [1, 5].
- Clinical presentation: pain, itching/burning, swelling, restless leg syndrome, skin discoloration, skin thickening and inflammation, ulceration, varicosities [6] See Table 16.1.
- Ulceration commonly along medial malleolus [5].
- Confirm retrograde reflux on diagnostic testing [1, 5].
- Conservative management: first step in management which includes compression therapy, leg elevation, Unna boots [1, 5].
- Surgery for complicated CVI or cases refractory to medical treatment. Must rule out DVT prior to surgery [1, 5].
- Surgical approach: sclerotherapy, endovenous ablation, ligation, and stripping for superficial and perforator systems [1, 5] (Table 16.1)

Superficial Thrombophlebitis (ST)

- Risk factors: venous stasis from chronic venous insufficiency; endothelial damage from cannulation, vein stripping, or other venous trauma; age > 60, pregnancy, elevated estrogen level, tobacco or IV drug use, vasculitis, hypercoagulable disease [7, 8].
- May be sterile or infected, commonly affects large vessels such as GSV or cephalic vein [7].

Table 16.1 CEAP classification table. Gold standard for scoring disease severity in chronic venous insufficiency using four parameters: clinical (C), etiologic (E), anatomic (A), and pathophysiologic (P) determinants [6]

Clinical classification	Etiologic classification	Anatomic classification	Pathophysiologic classification
C_0: No visible or palpable signs of venous disease	Ec: Congenital	As: Superficial veins	Pr: reflux
C_1: Telangiectasias or reticular veins	Ep: Primary	Ap: Perforator veins	Po: Obstruction
C_2: Varicose veins	Es: Secondary (postthrombotic)	Ad: Deep veins	Pr,o: Reflux and obstruction
C_3: Edema	En: No venous cause identified	An: No venous location identified	Pn: No venous pathophysiology identified
C_{4a}: Pigmentation or eczema			
C_{4b}: Lipodermatosclerosis or atrophie blanche			
C_5: Healed venous ulcer			
C_6: Active venous ulcer			
S: Symptomatic including ache, pain, tightness, skin irritation, heaviness, muscle cramps			

- Symptoms: pain, skin erythema and edema, palpable cord [7, 8].
- Migratory thrombophlebitis marker for underlying malignancy (Trousseau syndrome) [7, 8].
- Mondor disease is ST of the breast [7, 8].
- Damaged endothelium promotes platelet activation via thrombin and thromboxane a2, clot formation in early inflammatory phase. Late phase endothelial fibrotic changes [7, 8].

- GSV thrombophlebitis can progress to femoral vein leading to DVT (20%) or PE (4%) [7–9].
- Treatment is based on location and clinical severity. Conservative management with NSAIDs, warm compress, elevation of the affected extremity, gradient compression stocking [7–9].
- Expansive thrombus >5 cm in size or < 3 cm from confluence of the superficial inguinal veins should receive 6 wks of prophylactic anticoagulation (fondaparinux or LMWH) [7–9].
- If significant varicosities present, consider phlebectomy as adjunct to above therapies [7–9].

Deep Venous Thromboembolic (DVT) Disease

- Symptoms: calf pain and swelling.
- Increased risk with Virchow's triad (venous stasis, hypercoagulability, endothelial injury).
  - Risk factors: advanced age, immobilization, travel, history of venous thromboembolism, malignancy, surgery, trauma, pregnancy, oral contraceptives, and hormonal therapy [1].
- Diagnosis: duplex ultrasonography.
- Treatment: if no contraindications, start anticoagulation immediately for a minimum of 3–6 months.
  - Heparin bridged to vitamin K antagonist (warfarin).
  - Direct-acting oral anticoagulants (DOACs).

Post-thrombotic Syndrome (PTS)

- Caused by ambulatory venous hypertension (elevated venous pressure during exercise) secondary to venous valvular incompetence (reflux) and/or luminal obstruction.
- Swelling, pigmentation, lipodermatosclerosis followed by dermal breakdown.
- Ileofemoral DVT (IFDVT) causes the most severe PTS with decreased quality of life.

  - If treated by anticoagulation alone, 40% will develop venous claudication and up to 15% will develop venous ulceration within 5 years [1].
  - If treated by thrombolysis, improved quality of life. The greater the degree of lysis, the fewer symptoms of PTS observed. [1].

Vena Cava Interruption

- Inferior vena cava (IVC) filters are effective in preventing the complication of PE but not in preventing DVT recurrence.
- Recommend IVC filter placement for documented venous thromboembolism (VTE) with a contraindication to anticoagulation, complication of anticoagulation, or recurrent VTE despite therapeutic anticoagulation [1].
  - Contraindications to or complication of anticoagulation includes the need for major surgery, intracranial hemorrhage, pelvic or retroperitoneal hematoma, ocular injury, solid intraabdominal organ injury, uncorrected major coagulopathy, coagulation disorder, peptic ulcer disease [1].
- Permanent versus retrievable filter.
  - With retrievable filters, must create a removal plan when it is no longer indicated such as when the patient can be started on anticoagulation.
- Possible complications of IVC filter placement: DVT at the insertion site, IVC thrombosis, recurrent PE, and filter erosion, fracture, or migration.

Surgical and Interventional Treatment with Venous Thrombolysis and Thrombectomy

- Usually reserved for patients with phlegmasia cerulea dolens (painful, swollen blue leg, possible gangrene), massive iliofemoral DVT, or those who fail therapeutic anticoagulation.

- Thrombolytic drugs activate plasminogen to form plasmin, which dissolves thrombi.
- Candidates for thrombolysis should have symptoms for <14 days (new clot), good functional status, and low bleeding risk.
- Systematic thrombolysis versus catheter-directed thrombolysis (CDT).
  - CDT has a decreased risk of bleeding as it can dissolve clots faster and with lower doses compared to systematic thrombolysis.

Options for Thrombectomy

- Endovascular mechanical thrombectomy uses catheter extraction or fragmentation [1].
- Pharmacomechanical thrombolysis combines catheter directed thrombolysis with mechanical extraction/fragmentation and reduces the risk of bleeding [1].
- Operative thrombectomy:
  - Longitudinal venotomies of the common femoral vein (CFV) and distal posterior tibial vein with passage of a balloon catheter [1].
  - Once the CFV venotomy is closed, an end-to-side arteriovenous fistula (AVF) is constructed by anastomosing the amputated end of the proximal saphenous vein to the side of the superficial femoral artery [1].
  - The purpose of the AVF is to increase venous velocity but not venous pressure [1].

Iliocaval Venous Obstruction (ICVO)

- Pathophysiology:
  - Vein wall injury with neointimal hyperplasia leading to venous stenosis and possible thrombus formation.
  - Endoluminal obstruction from a foreign device (i.e. IVC filter) or thrombus.

- May result in venous hypertension, venous insufficiency, and lower extremity DVT.

May-Thurner Syndrome (Also Referred to as Iliac Vein Compression Syndrome)

- Extrinsic venous compression by the arterial system against bony structures in the iliocaval venous territory, most commonly of the left common iliac vein between the right common iliac artery and the fifth lumbar vertebrae [1].
- Risk factors: female, postpartum, multiparous, oral contraceptives, individuals with spinal abnormalities, prior aortoiliac vascular stent placement.
- Most are asymptomatic, but symptoms include acute extremity pain and swelling, venous claudication, chronic development of venous insufficiency.
- Diagnosis: clinical exam, duplex ultrasonography, CT/MR venography.
  - Intravascular US for definitive diagnosis as it shows the morphology of the intraluminal thickening and degree of stenosis [1].
- Treatment:
  - No or mild symptoms without DVT: conservative management with compression stockings as needed [1].
  - Moderate-to-severe symptoms without DVT: percutaneous angioplasty and stenting of the affected segment followed by compression stockings and antiplatelet therapy [1].
  - Suspected MTS with DVT: anticoagulation and catheter-directed or pharmacomechanical thrombolysis. If stenosis present, consider angioplasty and stenting [1].
- Open surgical treatment such as open venous angioplasty or venous bypass has worse outcomes compared to percutaneous intervention.
  - If thrombolysis is contraindicated, start with open thrombectomy via a common femoral venotomy prior to percutaneous angioplasty and stenting.

Nutcracker Syndrome (Also Referred to as Left Renal Vein (LRV) Entrapment)

- External compression disorder of the LRV most commonly between the abdominal aorta and superior mesenteric artery (SMA) [1].
- Risk factor: Females, young age.
- Symptoms of gross or microscopic hematuria, left flank pain, orthostatic proteinuria.
- Diagnosis:
  - Doppler ultrasonography, CT angiography, and magnetic resonance imaging.
  - "Beak sign" caused by narrowing of the LRV between the aorta and SMA [1]
  - Presence of pelvic venous collateralization.
- Treatment:
  - If <18yo typically treated conservatively as further development and weight gain widens the acute aortomesenteric angle and relieves the compression [1].
  - If >18yo, symptomatic, and imaging studies show renal vein compression with pelvic collaterals, consider operative treatment which includes LRV transposition, gonadal vein transposition, endovascular stent grafting of LRV [1].

Venous Aneurysms

- Dilation 2–3× of normal vein diameter. Rare, usually asymptomatic [1].
- Primary aneurysms from inherent weakness in the venous wall due to inherited conditions (e.g. Klippel-Trenaunay syndrome) vs secondary aneurysms acquired (e.g. trauma, mechanical stress) [1].
- Histology: venous intima is thickened or fibrosed. Media attenuated or absent, lack of smooth muscle cells. Matrix metalloproteinases are expressed at higher levels [1].

- Usually asymptomatic, complications include thrombosis, embolization, rupture, mass effect, pain [1].
- Diagnosis by US, CT, MRI. Venography is not indicated for primary diagnosis [1].

Lower Extremity Venous Aneurysm

- Superficial Aneurysms [1].
  - If symptomatic, tx with ligation and excision after ensuring the deep system is intact.
  - Perforating venous aneurysms rare. Diagnosed w/ US >9 mm.
- Deep Venous Aneurysms [1].
  - Popliteal aneurysms are most common and more likely to have complications.
  - 45–80% discovered incidentally w/ work up for PE
  - Treatment.

    when >20 mm or symptomatic. Surgical resection with lateral venorrhaphy, resection with primary anastomosis or saphenous vein interposition grafting.

    Anticoagulation for 3–6 months after procedures.

Abdominal Venous Aneurysms

- Inferior Vena Cava [1].
  - >5 cm considered aneurysmal. Rare and infrequently symptomatic.
  - Gradman and Steinberg classification system, Types 1–4.
  - Type 2–4 more frequently w/ thrombosis requiring surgical intervention.
- Visceral Venous Aneurysms (portal, mesenteric, renal) [1].
  - Half with non-focal abdominal pain, 20% with thrombus, 30% incidental findings.
  - Aneurysm when diameter > 15 mm or 19 mm in cirrhotics.

  - Treat if >3 cm, symptomatic, or if complications present such as enlarging aneurysm, thrombus, rupture, pain. For splenic aneurysms, tx women of child bearing age.
  - Rule out LVR entrapment or spontaneous splenorenal shunt first in renal vein aneurysms. Surgical repair with aneurysmectomy or nephrectomy.

Internal Jugular and Upper Extremity Venous Aneurysms

- Often mistaken for soft tissue mass. Careful exam with compression of the mass in dependent and elevated positions. US for definitive diagnosis [1].
- Treatment for symptomatic or cosmetic lesions w/ aneurysmectomy and venous reconstruction. Asymptomatic can be monitored [1].

Venous Reconstruction in Nonvascular Surgical Oncologic Procedures

- Pancreatic tumor resection involving tumor invading the portal vein (PV) or superior mesenteric vein (SMV) was once a contraindication for resection, now more resection and reconstruction options have been shown to be safe [1].
- Tumor involvement of the SMV is best seen on CT portal venous phase [1].
  - Tumor length > 5 mm, no fat plane between tumor and vessel, venous occlusion with collateral formation, "teardrop sign."
  - Circumferential involvement of the vessel >180° indicates unresectable tumor.
- Possible survival benefit with reconstruction if no residual disease left [1].
- Right anterolateral wall most common area of PV/SMV involvement [1].

- Reconstruction options [1].
  - Primary end-to-end anastomosis: luminal narrowing >30% and length of vein involved <2 cm. Splenic vein ligation involved in 78%.
  - Lateral venorrhaphy: luminal narrowing <30%.
  - Patch angioplasty: 0-50% circumference involvement and end-to-end not possible.
  - Interposition grafting: Circumference involvement >30% and > 2 cm length involvement.
- Portal vein thrombosis risk factors: preoperative chemo, pre-op radiation, increased operation time, prosthetic interposition graft. Thrombosis can cause ascites [1].

IVC Reconstruction

- Vascular leiomyosarcoma most commonly involves the IVC but is rare. Complete resection only option for cure [1].
- IVC invasion may occur from renal, adrenal, hepatic, GI, or retroperitoneal malignancy [1].
- 2–16% of renal cell carcinoma (RCC) involves the IVC through tumor spread from the renal vein [1]
- Surgical reconstruction planning with CT scan with arterial and venous phases. MRI has high sensitivity for IVC wall invasion with RCC [1].
- Neves and Zincke Classification of tumor thrombus [1].
  - Level 1: <2 cm extension into IVC from left renal vein.
  - Level 2: >2 cm extension.
  - Level 3: Extents to retrohepatic IVC.
  - Level 4: Extends to supradiaphragmatic IVC, right atrium.
- Surgical Approaches [1].
  - Often midline laparotomy; preferable if cardiopulmonary bypass (CPB) w/sternotomy required.
  - If extensive IVC exposure needed (e.g. for retrohepatic exposure), retrohepatic and suprahepatic IVC exposure best through right thoracoabdominal seventh, eighth, or ninth space.

  - Intraop US used to delineate tumor relation to vasculature.
  - IVC temporary occlusion can be performed to see if patient can hemodynamically tolerate. If not, CPB may be option.
- Repair methods [1].
  - Primary repair when wall resection will result in <50% narrowing.
  - Patch angioplasty when wall resection causes >50% narrowing.
  - Interposition grafting when circumferential segmental resection required.
    - Femoral vein, cryopreserved vena cava, aortic homograft, prosthetic grafts all used. Many prefer ePTFE.
    - Graft diameter ~ 14–20 mm.
    - 24% require renal vein reimplantation and 2% hepatic vein reimplantation.
  - IVC ligation should be avoided, 50% complication rate with acute renal failure and lower extremity edema. Ligation a possibility with collateral formation following chronic obstruction.
  - Palliative IVC bypass when the tumor is unresectable.
    - Via right thoracoabdominal exposure seventh, eighth, or ninth space.
    - 12–18 mm ePTFE conduit
    - Proximal anastomosis at patent cephalad portion of IVC. Distal at the suprahepatic IVC. Right atrium a possibility.
    - IVC filter often placed in the conduit prophylactically for PE.
  - IVC resection with interposition graft with 80–100% patency rate at 9 months—5 years.
  - IVC graft infection risk from perforated diverticulitis, bile leak, duodenal leak.

Questions and Answers

1. What is the treatment approach to chronic venous insufficiency?
2. In patients with DVT, what is the primary aim of medical and surgical management?
3. A patient is undergoing pancreaticoduodenectomy for a pancreatic head mass. Intra-operatively it is decided that PV/SMV resection and reconstruction are going to be necessary to achieve pancreatectomy. On evaluation it appears about 1.3 cm of vein will be involved in resection and is predicted that there would be about 40% luminal narrowing. Which of the following is the best reconstructive option?

Answer: 1 Conservative management first with compression therapy, leg elevation, +/− unna boots. If refractory to this, proceed with suitable surgical intervention such as sclerotherapy, endovenous ablation, ligation, and stripping.

Answer: 2 To prevent transformation of DVT into life threatening PEs.

Answer: 3 Primary end-to-end anastomosis (correct).

References

1. Sidawy A, Perler B. Rutherford's vascular surgery and endovascular therapy. Philadelphia, PA: Elsevier; 2019.
2. Meissner M, Moneta G, Burnand K, Gloviczki P, Lohr J, Lurie F, et al. The hemodynamics and diagnosis of venous disease. J Vasc Surg. 2007;46(6):S4–S24.
3. Gray H, Lewis W. Chapter VII, the veins of the upper extremity and thorax. In: Anatomy of the human body. 20th ed. Philadelphia: Lea & Febiger; 2000. p. 660–4.
4. Krishnan S, Nicholls S. Chronic venous insufficiency: clinical assessment and patient selection. Semin Intervent Radiol. 2005;22(03):169–77.

5. Nicolaides A. Investigation of chronic venous insufficiency. Circulation. 2000;102:20.
6. Eklöf B, Rutherford R, Bergan J, Carpentier P, Gloviczki P, Kistner R, et al. Revision of the CEAP classification for chronic venous disorders: consensus statement. J Vasc Surg. 2004;40(6):1248–52.
7. Scott G, Mahdi AJ, Alikhan R. Superficial vein thrombosis: a current approach to management. Br J Haematol. 2015;168(5):639–45.
8. Di Nisio M, Wichers IM, Middeldorp S. Treatment for superficial thrombophlebitis of the leg. Cochrane Database Syst Rev. 2013;2(2):CD004982. https://doi.org/10.1002/14651858.CD004982.pub5/full.
9. Kearon C, Akl EA, Comerota AJ, et al. Antithrombotic therapy for VTE disease: antithrombotic therapy and prevention of thrombosis, 9th ed: American College of Chest Physicians Evidence-Based Clinical Practice Guidelines. Chest. 2012;141(2 Suppl):e419S–94S.

17 Vascular Access

Beatriz Valdovinos Leong
and Theodore H. Teruya

Preoperative Evaluation

1. Timing of access placement
   (a) SVS guidelines and NKF-KDOQI recommend patients be referred to a vascular surgeon for permanent dialysis access when creatinine clearance is <25 mL/min (CKD stage 4). The stages of CKD based on creatinine clearance (CrCl) or glomerular filtration rate (GFR) are as follows (adopted from NKF KDOQI guidelines):
      - Stage 1 (CrCl >90 mL/min) kidney damage with normal or high GFR.
      - Stage 2 (CrCl 60–89 mL/min) mild kidney dysfunction.
      - Stage 3 (CrCl 30–56 mL/min) moderate kidney dysfunction.
      - Stage 4 (CrCl 15–29 mL/min) severe kidney dysfunction.
      - Stage 5 (CrCl <15 mL/min) kidney failure or end stage renal disease.

   (b) Access creation should be performed as soon as possible after referral.

B. V. Leong (✉) · T. H. Teruya
Department of Surgery, Loma Linda University, Loma Linda, CA, USA
e-mail: Beleong@llu.edu; Tteruya@llu.edu

A. Murga et al. (eds.), *The Vascular Surgery In-Training Examination Review (VSITE)*,
https://doi.org/10.1007/978-3-031-24121-5_17

- Placement should occur 6 months prior to initiation of dialysis to allow for autogenous access maturation.
- When an autogenous access is not possible, graft placement should occur 3–6 weeks prior to initiation of HD.

2. Medical assessment
   (a) **History:** Identify the dominant extremity, any history of central lines, tunneled lines, pacemakers/defibrillators, history of previous accesses/access related interventions, comorbid conditions, and medications. A history of arterial diseases should be noted.
   (b) **Physical exam**: Note pulse examination at brachial, radial, ulnar arteries, make note of palmar arch patency, note visible venous examination, look for prominent venous collaterals and edema both of which may suggest central venous stenosis [1].
   (c) Several demographics have an effect on autogenous access patency, most of which play a negative role.
      - **Age:** ESRD patients have a decreased life expectancy compared to the general population; increasing age also carries a higher risk for access creation failure. A meta-analysis looking at patients aged 50–70 years old demonstrated a significantly higher rate of primary failure in autogenous radio-cephalic AVF (RC-AVF) compared to younger patients (OR 1.8) [2].
      - **Diabetes mellitus (DM):** DM patients tend to have more arterial calcifications and atherosclerosis (rendering arteries less compliant); studies looking at DM are mostly retrospective, observational reports with similar outcomes, DM has a negative effect on access patency, some studies suggest increased risk of steal syndrome [3, 4].
      - **Smoking**: Increased early and late failures in smokers, smoking cessation should be encouraged [5].
      - **Medications**: Primarily observational studies with conflicting outcomes,
        - Dialysis Outcomes and Practice Patterns Study (DOPPS): [6].

Higher patency (RR 0.56) in patients taking ACE inhibitor,

Higher patency in prosthetic grafts (RR 0.86) in patients on calcium channel blocker (CCB),

Higher secondary patency (RR 0.7) in patients on aspirin,

Decreased primary patency (RR 1.33) in patients on Coumadin.

- USRDS study: Decreased patency with anti-platelets [7].
- ARBs combined w/anti-platelet: increased autogenous patency [8].

(d) **Arterial assessment:** An abnormal pulse examination should prompt segmental pressure examination and duplex. Ideally there should be no pressure gradient noted between the upper extremities; additionally, the arterial diameter should be a minimum of 2 mm [9].

(e) **Venous assessment:** Venous mapping of bilateral upper extremities should be obtained. Veins are examined for diameter, distensibility, continuity, thrombosis, stenosis, sclerosis.

- Vein diameter has been studied for rates of maturation and technical success:
  - Minimum vein 2.0 mm (maturation rate 76%) [10].
  - Minimum vein 2.5 mm (maturation rate 83%) [9].
  - Minimum vein 3.0 mm (maturation of 84% and technical success of 90%) [11].
- Prominent venous collaterals, upper extremity edema, a history of previous central venous catheters, or multiple accesses in the same arm should all prompt evaluation for central venous stenosis. This may be done via duplex ultrasound or venography. Venography has the advantage of allowing the opportunity for treatment in the same setting.

Selection of Access Location

There are a variety of access options and configurations (Fig. 17.1) a proposed algorithm of access location selection is provided (Fig. 17.2). Guideline 2 of the National Kidney Foundation's (NKF) clinical practice guidelines for hemodialysis vascular access selection specifically delineates the type and preferred location of access. The upper extremity offers more locations for cannulation and it also carries lower infection rates compared to lower extremity, thus the upper extremity is preferred over lower extremity/chest location. The non-dominant hand is preferred over the dominant hand. The best and most distal location is selected first to preserve more proximal locations for future access. Autogenous accesses are preferred over prosthetic ones due to lower infection rates and superior cumulative patency.

Forearm

The cephalic vein is preferred over the basilic vein, radial artery inflow is used first due to preference for cephalic vein and its proximity; if the fistula is unable to be created in the wrist (Fig. 17.3) or more distally in the snuffbox, a transposition may be performed to either ulnar or radial inflow. Lastly if no forearm vein is available a forearm prosthetic loop graft is an option (Fig. 17.4).

Upper Arm

The upper arm cephalic vein is the preferred vein if the size is adequate. Radial or brachial inflow is acceptable (Fig. 17.5). If the cephalic vein is too deep a transposition or superficialization surgery may be required. The upper arm basilic vein is also an option if cephalic vein is not available. The basilic vein usually lies medially in the upper arm, is deeper than the cephalic vein, and usually has more branches, thus transposition is nearly always required

Forearm

Autogenous

- Posterior radial branch–cephalic wrist direct access (snuffbox fistula)
- Radial-cephalic wrist direct access (Brescia-Cimino-Appel fistula)
- Radial-cephalic forearm transposition
- Brachial (or proximal radial)–cephalic forearm looped transposition
- Radial-basilic forearm transposition
- Ulnar-basilic forearm transposition
- Brachial (or proximal radial)-basilic forearm looped transposition
- Radial-antecubital forearm indirect femoral vein translocation
- Brachial (or proximal radial)-antecubital forearm indirect looped femoral vein translocation
- Radial-antecubital forearm indirect saphenous vein translocation
- Brachial (or proximal radial)-antecubital forearm indirect looped saphenous vein translocation

Prosthetic

- Radial-antecubital forearm straight access
- Brachial (or proximal radial)-antecubital forearm looped access

Upper Arm

Autogenous

- Brachial (or proximal radial)-cephalic upper arm direct access
- Brachial (or proximal radial)-cephalic upper arm transposition
- Brachial (or proximal radial)-basilic upper arm transposition
- Brachial (or proximal radial)-brachial vein upper arm transposition
- Brachial (or proximal radial)-axillary (or brachial) upper arm indirect femoral vein translocation
- Brachial (or proximal radial)-axillary (or brachial) upper arm indirect saphenous vein translocation

Prosthetic

- Brachial (or proximal radial)-axillary (or brachial) upper arm straight access

Adapted from Sidawy AN, Gray R, Besarab A, et al. Recommended standards for reports dealing with arteriovenous hemodialysis accesses. *J vasc Surg.* 2002;35:603-610.

Fig. 17.1 Varying types and locations of arteriovenous access for hemodialysis. (Reproduced with permission from Rutherford's Vascular Surgery and Endovascular Therapy)

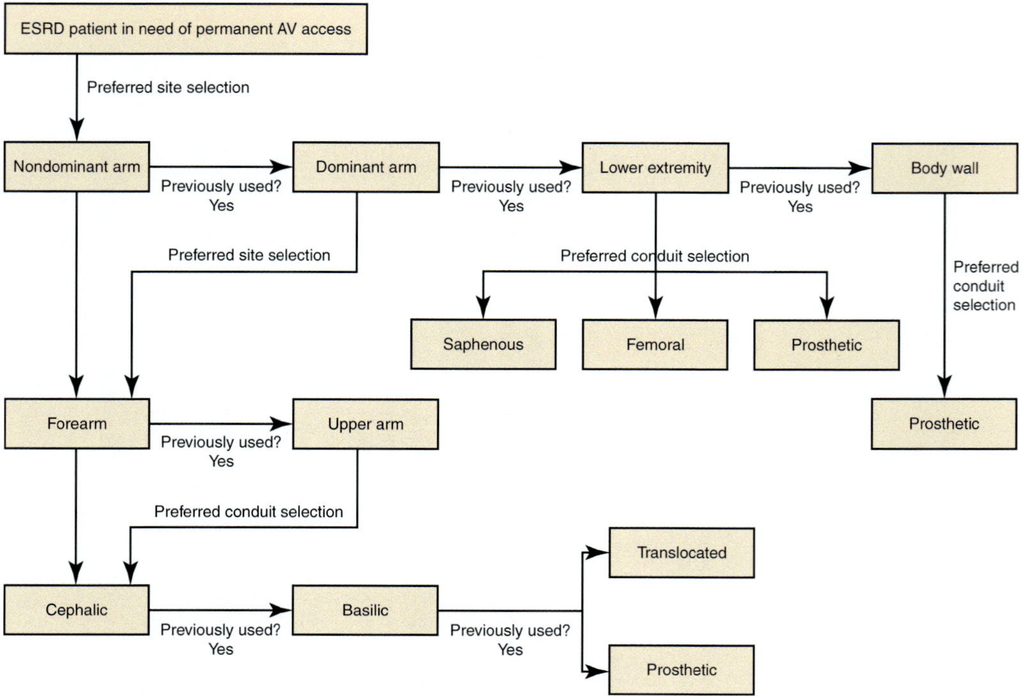

Fig. 17.2 Algorithm for selection of access placement location and type of access. (Reproduced with permission from Rutherford's Vascular Surgery and Endovascular Therapy)

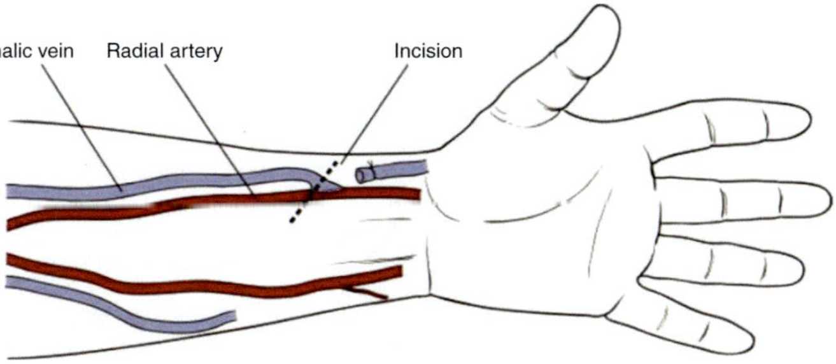

Fig. 17.3 Radial to cephalic arteriovenous fistula at the wrist. (Reproduced with permission from Atlas of Vascular Surgery and Endovascular Therapy)

(Fig. 17.6). Transposition of the basilic vein can be done in a single stage or in two stages after allowing time for maturation. If no acceptable upper arm vein is available a prosthetic graft may be placed in the upper arm as well, selecting the distal most inflow, brachial artery, and with usually axillary vein for outflow yielding a "C configuration" (Fig. 17.7), or with axillary inflow and axillary outflow in a "loop configuration."

Chest

Chest wall access usually involves use of prosthetic loop grafts such as axillary/axillary grafts (Fig. 17.8) or brachial-jugular straight grafts and is reserved for patients who have failed most or all arm access. A unique access reserved for patented with recalcitrant central stenosis is a unique prosthetic with a single arterial anastomosis and catheter-like outflow component placed in the sinoatrial junction, a Hemodialysis Reliable Outflow (HeRO) (Fig. 17.9).

Complex Access

Procedures, indications, contraindications, and anatomic requirements are compiled into Table 17.1.

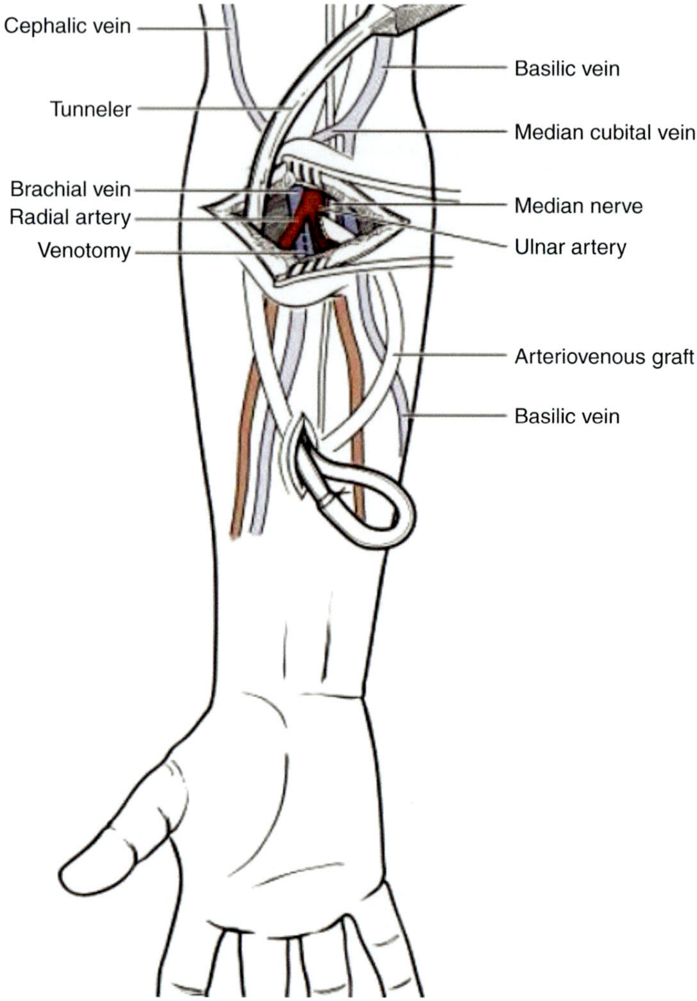

Fig. 17.4 Forearm loop arteriovenous graft. (Reproduced with permission from Atlas of Vascular Surgery and Endovascular Therapy)

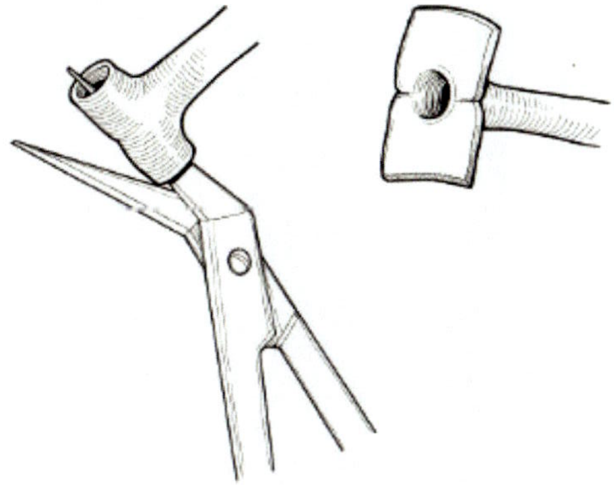

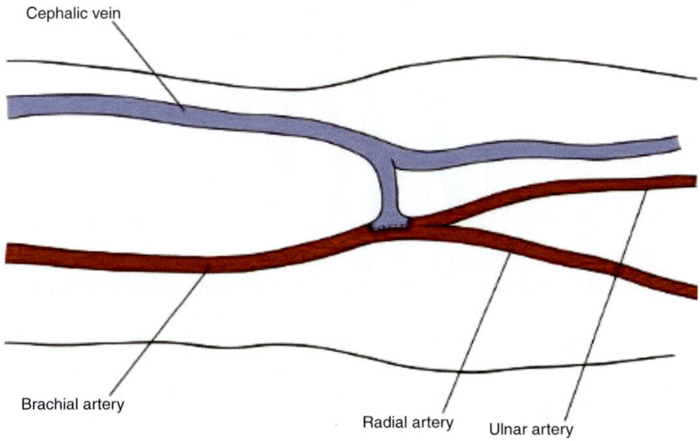

Fig. 17.5 Antecubital fossa brachial—cephalic/antecubital vein arteriovenous fistula creation. (Reproduced with permission from Atlas of Vascular Surgery and Endovascular Therapy)

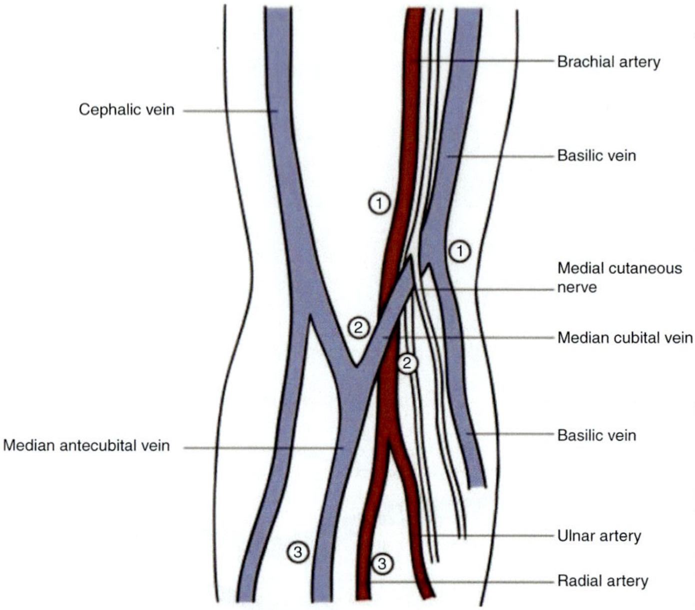

Fig. 17.6 The most common sites for anastomosing the basilic vein to the brachial artery (1). The basilic vein is divided at the entry of the median cubital into the basilic vein and transposed to the brachial artery in one stage (2). The basilic vein is divided into the antecubital fossa and anastomosed to the distal brachial artery. This may be done in one- or two-stage transposition procedures (3). A side-to-side anastomosis is created between the median antecubital, cephalic, or median cubital vein and the proximal radial artery. No second stage may be necessary if retrograde venous valve destruction results in maturation of forearm veins. If it does not, a second stage cephalic or basilic vein transposition is needed. (Reproduced with permission from Atlas of Vascular Surgery and Endovascular Therapy)

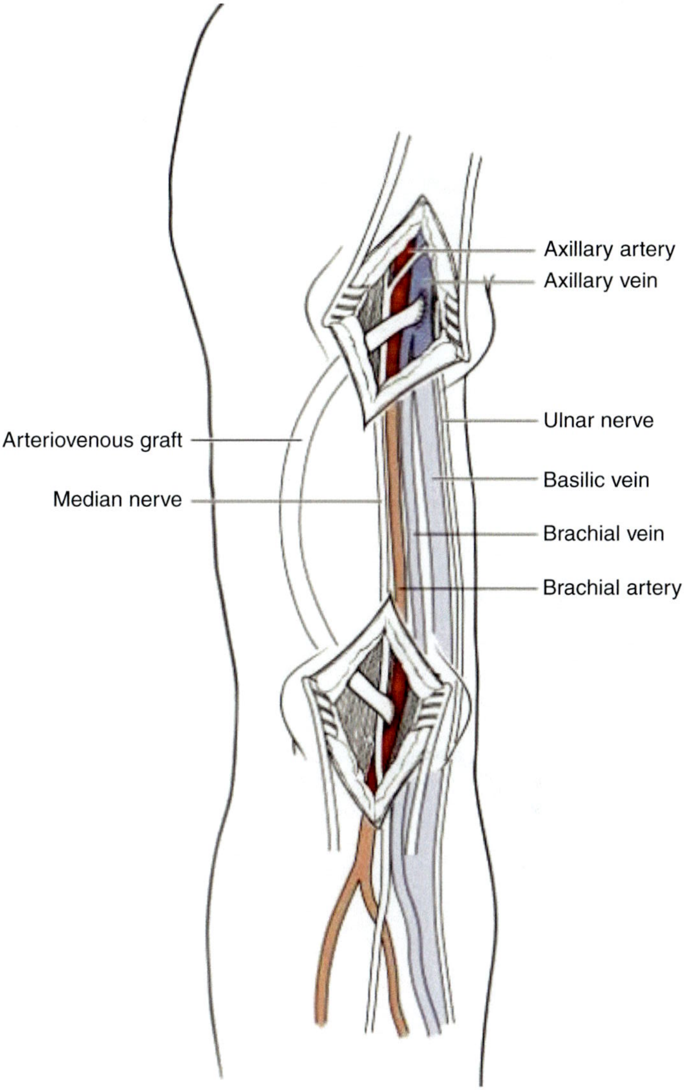

Fig. 17.7 A right upper arm brachial artery to axillary vein interposition graft. A gradual arch configuration increased the length of the cannulation segment. (Reproduced with permission from Atlas of Vascular Surgery and Endovascular Therapy)

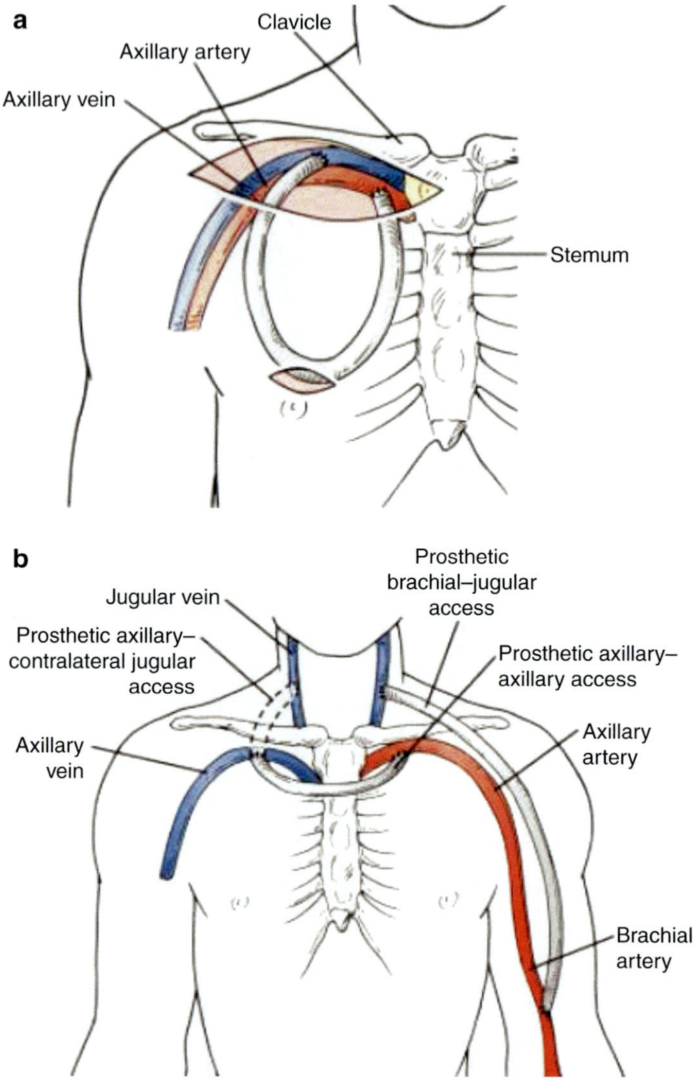

Fig. 17.8 (**a**) Prosthetic axillary artery-axillary loop graft. By situating the venous limb of the graft laterally on the chest wall and angling the venous anastomosis toward the central veins, subsequent percutaneous angioplasty is facilitated should a stenosis develop. (**b**) Prosthetic chest wall and cervical straight access options. (Reproduced with permission from Rutherford's Vascular Surgery and Endovascular Therapy)

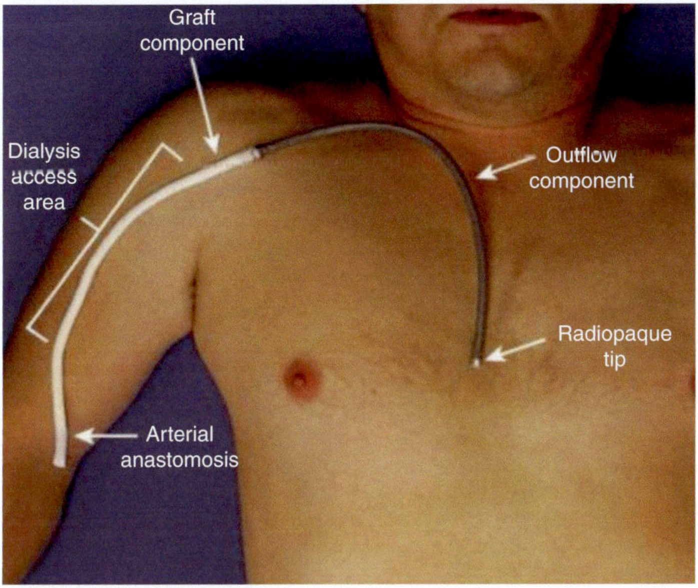

Fig. 17.9 Placement of a device for hemodialysis reliable outflow (HeRO) vascular access. The silicone catheter component of the HeRO device is placed into the central veins using a similar technique to that of placing a tunneled dialysis catheter. To facilitate passage of the catheter component of the HeRO device, it may be necessary to dilate the tract with an over-the-wire angioplasty balloon. A tunneling device is used to pass the silicone catheter from the neck incision to the counter incision at the deltopectoral groove. An end-to-side anastomosis between the graft component and the distal brachial artery is performed and the graft is tunneled retrograde to the incision at the deltopectoral groove. Silicone catheter and graft components are connected using the titanium connector. (Reproduced with permission from Rutherford's Vascular Surgery and Endovascular Therapy)

Table 17.1 Complex access, procedures, anatomic requirements, indications, and contraindications. (Adapted with permission from Rutherford's Vascular Surgery and Endovascular Therapy)

Access procedure	Anatomic requirement	Clinical situation	Contraindication (relative)
Autogenous femoral vein transposition	Patent femoral vein >3 mm, Patent SFA (without calcification)	Pediatric/young patients Hypercoagulable patients with no other available site Patients who are high risk for infection, immunosuppressed, of have multiple access infections	Thigh obesity Elderly/fragile patents High risk for limb related ischemia of leg
Prosthetic mid-thigh loop femoral to femoral access	Patent femoral of common femoral vein Patent SFA or CFA (without calcification)	Elderly patients or those who have distinct medical comorbidities	Patient is high risk for infection (poor hygiene, immunosuppressed, multiple previous infections, morbidly obese)
Prosthetic chest wall access	Patent axillo-subclavian artery and vein No central stenos	Morbidly obese High risk for limb ischemia	Candidates for autogenous or prosthetic thigh access
Tunneled dialysis catheter	Patent central vein	Medically fragile patients, limited life expectancy (<6 months) Patients who have exhausted all other access	Candidates for alternative access
Hemodialysis reliable outflow access (HeRO)	Ability to access a central vein Brachial artery >3 mm	Central venous stenosis/occlusion that precludes upper extremity access Patients relegated to catheter for access	Active infection SBP <100 mmHg EF <20%

Selection of Type of Access

Autogenous Vs. Prosthetic

1. Autogenous accesses are preferred over prosthetic ones due to lower infection rates and superior patency; however, one must carefully evaluate the patient's comorbidities and make an informed decision as the overall goal is to minimize catheter days. If the autogenous vein requires a transposition or superficialization, this may be done in a single stage or two stages. A single stage technique allows for a single anesthetic; however, the tradeoff is risk of failure to mature despite an extensive dissection. A two-stage procedure requires two anesthetics; however, before the second stage, one can ensure the fistula is ready by obtaining an access and evaluating flows. Judgment should be applied when deciding to perform single vs. two stage transpositions, in particular in veins smaller than 4 mm [12].
2. Primary patency for autogenous AVF ranges from 43 to 85% at one year [13] and 40–69% at two years [14]. Prosthetic grafts require more interventions per time unit to have similar patency compared to autogenous access (Fig. 17.10) [14].
3. Prosthetic grafts are preferentially made of ePTFE, which is supplied in thin walled, extended stretch, external rings, tapered, and heparin coating (none of these properties has been shown to be superior to the others). Standard wall grafts can be accessed as early as 2 weeks postoperatively which still requires the use of a central venous catheter. The "early cannulation" grafts are configured to have an additional hemostatic layer (foregoing the necessary formation of an autogenous pseudo-capsule around the graft to aid in hemostatic after decannulation of standard wall grafts) and can be cannulated as early as 24 h after surgery [15]. The primary advantage prosthetic grafts have over autogenous access is the lower primary failure rates; however, some of these failures can be mitigated by ensuring one has an adequate artery and adequate vein for access creation [16].

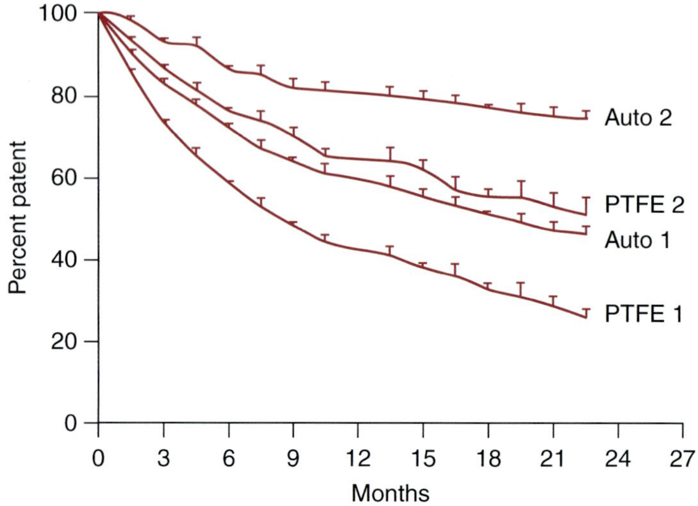

Fig. 17.10 Primary and secondary patency rates of autogenous and prosthetic arteriovenous accesses. PTFE, Polytetrafluoroethylene. (Reproduced with permission from Rutherford's Vascular Surgery and Endovascular Therapy)

(a) **Measuring access function**: Autogenous access should be ready for cannulation twelve weeks postoperatively and in rare cases earlier, and a graft should be ready for access at approximately 2 weeks. A physical examination demonstrating an easily palpable AVF/AVG, that is not too deep and has a readily palpable thrill for a length of at least 10 cm (allowing two access needles) is ideal. A practical rule to follow is the "Rule of 6's" where 6 weeks after an autogenous fistula has been placed the fistula should be able to support a blood flow of 600 mL/min, be at least 6 mm in diameter and be no more than 6 mm deep for successful cannulation and function for dialysis. Occasionally if these criteria are not met a dialysis access ultrasound should be performed to evaluate the flow, depth, and look for branches that may be impeding maturation or hindering access. Failing access may need secondary procedures, including open or endovascular procedures (such as balloon assisted maturation "BAM"), branch ligation, or superficialization to achieve successful assisted primary patency. Up to 69% of failing arteriovenous fistulas can achieve functional maturation via secondary procedures [17].

(b) **Detection of access failure**: Routine access monitoring is preferred, a monthly evaluation at dialysis centers is ideal. A flow <600 mL/min, rapid decrease in flow over time (over 25% reduction) should be further assessed with a formal duplex US of the fistula. Ultrasound findings should guide intervention but are often followed by fistulogram. Additional clinical signs of a potentially failing access include prolonged bleeding after needle decannulation, recirculation of blood in the fistula, evaluation of physical findings such as arm swelling, thinning of skin, or ulcerations of the skin around the access site, absence or decreased thrill, should all prompt a fistulogram with interventions.

(c) **Clinical vs. imaging**: Clinical evaluation for access failure is often the only thing necessary with a thorough palpation examination noting decreased or absence of a thrill. If the fistula or graft is pulsatile, there may be distal obstruction. The presence of extremity edema, facial edema, prominent chest wall or arm collaterals may indicate central stenosis or occlusion. Access ultrasound may be helpful in identifying flow issues, as well as areas of stenosis, and can help guide interventions.

(d) **Assessment during dialysis**: Access flow, pressure, or resistance can all be used to identify potentially failing accesses. Adequate flow is necessary for the dialysis machines to function effectively, machines in the USA typically have minimum flow rates of 350–500 mL/min. Recirculation during dialysis suggests an increase in venous pressure and ineffective dialysis. Venous pressure measurements may identify stenosis early, and the trends over time may be the most predictive of access issues [18]. Flow measurement is another quite useful measurement obtained at dialysis sessions, flow rates below 600–800 mL/min predict thrombosis in prosthetic access, this value is less well defined in autogenous access however KDOQI guidelines recommend intervention if the flow rates are lower than 900 mL/min, and monthly assessments [19].

Mechanisms of Access Failure

1. **Flow limitation**: Flows of 1000–1200 mL/min are required to avoid recirculation as modern dialysis machines may have speeds nearing 500 mL/min [20]. Cardiac output must also be assessed as decreased cardiac output may be associated with decreased flow with dialysis, and marginal fluid removal during dialysis leading to the requirement of longer dialysis sessions [21].
2. **Venous outflow stenosis**: The most common cause of recirculation is venous outflow stenosis which limits the flow through the access.
3. **Arterial inflow stenosis**: arterial inflow limitations also results in recirculation, low flows, longer dialysis sessions, and is a common mode of access failure.
4. **Cannulation location**: A very important cause of recirculation is the location of the cannulas, specifically inadequate distance between the needles. Repeated access at the same location will lead to pseudoaneurysm formation, which if large enough can also lead to recirculation as well as other complications such as ulceration, bleeding, and thrombosis.
5. **Central venous occlusion.**
   (a) **HeRO:** Patients who have significant central venous occlusions/stenosis precluding adequate functional access in upper extremity may be candidates for the hemodialysis reliable outflow (HeRO) device (Fig. 17.9). The device has two components: a conventional (or early access) prosthetic graft connected to the brachial artery and a venous outflow component, a 19 Fr silicone catheter reinforced with nitinol braid to prevent kinking, that is placed at the sinoatrial junction under fluoroscopic guidance.

Interventions for Failing and Thrombosed Access

1. Open surgical techniques
   (a) **Revisions for stenosis:** Open surgical revision of a stenotic segment improves outflow and function, careful identification of all culprit lesions must be done prior to operation to ensure all lesions are addressed. Surgical revision may involve interpositions or patch repairs; however, central lesions are less accessible and endovascular interventions are preferred.
   (b) **Revisions for other issues:** Multiple outflow veins may limit the maturation of an autogenous fistula and can also limit the length of sites available for cannulation thus branch ligations are occasionally needed. Deep veins are also inaccessible; thus, transposition or superficialization may be needed.
2. **Endovascular techniques**: Specific approach to intervention is dictated by specific issues identified on pre-procedural imaging. AV access US should be obtained to aid in characterizing the issue.
   (a) **Balloon angioplasty:** The most commonly performed intervention, typically required high-pressure balloons, longer inflation times at least 2–3 min, recurrent stenosis is common.
   (b) **Balloon assisted maturation "BAM"**: Initially described in 2001, involves serial dilation of the outflow vein with progressively larger balloons to achieve a certain diameter, reported success rates of 97%, with primary 1 year patency of 39% and secondary patency 79% [22].
   (c) **Stenting**: Stents are indicated for refractory stenosis, dissections, or ruptures after angioplasty. In-stent restenosis is very common with bare metal stents, but also occurs at lower rates with the use of covered stents [23]. Covered stents have also been used to salvage graft from pseudoaneurysm as an alternative to interposition graft placement as they are amenable to continued access for dialysis with similar patency to autogenous grafts, and similar rates of infection [24].

   (d) **Hybrid Approach**: The most versatile approach to complete treatment of a malfunctioning access, as often there may be multiple issues contributing to access failure (i.e., central stenosis with aneurysmal AVF).
3. Thrombosed access:
   (a) **Autogenous access**: Open surgical thrombectomy is an option although the venous endothelium can be damaged with balloon thrombectomy and re-generate intimal hyperplasia. Percutaneous mechanical thrombectomy is reported to have good technical success, highly versatile, and currently the preferred initial mode of approaching a thrombosed fistula with acute thrombosis, although long term studies are still lacking [25].
   (b) **Prosthetic access:** These accesses tend to thrombose more frequently than autogenous access, with intimal hyperplasia at the venous anastomosis being the primary culprit.
   (c) **Thrombolysis**: Percutaneous thrombolysis with the injection of thrombolytics locally with balloon occlusion of the arterial and venous anastomosis. In the "lyse-and-wait" technique, the patient gets tPA infused in a monitored setting and is taken to the interventional suite after flow has returned [26]. Alternatively "lyse-and-go" has also been used although patients are taken for intervention immediately after lytic injection. A relatively frequent complication from percutaneous thrombectomy is pulmonary embolism. Several commercially available thrombectomy devices are available such as the Arrow-Trerotola device, Hydrolyser (Cordis), Angiojet (Boston Scientific), and Indigo (Penumbra) devices. Reported complications for mechanical thrombectomy remain low ~3%; however, care must be taken to ensure all instructions are followed carefully, blood loss is monitored, and hemolysis is considered.

Non-thrombotic Complications

KDOQI guidelines recognize there are multiple and fairly frequent access complications, they also publish guidelines for surveillance and early intervention for potentially failing access [27].

1. **Bleeding**: Prolonged needle site bleeding, easy bruising (platelet dysfunction, chronic anemia) in addition to peptic ulcer bleeding, spontaneous retroperitoneal bleeding, hemorrhagic stroke, and conversion of ischemic stroke to hemorrhagic stroke are also more common in dialysis patients compared to general population [28]. Persistent access bleeding should be evaluated for mechanical causes such as venous outflow stenosis, as well as for other causes such as infection and pseudoaneurysm.
2. Treatment: Active bleeding:
   - (a) Desmopressin: induces rapid release of autologous von Willebrand factor (vWF) and Factor VIII; tachyphylaxis after second dose.
   - (b) Platelet transfusion: works immediately, lasts 4–5 h.
   - (c) Cryoprecipitate (plasma rich in fibrinogen, vWF, Factor VIII, works in minutes, lasts up to 24 hrs (rarely cause anaphylaxis or hemolysis).
3. Elective Surgery:
   - (a) Erythropoietin [29] corrects anemia (takes several weeks) and also enhances platelet expression of GP-IIb/IIIa as well as platelet aggregation [30].
   - (b) Conjugated estrogens: increase vWF synthesis, reduced protein S, and nitrous oxide (NO), corrects bleeding time [31].
   - (c) Hemodialysis day prior to elective surgery: minimize uremia, maximize platelet function.
   - (d) Discontinuing anti-platelet medications 7 days prior to elective surgery.

4. **Infection**: second most common cause of death and loss of access [32]. Loss of access occurs due to infection at a rate 4.5% at one year for autogenous access and 19.7% for prosthetic access [33].
   (a) Grading: The SVS published reporting guidelines for location and severity of infections, as well as timing with early infections being <30 days after access creation, late >30 days,
   (b) Grade 0: no infection.
   (c) Grade 1: resolved with antibiotics.
   (d) Grade 2: loss of AV access due surgical intervention.
   (e) Grade 3: loss of limb.
5. Bacteriology: staph aureus is most common, 25% due to gram-negative organisms, small percentage are polymicrobial.
6. Catheter-related infections: responsible for 2/3 of all access related infections; responsible for 80% of all bloodstream infections in hemodialysis patients, tunneled lines carry 13.6 times higher risk compared to fistulas for infection, non-tunneled carry a 32.6 times risk [34].
7. Treatment: Initiate broad spectrum antibiotics as soon as infection is suspected and after blood cultures are drawn, tailor the antibiotics to cultures as soon as possible.
   (a) Autogenous access: most autogenous access infections are due to cannulation issues and hematoma. Majority of these infections respond to a 2–4 week course of antibiotics. Autogenous access with intraluminal prosthetics (stents) behaves more like prosthetic access and requires a longer course of antibiotics, and occasionally excision [34].
   (b) Prosthetic: complex, attempts at salvage are reasonable, however failure to improve will require resection, often a full graft excision.
8. **Pseudoaneurysm and aneurysm**: create a challenge for cannulating the access, have increased risk of thrombosis, pain, bleeding, infection, and are aesthetically displeasing [35].
   (a) **Pseudoaneurysm** develops due to repetitive access in the same location, poor technique, or increased outflow resistance; they are more common in older grafts and

occur in 2–10% of polytetrafluoroethylene (PTFE) grafts [36].

- Open treatment: interposition graft or bypass around the lesion, fistula plication.
- Endovascular treatment: concomitant venogram to evaluate for central stenosis (present in up to 73%) [37]. Technical success rates are high; however, repeat interventions are common (20%), high rates of post-procedural infection 35%, and thrombosis 12%. Patients with skin erosions have an increased failure rate (OR 5.0).

(b) **Aneurysm:** occurs near areas of stenosis or occlusion,

- Post-anastomotic: proximalizes the anastomosis, stenotic segment angioplasty vs. serial dilation vs. patch.
- Mid/diffuse aneurysm: aneurysmorrhaphy after evaluation and treatment for central stenosis.

9. **Venous Hypertension:** Due to central venous stenosis or occlusion, causes significant disability due to access malfunction and extremity swelling. Some patients with central stenosis/occlusion have enough collaterals to remain asymptomatic thus the true prevalence of central venous stenosis is unknown.

(a) Etiology: Primarily due to having a history of catheters, multiple catheters, long duration of catheters. Most common with subclavian catheter access, followed by IJ location (80% of patients still initiating dialysis with catheter). Similarly, implantable devices such as PICC lines, long term central venous access lines, pacemakers, and defibrillators all can lead to the same neointimal fibromuscular hyperplasia; 10% of central venous occlusions are idiopathic, but thought to be due to increased blood flow with presence of ipsilateral access, valve presence with scarring, and natural anatomic narrowing.

(b) Treatment:

- Ligation: tolerated well, relieves swelling in most, but requires loss of access,
- Endovascular: percutaneous transluminal angioplasty (PTA) is recommended by KDOQI for symptomatic patients; however, the trauma of the angioplasty itself

will lead to further intimal hyperplasia development. Technical success rates are high, but primary patency drops to <50% at 6 months and 12–43% at 12 months [38]. Stent placement is reserved for refractory lesions, or lesions that have failed angioplasty multiple times.

- Open surgical: Direct reconstruction, decompression, or bypass. Open surgical treatment carries substantial morbidity and is reserved for patients who have failed endovascular options.

10. **Ischemic monomelic neuropathy (IMN)**: Occurs in 0.5% of access cases (access related to the brachial artery), results from ischemia to the nerve. Delayed recognition leads to irreversible, profound neurologic deficits in median, radial, and ulnar nerves. Treatment is early access ligation, or emergent augmentation of flow.
11. **Ischemic steal syndrome:** Access related hand ischemia (AHRI): described in 1969, access creation leads to hand blood flow reduction in nearly 80% of cases, while most do not develop symptoms [39]. Significant hand ischemia ranges from 1–2% with autogenous access at the wrist and 4–8% in those with brachial artery access [40]. Ischemia results from inadequate collateral blood flow, and inability of arteries to meet the higher demand.
    (a) Ischemia Severity Grading: [41].
    (b) Grade 0: No symptoms.
    (c) Grade 1: Mild-cool extremity, few symptoms, Flow augmentation with access occlusion.
    (d) Grade 2: Moderate-intermittent ischemia only during dialysis claudication.
    (e) Grade 3: Severe-ischemic pain at rest, tissue loss.
        - Risk factors: DM, PAD, CAD, brachial artery-based access, female gender, history of access related hand ischemia, multiple previous accesses, preoperative digital brachial index (DBI) <1.0, a DBI < 0.6% has 100% sensitivity and 18% PPV for predicting ARHI [42].

- Presentation: Hand coolness, paresthesia, numbness, burning pain, weakness, on examination cool extremity, pallor, cyanosis, absent pulse, deceased sensation, the pulse should increase with fistula compression.
- Work-up: Digital pressure, plethysmography (PPG), pulse oximetry, arterial duplex, angiography all with and without compression. Angiography helps identify etiology of hand ischemia.

12. Treatment:
    (a) Indications: Grades 1–2 do not require treatment. Treatment is indicated in those patients with grades 3–4 AHRI, or those with severe symptoms, progressive numbness or pain, pallor, diminished sensation, ischemic ulcers, gangrene, motor dysfunction, and hand atrophy, tissue loss.
    (b) Techniques:
    - **Banding/Flow limiting procedures:** creating stenosis in the access near the arterial anastomosis via plication, narrowing tie. Degree of banding is not precise, results variable.
    - **Proximalization**: Ligation of the anastomosis and conversion of the inflow to an arterial level more proximal, typically using a small prosthetic interposition graft (Fig. 17.11).
    - **Distal revascularization and interval ligation (DRIL)**: ligation of the native artery distal to the arterial anastomosis and creating an arterial bypass with inflow placed primal to the access inflow. Excellent long term results, quite invasive, hand is bypass dependent. (Fig. 17.12).
    - **Revision using distal inflow (RUDI):** Ligation of the fistula itself at the arterial anastomosis, with re-establishment of flow to a more distal artery via bypass, or translocation of a vein side-branch. (Fig. 17.12).

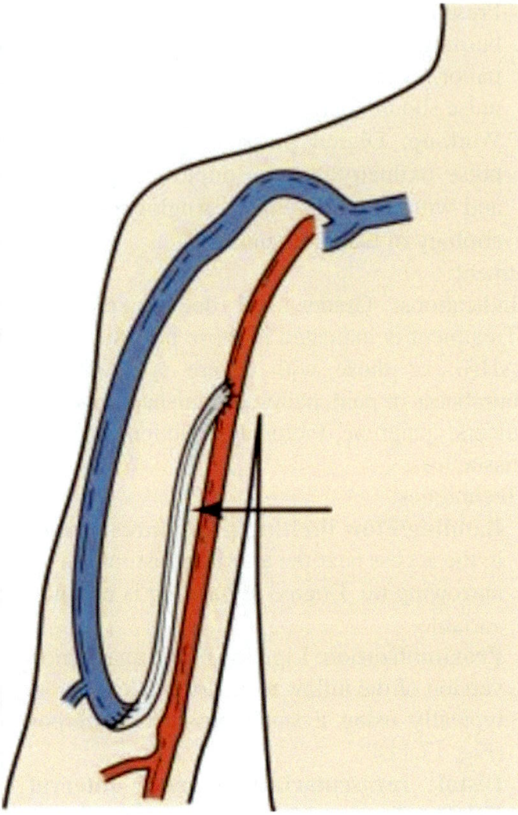

Fig. 17.11 Proximalization of arterial inflow, where the inflow to the arteriovenous graft is "proximalized" to originate more centrally. (Reproduced with permission from Rutherford's Vascular Surgery and Endovascular Therapy)

- **Distal radial artery ligation (DRAL)**: Flow reversal in radiocephalic AVF, leading to distal radial artery reversal of flow through the palmar arch, ligating the radial artery distal to the access preserves both the access and prevents digital steal.

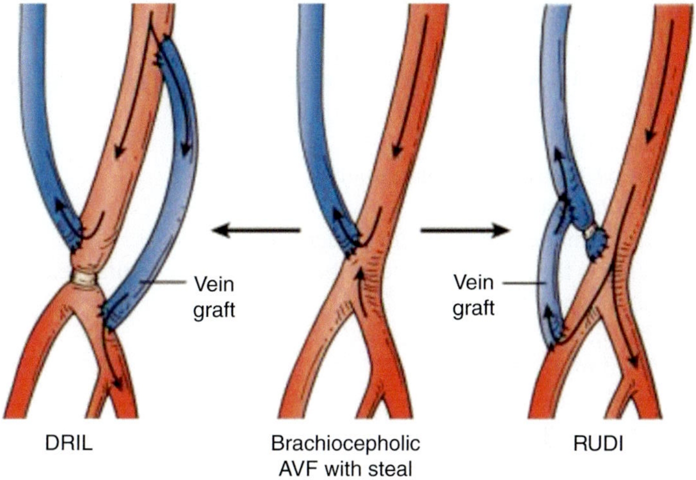

Fig. 17.12 The anatomic configurations of the DRIL and RUDI procedures are illustrated for the treatment of hand ischemia or steal syndrome after an autogenous brachiocephalic arteriovenous access. (Reproduced with permission from Rutherford's Vascular Surgery and Endovascular Therapy)

(c) **Coronary steal syndrome:** The internal mammary artery is a preferred conduit for coronary artery bypass grafting, patients with ipsilateral access may steal from the coronary circulation in setting of proximal subclavian artery stenosis.
- Work up: CTA to evaluate arch and proximal subclavian artery (may identify proximal subclavian artery stenosis), conventional angiogram demonstrating flow, correctable by fistula compression.
- Treatment: correction of stenosis.

Questions and Answers

1. Of the following, which are options for treatment of steal syndrome?
   (a) DRIL
   (b) Decreased dialysis session
   (c) Pain medications
   (d) Tunneled line catheter placement
2. What is the minimum size of the vein used for fistula creation
   (a) 6 cm
   (b) 3.5 cm
   (c) 3 mm
   (d) 1 mm
   (e) 0.1 cm

Answers: 1 (a), 2 (c)

References

1. Sidway AN, Spergel LM, Besarb A, et al. Clinical practice guidelines for the placement and maintenance of arterio-venous hemodialysis access. J Vasc Surg. 2008;48:2S–25S.
2. Lazarides MK, Georgiadis GS, Antonio GA, Staramos DN. A meta-analysis of dialysis access outcomes in elderly patients. J Vasc Surg. 2007;45:420–6.
3. Sedlacek M, Teodorescu V, Falk A, Vassalotti JA, Uribarri J. Hemodialysis access placement with preoperative noninvasive vascular mapping: comparison between patients with and without diabetes. Am J of Kid Disease. 2001;38(3):560–4.
4. Konner K, Hulbert-Shearon TE, Royrs EC, Port FK, Tailoring the initial vascular access for dialysis patients. Kidney Int. 2002;62:329–38.
5. Wetzig GA, Cough IR, Furnival CM. One hundred cases of arteriovenous fistula for hemodialysis access: the effect of cigarette smoking on patency. Aust NZ J Surg. 1985;55:551–4.
6. Saran R, Dykstra DM, Wofe RA, Gillespie B, Held PJ, Young EW. Association between vascular access failure and the use of specific drugs: the dialysis outcomes and practice patterns study (DOPPS). Am J Kidney Dis. 2002;40:1255–63.
7. Yevzlin AS, Conely EL, Sanchez RJ, Young HN, Becker BN. Vascular access outcomes and medication use: a USRDS study. Semin Dial. 2006;19(6):535–9.

8. Jackson RS, Sidway AN, Amdur RL, Khetarpal A, Macsata RA. Angiotensin receptor blocker and antiplatelet agents are associated with improved primary patency after arteriovenous hemodialysis access placement. J Vasc Surg. 2011;54:1706–12.
9. Silva MB, Hobson RW, Pappas PJ, et al. A strategy for increasing the use of autogenous hemodialysis access procedures: impact of preoperative noninvasive evaluation. J Vasc Surg. 1998;27(2):302–8.
10. Mendez RR, Farber MA, Marston WA, Dinwiddie LC, Keagy BA, Burnham SJ. Prediction of wrist arteriovenous fistula maturation with preoperative vein mapping with ultrasonography. J Vasc Surg. 2002;36(3):460–3.
11. Huber T, Ozaki C, Flynn TC, et al. Prospective validation of an algorithm to maximize native arteriovenous fistulae for chronic hemodialysis access. J Vasc Surg. 2002;36(3):452–9.
12. Arroyo MR, Sideman MJ, Spergel L, Jennings WC. Primary and staged transposition arteriovenous fistulas. J Vas Surg. 2008;47:1279–83.
13. Choe HM, Lal B, Cerveira JJ, et al. Durability and cumulative functional patency of transposed and non-transposed arteriovenous fistulae. J Vasc Surg. 2003;38(6):1206–12.
14. Huber TS, Carter JW, Carter RL, Seeger JM. Patency of autogenous and polytetrafluoroethylene upper extremity arteriovenous hemodialysis accesses: a systematic review. J Vasc Surg. 2003;38(5):1005–11.
15. Glickman MH, Burgess J, Cill D, et al. Prospective multi-center study with 1-year analysis of new vascular grafts used for early cannulation in patients undergoing hemodialysis. J Vasc Surg. 2015;62:434–41.
16. Patel ST, Hughes J, Mills JL. Failure of arteriovenous fistula maturation: an unintended consequence of seeing dialysis outcome quality initiative guidelines for hemodialysis access. J Vasc Surg. 2003;38(3):439–45.
17. McLafferty RB, Pryor RW, Johnson CM, Ramsey DE, Hodgson KJ. Outcome of a comprehensive follow-up program to enhance maturation of autogenous arteriovenous hemodialysis access. J Vas Surg. 2007;45(5):981–5.
18. Dember LM, Holmberg EF, Kaufman JS. Value of static venous pressure for predicting arteriovenous graft thrombosis. Kidney Int. 2002;61(5):1899–904.
19. NKF-K/DOQI Clinical Practice Guidelines for Vascular Access: update 2000. Am J Kidney Dis. 2001;37:S137–81.
20. Weitzel WF, et al. Analysis of variable flow Doppler hemodialysis access flow measurements and comparison with ultrasound dilution. Am J Kidney Dis. 2001;38(5):935–40.
21. Hassell DH, et al. Optimizing dialysis dose by increasing blood flow rate in patients with reduced vascular-access flow rate. Am J Kidney Dis. 2001;38(5):948–55.
22. Powell S, Chan T. Augmented balloon-assisted maturation (BAM) for non-maturing dialysis arteriovenous fistula. J Vasc Access. 2011;12(1):9–12.

23. Anaya-Ayala JE, et al. Efficacy of covered stent placement for central venous occlusive disease in hemodialysis patients. J Vasc Surg. 2011;54(3):754–9.
24. Kim CY, et al. Analysis of infection risk following covered stent exclusion of pseudoaneurysm in prosthetic arteriovenous hemodialysis access grafts. J Vasc Interv Radiol. 2012;23(1):69–74.
25. Shatsky JB, et al. Single-center experience with the arrow-Trerotola percutaneous thrombectomy device in the management of thrombosed native dialysis fistulas. J Vasc Interv Radiol. 2005;16(2):1605–11.
26. Vogel PM, Bansal V, Marshall MW. Thrombosed hemodialysis grafts: lyse and wait with tissue plasminogen activation or urokinase compared to mechanical thrombolysis with the arrow-Trerotola percutaneous thrombolytic device. J Vasc Interv Radiol. 2001;12(10):1157–65.
27. KDOQI guidelines 2006 updates. http://www.kidney.org/progessionals/kdoqi/guideline_uphd_pd
28. Bos MJ, Koudstaal PJ, Hofman A, Breteler MM. Decreased glomerular filtration rate is a risk factor for hemorrhagic but not for ischemic stroke: the Rotterdam study. Stroke. 2007;38(12):3127–32.
29. Cases A, Escolar G, Reverter JC, et al. Recombinant human erythropoietin treatment improves platelet function in uremic patients. Kidney Int. 1992;42(3):668–72.
30. Gawaz MP, Dobs G, Spath M, Schollmeyer P, Gurland HJ, Mujais SK. Impaired function of platelet membrane glycoprotein IIb/IIIa in end-stage renal disease. J Am Soc Nephrol. 1994;5(1):36–46.
31. Livio M, Mannucci PM, Vigano G, et al. Conjugated estrogens for the management of bleeding associated with renal failure. N Engl J Med. 1986;315(12):731–5.
32. Mailloux LU, et al. Mortality in dialysis patients: analysis of the cause of death. Am J Kidney Dis. 1991;19:326–35.
33. Churchill D, et al. Canadian hemodialysis morbidity study. Am J Kidney Dis. 1992;19:214–34.
34. Stevenson KB, et al. Epidemiology of hemodialysis vascular access infections from longitudinal infection surveillance data: predicting the impact of the KKF-DOQI clinical practice guidelines for vascular access. Am J Kidney Dis. 2002;39:549–55.
35. Barshes NR, et al. Endovascular repair of hemodialysis graft-related pseudoaneurysm: an alternative treatment strategy in salvaging failing dialysis access. Vasc Endovasc Surg. 2008;42:228–34.
36. Moszkowicz A, et al. Occlusion of rapidly expanding hemodialysis graft with placement of a stent graft. Semin Interv Radiol. 2007;24:34–7.
37. Florescu MC, et al. Endovascular treatment of arteriovenous graft pseudoaneurysms, indications, complications and outcomes: a systematic review. Hemodial Int. 2014;18:785–92.

38. Surowiec SM, Fegley AJ, Tanski WJ, et al. Endovascular management of central venous stenosis in the hemodialysis patients: restyle of percutaneous therapy. Vasc Endovasc Surg. 2004;38(4):249–354.
39. Papasavas PK, Reifsnyder T, Birdas TJ, Caushaj PF, Leers S. Prediction of arteriovenous access steal syndrome utilizing digital pressure measurements. Vasc Endovasc Surg. 2003;37(3):179–84.
40. Morsy AH, Kulbaski M, Chen C, Isiklar H, Lundsmen AB. Incidence and characteristics of patients with hand ischemia after hemodialysis access procedure. J Surg Res. 1998;74(1):8–10.
41. Sidway AN, Gray R, Besarb A, et al. Recommended standards for reports dealing with arteriovenous hemodialysis accesses. J Vasc Surg. 2002;35(3):603–10.
42. Goff CD, Sato DT, Bloch PH, et al. Steal syndrome complicating hemodialysis access procedures: can it be predicted? Ann Vasc Surg. 2000;14(2):138–44.

18 Non-Atherosclerotic Vascular Disease

Kristine Bonnick and Allen Murga

Non-atherosclerotic Vascular Disease

Systemic vasculitis is a broad group of disorders which share common pathophysiology, blood vessel inflammation leading to mural damage (see Fig. 18.1). Classification is based on 2012 Chapel Hill Consensus Conference nomenclature of vasculitides which is based on vessel size [1, 2].

Large Vessel Disease

Giant Cell Arteritis (GCA)

- Clinical characteristics:
  - Fevers, fatigue, weight loss, headache, tender temporal artery and scalp, absent temporal artery pulse, optic neuritis, diplopia, amaurosis fugax, blindness, and jaw claudication.
  - Amaurosis fugax is the strongest predictor of future blindness.

K. Bonnick (✉) · A. Murga
Department of Surgery, Loma Linda University, Loma Linda, CA, USA
e-mail: Kbonnick@llu.edu; amurga@llu.edu

A. Murga et al. (eds.), *The Vascular Surgery In-Training Examination Review (VSITE)*,
https://doi.org/10.1007/978-3-031-24121-5_18

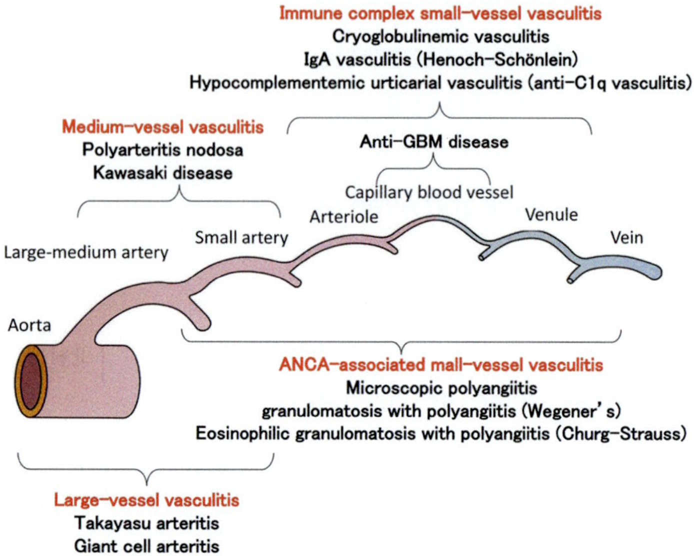

Fig. 18.1 Systemic Vasculitis. Reproduced with permission from 2012 Revised International Chapel Hill Consensus Conference Nomenclature of Vasculitides

- Etiology:
  - The exact etiology is unknown but there is some association with HLA-DRB104 gene.
  - Also noted that t-cell cytokine IFN-gamma is expressed in GCA.
- Risk factors:
  - Polymyalgia rheumatic.
  - Family history, race, age, and sex.
- Diagnosis:
  - At least 3 of 5 criteria must be present for the diagnosis of GCA [3].

    Age at disease onset >50.

    New headache.

    Temporal artery abnormality.

    Elevated erythrocyte sedimentation rate ESR.

    Abnormal artery biopsy.

  - Gold standard remains temporal artery biopsy; artery should be 2–3 cm in length [4].
  - Biopsies should be obtained ideally prior to starting steroids.
- Treatment:
  - Corticosteroid therapy is considered the standard of care.
  - Dosing: Initial 40–60 mg daily; with visual loss intravenous steroid should be considered.

    Inflammatory markers should be followed closely to tailor tapering of steroids.
  - Low dose aspirin is also recommended to reduce cardiovascular events.
  - Surgical interventions are rarely required.

Takayasu Arteritis ("Pulseless Disease")

- Clinical characteristics:
  - Fevers, weakness, fatigue, arthralgia, hypertension, weight loss, carotidynia, unequal pulses or absent pulses and unequal BP in extremities, bruits, limb claudication, neurogenic syncope, TIA, visual disturbances, middle aortic syndrome.
- Epidemiology:
  - Most often occurs in people ages 18–40 years and affects women more frequently than men.
  - More common in patients from East Asia and the incidence varies by geographic location.
- Etiology:
  - Increased susceptibility in patients with gene mutation in the HLA-A, -D and -DR.
  - Immune-mediated mechanism.
- Diagnostic Criteria:
  - The 1990 American College of Rheumatology diagnostic criteria were created with a sensitivity of 90.5% and a specificity of 97.8% if at least three of the six criteria were met as described by Arend et al. [5].

  - General inflammatory markers are frequently followed consisting of erythrocyte sedimentation rate (ESR), C-reactive protein (CRP), and interleukin-6 (IL-6).
  - All forms of imaging have been used to assess vessels affected by Takayasu.

    Digital subtraction angiography remains the "gold standard" for evaluation of vascular lesions.

    Lesion characteristics of TA include: stenosis, short, segmental or long and diffuse occlusion/stenosis, aneurysmal dilation.
- Treatment:
  - Medical management:

    Glucocorticoids are first line agents and can be tapered if improvement in disease.

    In patients without remission with glucocorticoids other agents can be added.

    - Methotrexate, cyclophosphamide, azathioprine, or mycophenolate mofetil.

    In patient with refractory disease anti-TNF therapy can be added.

    - Infliximab (Remicade) and adalimumab (Humira).

    Anti-IL-6 therapy has also been used to induce remission.

    - tocilizumab,
  - Surgical management:

    Approximately 50% of patients that develop Takayasu's arteritis in the United States will need surgery as discussed by Ehlert and Abularrage [6].

    Interventions should be performed when patient in the quiescent phase as discussed by Ehlert and Abularrage [6].
  - Indications for surgical intervention include:

    Hypertension in setting of renal artery stenosis.

    Lifestyle limiting ischemia.

    Cerebral ischemia.

    Cardiac ischemia.

    Severe aortic coarctation.

    Aortic regurgitation.
    Progressive aneurysmal enlargement.
  - Endovascular options.
    Percutaneous transluminal angioplasty.
    Bare metal stents
    Covered stents.
    Drug coated balloons and stents.
  - Open surgical treatment.
    Mainstay in the treatment of problems associated with Takayasu's.
    - Common carotid bypass, typically performed for stroke prevention.
    - Upper extremity bypass for subclavian and axillary lesions.
    - Coronary artery bypass.
    - Aortic bypass surgery with revascularization of the visceral arteries if needed.

Medium Vessel Disease

Polyarteritis Nodosa (PAN)

- Clinical characteristics:
  - Will present with constitutional symptoms: fevers, fatigue, weight loss.
  - Skin lesions-including palpable purpura, livedo reticularis.
  - Hypertension with proteinuria and hematuria often microscopic.
  - Peripheral neuropathy, mononeuritis multiplex, abdominal pain.
- Etiology:
  - Can be either idiopathic or secondary to infection including hepatitis B and HIV.
  - Also can be associated as a paraneoplastic manifestation-hairy-cell leukemia.
- Pattern of Involvement:
  - Mainly affects medium sized vessels and causes segmental necrotizing vasculitis, spares large vessels.

- Diagnostic criteria:
  - No diagnostic serologic tests for PAN.
  - Can have elevated inflammatory markers, ESR and CRP.
  - Rheumatoid factor, cryoglobulins, antinuclear antibodies, and ANCA should be negative.
  - As described by Lightfoot et al. in Table 18.1 [7] diagnosis is based on presence of 3 out of the 10 criteria established by the American college of Rheumatology.

Table 18.1 American College of Rheumatology Diagnostic Criteria for Polyarteritis Nodosa. (Taken from Rutherford's Vascular Surgery and Endovascular Therapy 9th ed. Ch.137. p. 1801)

Criterion	Definition
Weight loss >4 kg	Loss of at least 4 kg since illness began without dieting or other confounding factors
Livedo reticularis	Mottled reticular pattern over the skin of extremities or torso
Testicular pain or tenderness	Pain or tenderness of the testicles not due to infection, trauma, or other causes
Myalgias, weakness or leg tenderness	Diffuse myalgias or weakness of muscles, tenderness of leg muscles
Mononeuropathy or polyneuropathy	Development of mononeuropathy, multiple mononeuropathies, or polyneuropathy
Diastolic BP >90	Development of hypertension with diastolic BP >90 mmHg
Elevated BUN or creatinine	Elevation of BUN >40 mg/dL or creatinine >1.5 mg/dL
Hepatitis B infection	Presence of Hepatitis B Surface antigen or antibody in serum
Arteriographic abnormality	Arteriogram showing aneurysms or occlusions of visceral arteries not due to arteriosclerosis, fibromuscular dysplasia, or noninflammatory causes
Biopsy of small or medium-sized artery demonstrating polymorphonuclear neutrophils	Histologic changes showing presence of granulocytes, and or mononuclear leukocytes in vessel wall

- Treatment:
  - Hepatitis associated PAN-start antiviral therapy prior to immunosuppression.
  - PAN not viral associated:
    Mild and isolated cutaneous disease-monotherapy with prednisone.
    Moderate to severe-induction therapy using steroid and cyclophosphamide, followed with remission medication using methotrexate or azathioprine.

Buerger's Disease

- Clinical presentation:
  - Most common presentation is lower extremity claudication.
  - In severe case can present with digital ischemia in the form of rest pain, ulceration or gangrene in either lower or upper extremities.
- Epidemiology:
  - Strong association with tobacco exposure.
  - Predominantly found in young men between the ages of 18–55 year old.
  - Also it is more prevalent in people from middle east background.
- Pattern of involvement: medium sized vessels often infrapopliteal or brachial arteries.
- Diagnostic criteria:
  - Usually diagnosis of exclusion.
  - Smoking history, onset before 50 absence of atherosclerotic risk factors.
  - Echocardiogram to rule out any infections process.
  - Non-invasive testing demonstrating abnormal digital patterns.
  - Angiography will demonstrate normal proximal vessels without atherosclerosis with collateralization around areas of occlusion.
    Usually collaterals will appear as spider web or corkscrew.

- Treatment:
  - The most important treatment is smoking cessation.
  - Calcium channel blockers or pentoxifylline can be useful.
  - Exercise for claudication symptoms.
  - Often amputation is required.

Kawasaki Disease

- Clinical presentation:
  - High grade fevers, conjunctivitis, erythema, rash and edema of the hands and feet and lymphadenopathy in the acute phase.
  - Postacute phase patients can present with coronary artery dilation and aneurysm leading to myocardial infarction.
- Etiology:
  - Unknown etiology but presumed multifactorial with infection and genetic predisposition playing a role.
- As described by Kawasaki [8] diagnostic criteria:
  - Fever greater than 5 days with a peak of greater than 104F and four or more of the following features:

    Polymorphic rash.

    Bilateral conjunctival erythema.

    Changes in mucosal membranes in oral cavity (strawberry tongue, cracked lips, erythema).

    Cervical lymphadenopathy >1.5 cm.

    Changes in extremities (erythema of palms and soles).
  - Elevated inflammatory markers, leukocytosis and thrombocytosis are common lab findings.
  - Routine echocardiography.
- Pattern of involvement:
  - Coronary artery aneurysms, systemic arteritis particularly iliac arteritis.
- Treatment:
  - IV immunoglobulin and aspirin therapy.
  - Surgical Intervention: Coronary artery bypass and percutaneous angioplasty, cardiac transplantation is reserved for severe ischemic heart disease.

Small Vessel Disease

Eosinophilic Granulomatosis with Polyangiitis (Churg-Strauss Syndrome)

- Clinical presentation:
  - Often a three stage process.
  - Initially will present with allergic rhinitis, asthma, nasal polyposis, and recurrent fevers.
  - Followed by development of pulmonary infiltrates, eosinophilia, chronic eosinophilic pneumonia, gastroenteritis.
  - Palpable purpura and subcutaneous nodules are often present.
  - Late stage will present with myocarditis, valvular insufficiency, and systemic vasculitis.
- Etiology:
  - Pathogenesis is unknown.
  - Suggestion of a link to cytokine pathways that stimulate eosinophils.
  - Leukotriene inhibitors may contribute to pathogenesis.
- Pattern of involvement:
  - Affects mainly the small and medium-sized vessels and associated with eosinophilia.
- Diagnostic criteria:
  - Inflammatory markers (CRP and ESR) are often elevated and pANCA is positive.
  - According to Masi et al. [9] there need to be at least 4 of 6 criteria must be present:

    asthma, eosinophilia, mononeuropathy or polyneuropathy, non-fixed pulmonary infiltrates, paranasal sinus abnormalities or biopsy finding eosinophilic infiltrates,
- Treatment:
  - Induction therapy with IV steroids, along with cyclophosphamide or rituximab.

Wegener's Disease (Granulomatosis with Polyangiitis)

- Clinical presentation:
  - Chronic sinusitis, epistaxis, chronic purulent nasal drainage.
  - Chronic inflammation of the auditory canal which can cause acute or chronic otitis media.
  - Central nervous system involvement includes cranial neuropathies, spinal cord lesions, pituitary involvement.
  - Pulmonary involvement includes nodules and infiltrates, can form granulomas.
- Epidemiology:
  - Mean age of diagnosis is 40 s.
  - More common in Caucasian.
- Pattern of Involvement:
  - Primarily involves upper and lower respiratory tract and kidneys.
- Diagnostic criteria:
  - c-ANCA positivity with PR-3 specificity.
  - Screening urinalysis to evaluate for proteinuria, casts, hematuria or pyuria.
  - Tissue diagnosis gold standard.
- Treatment:
  - Involves a combination of high dose steroids and either cyclophosphamide or rituximab.
  - Limited disease can be treated with steroids and either methotrexate or mycophenolate mofetil.

Radiation Induced Arterial Disease

- Clinical presentation:
  - Can present similar to symptoms of atherosclerosis.
    Transient ischemic attacks, amaurosis fugax, stroke, mesenteric angina, claudication, embolization, or aneurysm formation.

  - Presentation can be delayed for decades from initial radiation exposure.
- Epidemiology:
  - External radiation used for treatment of malignancies can lead to inflammation and fibrosis of vessels over time.
- Pattern of Involvement:
  - Early phase, there is endothelial damage, intimal thickening, and smooth muscle fibrosis.
    Intimal thickening and proliferation, medial hyalinization, proteoglycan deposition, and cellular infiltration of the adventitia.
  - Later phase will lead to calcification and atherosclerosis formation.
- Diagnostic criteria:
  - Similar to typical atherosclerosis workup noninvasive including duplex.
  - Angiography.
- Treatment:
  - As a result of poor wound healing endovascular is preferred method to manage lesions.

Popliteal Entrapment Syndrome (PAES)

- Clinical presentation:
  - Affects mostly young healthy, physically active males.
  - Typical presentation is lower extremity claudication, which could be atypical or paradoxical.
  - Paresthesia, cramping, swelling, feeling of fullness, acute limb ischemia, chronic limb ischemia.
  - Pedal pulses are normal at rest, but will diminish with passive dorsiflexion or active plantar flexion of the foot.
  - Typically, will present as unilateral.
- Etiology:
  - The lower extremity artery system arises from the axial and external iliac arteries.
  - Both gastrocnemius muscle heads originate from the proximal tibia and they both migrate during development.

- Classification of PAES (see Fig. 18.2) [10]:
  - **Type I**: Popliteal artery entrapped medially under the head of the gastrocnemius with normal attachment of the gastrocnemius muscle.
  - **Type II**: Medial displacement of the artery and entrapment by abnormal attachment of the medial head of the gastrocnemius muscle to the lateral aspect of the medial femoral condyle.
  - **Type III**: Abnormal muscle flap or band from the medial or lateral femoral condyle. Can also occur when there is a double origin of the gastrocnemius muscle that can surround and compress the popliteal artery.
  - **Type IV**: Persistence of fetal artery deep to the popliteus muscle.

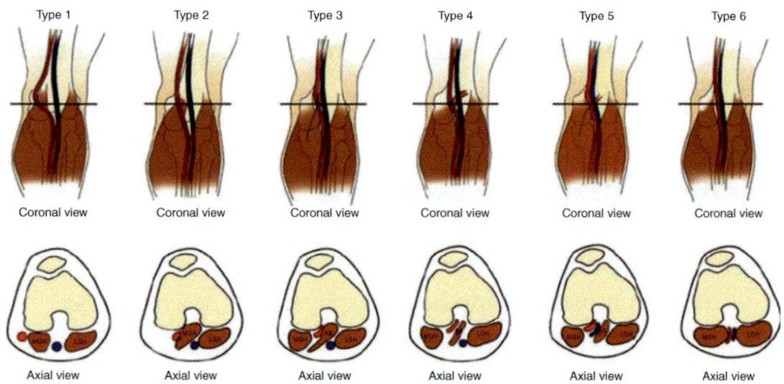

Fig. 18.2 Popliteal artery entrapment Syndrome Classification. Coronal and axial views of different types of popliteal artery entrapment syndrome (PAES) (*LGH* lateral gastrocnemius head, *AS* accessory slip of MGH, *PM* popliteus muscle). Type 1: normal attachment of MGH, medial course of PA. Type 2: lateral attachment of MGH, PA medially deviated. Type 3: PA between accessory slip of MGH. Type 4: PA posterior to PM. Type 5: any PAES involving papliteal vein (type 3 in this case). Type 6: hypertrophied gastrocnemius muscles entrapping normally localized PA (with permission from Kim et al.) (Reproduced with permission from Popliteal artery entrapment syndrome: morphological classification utilizing MR imaging. September 2006, Volume 35, Issue 9, pp. 648–658; Fig. 18.3)

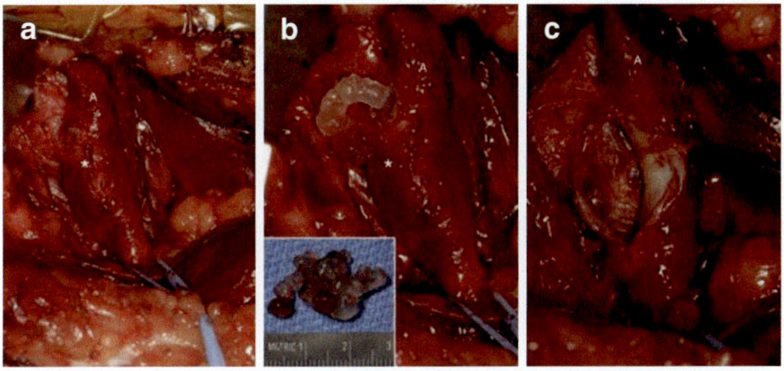

Fig. 18.3 Adventitial Cystic Disease. (**a**) Cystic adventitial disease of the popliteal artery. (**b**) Incision of adventitia with drainage of mucoid material (inset). (**c**) The popliteal artery after evacuation of mucoid cyst. (Taken from Rutherford's Vascular Surgery and Endovascular Therapy ninth ed. Ch 143. p. 1901)

  - **Type V**: Entrapment of both popliteal artery and vein.
  - **Type VI**: Symptoms of PEAS without anatomic abnormality. Type VI is thought to be related to hypertrophy of the gastrocnemius muscle or a particularly lateral attachment of the medial head of the gastrocnemius muscle to the medial femoral condyle.
- Diagnostic evaluation:
  - Exercise treadmill testing.
  - Duplex study with provocative maneuvers initial diagnostic tool of choice (passive dorsiflexion or active plantar flexion).
  - Computed tomography and magnetic resonance imaging, useful if vessel is disease and or occluded.
  - Angiography remains gold standard in particular if the following angiographic findings are present:

    Medial deviation of the proximal popliteal artery.

    Focal occlusion of the popliteal artery.

    Post-stenotic dilation of the distal popliteal artery.
- Treatment:
  - For the symptomatic patient surgical intervention is warranted.
  - Approach to surgery is based on anatomy, presentation, and patency of artery.

Table 18.2 Treatment options for Popliteal Artery Entrapment Syndrome. (Taken from Rutherford's Vascular Surgery and Endovascular Therapy 9th ed. Ch. 143. p. 1898)

Status of Artery	Entrapment Type	Operation	Surgical Approach
Normal	I and II	Myotomy	Medial
	III and IV	Myotomy	Posterior
	V	Myotomy	Medial or posterior
	VI	Myotomy if symptomatic	Medial or posterior
Abnormal (occluded, stenosed, or poststenotic dilatation or aneurysm)	I to VI	Decompression and arterial resection and replacement or exclusion and bypass	Medial or posterior

- Early intervention allows for limited surgery to the muscle rather than arterial reconstruction.
- Endovascular intervention is of limited use as muscular anatomy is still present without any myotomy.
- Management options for PAES (see Table 18.2) [11]

Adventitial Cystic Disease (ACD)

- Clinical presentation:
  - Typical presentation is young male with sudden onset of calf claudication with short distances.
  - Typically, unilateral, with recovery time being prolonged.
  - Diminished pedal pulses, audible bruit in the popliteal fossa.
  - Pedal pulses present at rest that may disappear with hip or knee flexion.
- Epidemiology:
  - Most commonly involved arteries are popliteal artery, external iliac, and femoral arteries.
  - Affects males 5 to 1 ratio and they are in their 40 s.
- Etiology:

  - Exact cause remains unclear and controversial.
  - Theories for ACD cause include:
    - Repetitive trauma: repetitive flexion and extension of the knee joint causes injury to the artery and cystic degeneration.
    - Ganglion: synovial cysts tract along arterial branches and implant in the adventitia.
    - Systemic disorder: systemic mucinous or myxomatous degenerative conditions lead to ACD.
    - Developmental: ACD occurs when mesenchymal mucinous cells are implanted in the adventitia of vessels during development.
    - Articular (synovial): synovial fluid from adjacent joints egresses and dissects along the adventitia of related vessels.
- Pathology:
  - Adventitial cysts are filled with gelatinous mucoid material (see Fig. 18.3).
  - Cyst contents are clear or yellow and typically unilocular.
- As described by Forbes and Kayssi [11] diagnostic criteria:
  - Ankle-brachial indices are normal at rest but drop after exercise.
  - Doppler ultrasound should be initial screen tool.
  - CTA or MRI can be used to further evaluate and differentiate popliteal arterial disease.
  - Angiography remains the gold standard for diagnosing ACD can demonstrate how cyst affects lumen.
- Treatment:
  - Typically separated into resection versus non-resection.
    - Resection: typically used in cases where artery is occluded.
      - Artery explored via a posterior approach and extent of resection depends on length of artery that is involved, with artery typically be reconstructed with vein.

Non-resection- non-occlusive stenosis.

- Transluminal angioplasty: uncommon.
- Cyst aspiration: cyst content can be viscous and difficult to completely aspirate, high recurrence rate.
- Cyst excision and evacuation.

Exercise-Related External Iliac Endofibrosis

- Clinical presentation:
  - Exercise induced claudication.
  - Typically seen in competitive bicyclists.
- Epidemiology:
  - Rare cause of arterial stenosis classically seen in young athletes.
  - Occurs in both men and women.
  - Both external iliac arteries can be affected.
- Etiology:
  - It is thought to be related to repetitive trauma to the vessel by stretching and compression, which can then lead to development of fibrosis and thickened artery wall.
- Diagnostic criteria:
  - Workup should include immediate post-exercise ABI's and duplex ultrasonography.
  - CTA or MRA can help evaluate and serve for surgical planning.
- Treatment:
  - Surgical management:
- Bypass, endarterectomy with patch, angioplasty, and stenting.

Behcet Syndrome

- Clinical presentation:
  - Typically presents with oral and genital ulcers, skin lesions, and uveitis.
  - Vascular presentation at young age, which include arterial and venous thrombosis, aneurysm especially in the pulmonary arteries and central vein thrombosis.

- Epidemiology:
  - Has been documented worldwide, but more common in middle eastern regions.
  - Young patients usually in 20 s to 40 s.
- Etiology:
  - Unknown but there is high prevalence in patients with HLA-B51 genotype.
- Diagnostic criteria:
  - International Criteria for Behcet's Disease [11]:

    Recurrent oral ulcerations at least three times in one year.

    Plus two of the following:
    - Recurrent genital ulcerations, uveitis or retinal vasculitis, erythema nodosum, acneiform nodules, positive pathergy test.
- Treatment:
  - Systemic immunosuppression with steroids and biologic agents.
  - For mucocutaneous lesions colchicine has been used.

Congenital Connective Tissue Syndromes

- Marfan's:
  - Clinical presentation:

    Ectopia lentis, aortic root dissection/dilation, dural ectasia, long bone overgrowth, marfanoid habitus.
  - Etiology:

    Autosomal dominant, Fibrillin 1 gene mutation.
  - Diagnostic criteria:

    In the absence of family history there are four criteria that diagnose.

    1. Aortic Root dilation Z score of greater or equal to 2 AND ectopia lentis.
    2. Aortic Root dilation Z score of greater or equal to 2 AND systemic score of 7 points or more.
    3. Aortic Root dilation Z score of greater or equal to 2 AND FBN1.

    4. Ectopia lentis AND a FBN1 mutation associated with Aortic Root dilation.

    In the presence of Family history.

    1. Ectopia lentis AND family history of Marfan syndrome.
    2. A systemic score of greater or equal to 7 points and family history of Marfan syndrome.
    3. Aortic Root dilation Z score greater or equal to 2 above 20 years old AND family history of Marfan syndrome.

  - Treatment.

    Medical: Beta adrenergic receptor blockade, HR <70, angiotensin II receptor antagonist.

    Surgical: Aortic root replacement- 5 cm, Aortic arch 5.5–6.0 cm and descending thoracic or TAAA 5.5–6.0 cm, infrarenal abdominal aortic aneurysm 5.0 cm.

- Ehlers-Danlos Syndrome.
  - Clinical presentation:

    Clubfoot, early onset varicose veins, gingival recession, family history, thin translucent skin, extensive bruising, joint hypermobility, aneurysm, AV fistula or dissections, spontaneous rupture of bowel or gravid uterus.

  - Etiology:

    Mutations in COL3A1 gene which produces defective type III procollagen.

  - Treatment:

    Medical: celiprolol reduces incidence of vascular ruptures in patients with EDS, Beta-adrenergic receptor blockade, HR <70, angiotensin II receptor antagonist.

    Surgical: Aortic root replacement- 5 cm, Aortic arch 5.5–6.0 cm and descending thoracic or TAAA 5.5–6.0 cm, infrarenal abdominal aortic aneurysm 5.0 cm.

- Loeys-Dietz Syndrome:
  - Clinical presentation:

    Craniofacial abnormalities, hypertelorism and artery aneurysm or/and tortuosity, bifid uvula.

- Etiology:
  Gene mutations in genes encoding TGF-beta receptors 1 and 2, SMAD3 genes.
- Treatment:
  Medical: Medical management- beta adrenergic receptor blockade and surveillance.
  Surgical: any aortic segment 4 to 5 cm or growth of the aneurysm more than 0.5 cm in 1 year.

• Stent grafts should not be used in the aorta of patient with connective tissue disorder.
• True aneurysms in Ehlers Danlos syndrome are rare and conservative management is recommended.
• Angiography should be avoided as patients are at highest risk of tissue fragility.

Questions and Answers

1. A 35y.o M smoker presents with sudden cyanosis of the second and third digits of the right hand with gangrene of the tip of the second digit. The remaining digits are not affected. Which of the following is true regarding his diagnosis?
   (A) Distal revascularization is indicated to preserve the digits
   (B) Embolic sources should be ruled out
   (C) Abstinence from tobacco does not induce disease remission
   (D) The disease affects only young men
2. A 43-year-old competitive amateur cyclist presents for evaluation of symptoms of burning left thigh pain approximately 5 miles into her ride. Her symptoms have progressed to include pain when walking rapidly up an incline or stairs but not on level ground. Which of the following regarding management is true?
   (A) Endovascular therapy should be attempted
   (B) If surgical management is indicated endarterectomy and vein patch repair of the external iliac should be performed
   (C) Exercise cessation is recommended
   (D) Surgical management should include musculotendinous release of the gastrocnemius muscle.

3. A 71-year-old female presents to the emergency department complaining of right eye blindness and headache that recently started. Her CRP and ESR are elevated. The gold standard for diagnosis is?
   (A) Inguinal lymph node biopsy
   (B) CTA of the head and neck
   (C) Temporal artery biopsy
   (D) MRI of the head
   (E) Greater auricular nerve biopsy

Answers: 1 (B), 2 (B), 3 (C)

References

1. Jennette JC. ClassificationNon-atherosclerotic vascular diseaseclassification is based on 2012 Chapel Hill Consensus Conference nomenclature of vasculitides which is based on vessel size NIH Public Access. 2014;17(5):603–6.
2. Guillevin L, Hagen EC, Hoffman GS, Jayne DR, Kallenberg CGM, Lamprecht P. Arthritis Rheum. 2013;65(1):1–11.
3. Dasgupta B, Borg FA, Hassan N, Alexander L, Barraclough K, Bourke B, et al. BSR and BHPR guidelines for the management of giant cell arteritis. Rheumatology (Oxford). 2010;49:1594–7.
4. Ness T, Bley TA, Schmidt WA, Lamprecht P. The Diagnosis and Treatment of Giant Cell Arteritis. Dtsch Arztebl Int. 2013;110(21):376–87.
5. Arend WP, Michel BA, Block DA, Hunder GG, Calabrese LH, Edworthy SM, Fauci AS, Leavitt RY, Lie JT, Lightfoot RW Jr. The American College of Rheumatology 1990 criteria for the classification of Takayasu arteritis. Arthritis Rheum. 1990;33(8):1129–34.
6. Ehlert BA, Abularrage CJ. Takayasu disease. In: Sidawy AN, Perler BA, editors. Rutherford's vascular surgery and endovascular therapy. 9th ed. Amsterdam: Elsevier; 2019.
7. Lightfoot RW Jr, Michel BA, Block DA, Hunder GG, Zvaifler NJ, McShane DJ, Arend WP, Calabrese LH, Leavitt RY, Lie JT. The American College of Rheumatology 1990 criteria for the classification of polyarteritis nodosa. Arthritis Rheum. 1990;33(8):1088–93.
8. Kawasaki T. Kawasaki disease. Proc Jpn Acad Ser B Phys Biol Sci. 2006;82(2):59–71.
9. Masi AT, Hunder GG, Lie JT, Michel BA, Block DA, Arend WP, Calabrese LH, Edworthy SM, Fauci AS, Leavitt RY. The American

College of Rheumatology 1990 criteria for the classification of Churg-Strauss syndrome. Arthritis Rheum. 1990;33(8):1094–100.
10. Kim HK, Shin MJ, Kim SM, Lee SH, Hong HJ. Popliteal artery entrapment syndrome: morphological classification utilizing MR imaging. Skelet Radiol. 2006;35:648–58.
11. Davatchi F, Assaad-Khalil S, Calamia KT, Crook J, Sadeghi-Abdollahi B, Schirmer M, et al. The international criteria for Behcet's disease (ICBD): a collaborative study of 27 countries on the sensitivity and specificity of the new criteria. J Eur Acad Dermatol Venereol. 2014;28(3):338–47.

Vascular Trauma

19

Anna Romagnoli and Megan Brenner

Initial Evaluation

Hard signs of vascular injury: active hemorrhage, expanding or pulsatile hematoma, bruit or thrill over wound, pulse deficit, signs of extremity ischemia [2].

- Proceed directly to operating room without time-consuming adjunctive studies.

Soft signs of vascular injury: history of arterial bleeding, proximity of wound to major vessel, non-pulsatile hematoma, neurologic deficit adjacent to named artery

- Additional workup:
  - Injured extremity index (IEI)/ankle-brachial index (ABI): ratio of highest systolic occlusion pressure in injured extremity (distal to injury) to the highest proximal vessel

A. Romagnoli
University of Maryland Shock Trauma Center, Baltimore, MD, USA
e-mail: anna.romagnoli@som.umaryland.edu

M. Brenner (✉)
University of California Los Angeles, Los Angeles, CA, United States
e-mail: m.brenner@ruhealth.org

A. Murga et al. (eds.), *The Vascular Surgery In-Training Examination Review (VSITE)*,
https://doi.org/10.1007/978-3-031-24121-5_19

systolic occlusion pressure in an uninjured extremity (usually brachial artery).
  - IEI >0.9 high NPV for vascular injury.
  - IEI ≤0.9 predictive of vascular injury, needs more workup [3, 4].
  - CT angiography NPV of 100% [5].
  - Catheter arteriography gold standard study.

Aortic Occlusion

Resuscitative thoracotomy with aortic cross-clamping: redistributes blood volume to myocardium and brain. In penetrating thoracic trauma provides direct access to injured organs, associated with ~20% survival rate [6]. <5% survival rate in setting of abdominal trauma [6].

- Operative approach: Supine anterolateral thoracotomy performed in fifth intercostal space.
  - Key points: dividing the sternum with Lebsche knife provides superior visualization of the midline structures. Take down inferior pulmonary ligament, taking care not to injure pulmonary vein. Incise mediastinal pleura the level of the diaphragm, blunt dissection of aorta to free from esophagus and prevertebral fascia. Clamp placed across aorta alone.

Supraceliac Aortic Control

- Operative approach: midline exploratory laparotomy.
  - Key points: Retract left lobe of liver to patient's right, open gastrohepatic ligament. Retract distal and esophagus, manually compress aorta. Divide right crus of diaphragm, pass clamp taking care to not injure posterior branches of vagus nerve.

Resuscitative endovascular balloon occlusion of the aorta (REBOA): Supports proximal pressure and controls hemorrhage equivalent with resuscitative thoracotomy [7, 8]. Improved survival to definitive intervention [9, 10], survival benefit [11]. Indications under investigation (Fig. 19.1).

- REBOA zones [12, 13].
  - Zone I: Left subclavian to celiac artery, indication subdiaphragmatic hemorrhage.
  - Zone II: Visceral aorta, indication NO occlusion.
  - Zone III: Lowest renal to aortic bifurcation, pelvic fracture, bleeding below aortic bifurcation.

Relative Contraindications to REBOA use: penetrating thoracic injury in cardiac arrest (unless REBOA used in conjunction

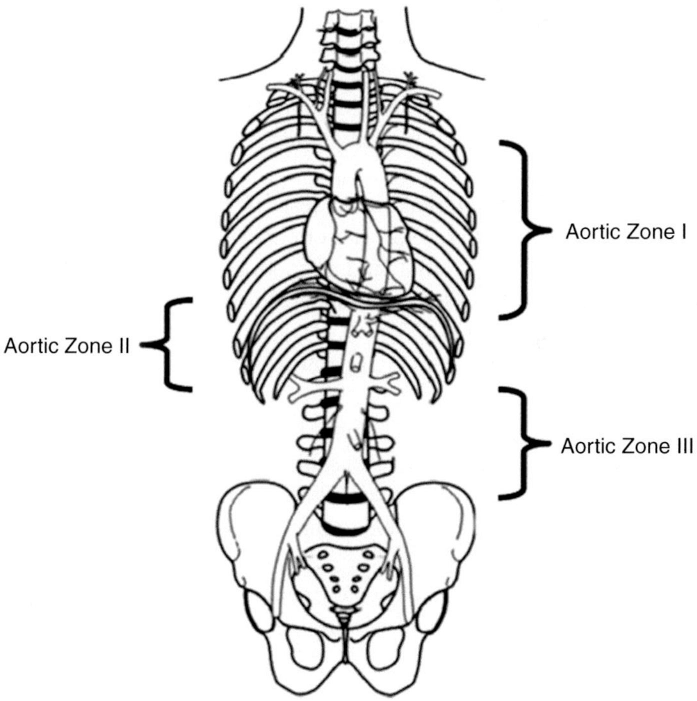

Fig. 19.1 REBOA zones of occlusion. (Taken from The Journal of Trauma and Acute Care Surgery. August 2013, volume 75 issue 2)

with ED thoracotomy) severe intrathoracic vascular hemorrhage (evidenced on CXR, CT placement, or ultrasound).

- Procedure: common femoral artery access, sheath placement, balloon position and inflation, management while occluded, balloon deflation, sheath removal, and post-resuscitation care.

Aortic Injury

Blunt thoracic aortic injury: uncommon but lethal (incidence <1% [14, 15]), second most frequent cause of mortality after blunt trauma [16, 17], 85% prehospital mortality [18].

- Mechanism: shear, torsion, pinch, stretch, and hydrostatic forces. >60% oat aortic isthmus, fixed descending thoracic aorta meets mobile arch [19].
- Presentation: ranges from asymptomatic to chest, back, or shoulder pain. Normal hemodynamics or obvious shock [20].
- Workup:
  - AP CXR initial diagnostic test of choice. Widening of mediastinum (Fig. 19.2) (>8 cm at level of aortic knob, left pleural effusion, first and second rib fractures, tracheal deviation, depressed left bronchus, indistinct aortic knob, or apical capping [21, 22]).
  - CTA 95–100% sensitivity, 99–100% negative predictive value [23–25].
  - Formal angiography, TEE and IVUS can be utilized.
- Blunt thoracic aortic injury classification [26, 27].
  - Grade I: Intimal tear; medical management.
  - Grade II: Intramural hematoma; medical management versus TEVAR.
  - Grade III: Pseudoaneurysm; treatment with TEVAR.
  - Grade IV: Full thickness injury with rupture; treatment with TEVAR.

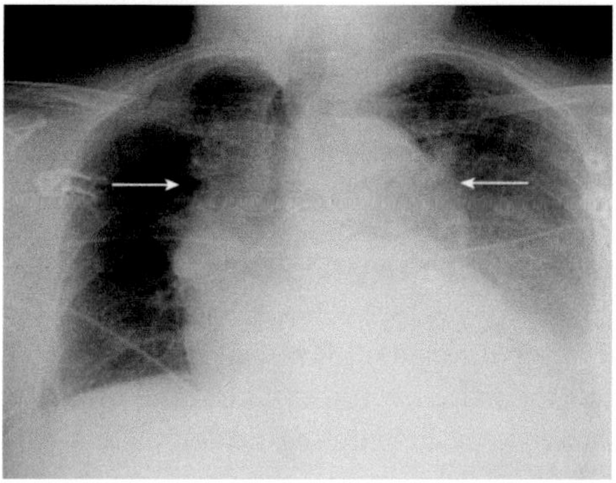

Fig. 19.2 AP CXR with widened mediastinum. (Taken with permission from Braunwald's Heart Disease, Ch 42, January 2022, p 196)

- Management.
  - Immediate medical management with aggressive blood pressure and heart rate control, SBP <100, HR <60 with intravenous beta blocker, consider addition of nitroprusside [28, 29].
  - Medical management alone may be adequate for grade I injuries [27], SVS guidelines recommend TEVAR for grade II injuries [27]; however, recent data suggests that only 5% of grade I and II injuries advance on serial injuries [30] and more selective management may be appropriate.
  - Urgent repair for grade II–IV injuries [27], TEVAR mainstay of treatment [27, 31].
  - Left subclavian artery coverage well tolerated without prophylactic carotid subclavian bypass [32].
  - Open repair indicated in absence of acceptable proximal landing zone or inability to support such a procedure at the facility in question.
- Timing.
  - SVS recommends urgent intervention [27].
  - TEVAR following 24 h period of hemodynamic optimization associated with improved survival [33].

- Complex polytrauma patient may have contraindications to maintaining hemodynamics within the above-mentioned parameters (traumatic brain and spinal cord injury) necessitating operative intervention.

Abdominal Aortic Injury (Fig. 19.3)

- Zones of retroperitoneum [34]: see Fig. 19.3.
  - Zone I: Abdominal aorta, IVC, visceral branches.
    Management: Penetrating-explore; Blunt-explore.
  - Zone II: Bilateral paracolic gutters, renal vessels, kidneys.
    Management: Penetrating-Explore; Blunt-Explore if expanding or pulsatile hematoma.
  - Zone III: Iliac arteries and veins.
    Management: Penetrating-explore; Blunt-explore if expanding or pulsatile hematoma.
- Abdominal aortic injury classification [26, 35] and management [36].
  - Grade I: Intimal tear/minimal aortic injury, imaging finding <10 mm in size, no contour abnormality on CTA, management includes blood pressure control, HR control, antiplatelet therapy.
  - Grade II: Large intimal flap, imaging finding >10 mm in size no contour abnormality on CT, management includes blood pressure and HR control, repeat imaging within 48 h.
  - Grade III: pseudoaneurysm, stent graft placement or open repair.
  - Grade IV: Rupture, extravasation of contrast, very high mortality, proximal control open or endovascular, can consider shunt with chest tube.
- Abdominal aortic zones [29].
  - Abdominal aortic zone I: from diaphragmatic hiatus to SMA.
    Approach: Laparotomy, through lesser sac or left medial visceral rotation with kocherization of duodenum, can present with contained hematoma, can be treated endovascularly.

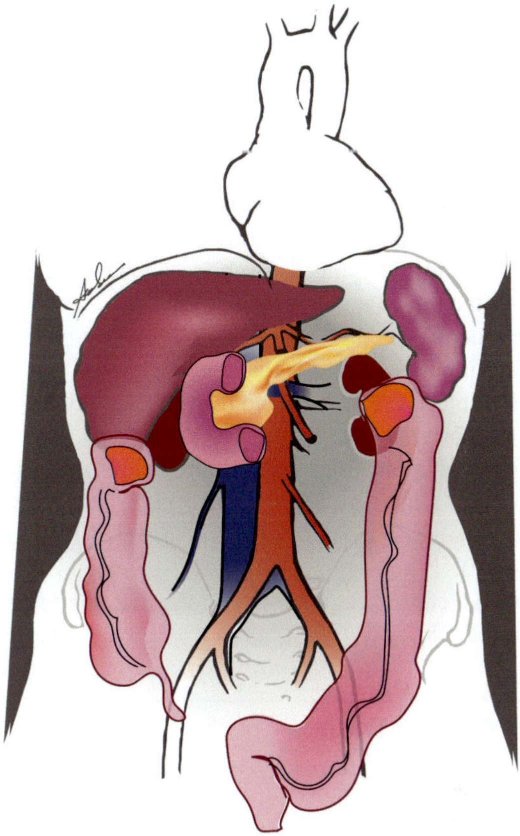

Fig. 19.3 *Zones of retroperitoneum*. (Illustration by © Sara B. Edwards, MD MS FACS Visceral Anatomy LLC)

- Abdominal aortic zone II: SMA to renal arteries.

  Approach:- Laparotomy with left medial visceral rotation with kocherization of duodenum, most lethal, obtain proximal control before opening hematoma.
- Abdominal aortic zone III: Infrarenal.

  Approach: Laparotomy, lift transverse mesocolon, eviscerate small bowel, takedown ligament of treitz to expose aorta, open peritoneum inferior to left renal vein, can be treated endovascularly.

- Timing: based on hemodynamic stability and concomitant injuries.

Iliac Artery Injury

- Operative approach: Midline laparotomy.
  - Key points: eviscerate small bowel to patient's right, open peritoneum overlying aortic bifurcation. Identify and preserve the ureter at pelvic brim.
- Management.
  - Small injuries: primary repair.
  - Large injuries: resection and reconstruction with prosthetic or autologous conduit.
  - Gross contamination: risk of later blow out after repair. Consider endovascular repair [37] or ligation and extra-anatomic bypass outside of infected field (fem-fem, ax-fem).
  - Damage control: ligation, well tolerated due to pelvic collaterals [38].

Visceral Arterial Trauma

Celiac Artery

- Operative approach: Midline laparotomy, left medial visceral rotation or through lesser sac.
- Management:
  - Small nondestructive injuries: primary repair.
  - Damage control: celiac can be ligated due to extensive collaterals with SMA [39, 40]; however, gallbladder ischemia may result so cholecystectomy must be performed [39, 41].

Superior Mesenteric Artery

- Fullen SMA zone classification [42].
  - Zone I: trunk proximal to first branch.

    Left medial visceral rotation or through root of mesentery beneath pancreas via lesser sac, maximal ischemia risk. Supplies jejunum, ileum, right colon.
  - Zone II: trunk between inferior pancreaticoduodenal and middle colic arteries.

    Left medial visceral rotation or through root of mesentery beneath pancreas via lesser sac, moderate risk of ischemia. Supplies small bowel and right colon.
  - Zone III: trunk distal to middle colic.

    Eviscerate small bowel to the patient's right and divide ligament of treitz or mobilize duodenum off SMA, minimal risk of bowel ischemia.
  - Zone IV: segmental branches.

    Exposed directly by opening the mesenteric hematoma, minimal risk of ischemia.
- Management.
  - Small injuries: primary repair.
  - Large or destructive injuries: patch angioplasty, interposition graft and reimplantation should be considered.
  - Damage control: Shunting is a viable option in unstable patients [43], ligation can be performed, but bowel ischemia may occur. Second look laparotomy is recommended if ligation is performed.

Inferior Mesenteric Artery

- Management.
  - Small injuries: primary repair.
  - Complex or destructive injuries: Ligation. Generally well tolerated, however in rare cases can result in colorectal ischemia especially in setting of premorbid atherosclerotic disease.

Carotid Injury: Carotid artery injury occurs in ~6% of all penetrating neck injury with 10–20% in-hospital mortality [44].

Blunt extracranial carotid injury: secondary to hyperextension, rotation, or flexion of the neck; vessel laceration from bony fracture; direct vessel impact [45]. Significant neurologic morbidity (60%) and mortality (19–43%) [45] with often times delayed symptom onset.

- Screening criteria: arterial hemorrhage from neck/nose/mouth, cervical bruit patient <50yo, expanding cervical hematoma, focal neurologic deficits, deficits inconsistent with head CT, stroke on CT or MRI, and high-energy transfer mechanisms with LeFort II or III fractures, cervical spine fractures involving C1–C3 and/or transverse foramen, skull base fractures involving carotid canal, cervical spine subluxation, near hanging with hypoxic-ischemic injury [46].
- Workup: CTA initial screening modality of choice, catheter based angiography with digital subtraction imaging is gold standard [47].
- Blunt cerebrovascular injury classification [48].
  - Grade I: Luminal irregularity of dissection/intramural hematoma with <25% luminal narrowing.
  - Grade II: Dissection or intramural hematoma less than or equal of 25% of lumen.
  - Grade III: Pseudoaneurysm.
  - Grade IV: Vessel occlusion.
  - Grade V: Vessel transection.
- Management.
  - Observation alone: consider only if absolute contraindications to other management strategies.
  - Grade I–IV: nonoperative management with antithrombotic (systemic heparin) or antiplatelet therapy (clopidogrel 75 mg or ASA 325 mg) recommended [49], although optimal regimen and duration are not known. Heparinization seems to be superior to antiplatelet agents in symptomatic patients [50].

  - Grade V: require immediate attempts at surgical control, open or endovascular [48, 49].
- Follow-up imaging: 7–10 days post-injury or change in exam [47].
  - With progressive vessel narrowing or pseudoaneurysm enlargement, endovascular stents should be considered [47].

Anatomic Zones (Fig. 19.4)

- Zones of neck [51]: Penetrating Trauma. Becoming historic, as most management decisions are now based upon clinical assessment of patient.
- Workup: CT Angiography, esophagoscopy, esophogram, bronchoscopy.
- Management.
  - Selective neck exploration for patients not in hemorrhagic shock with concern for injury after nonoperative workup.

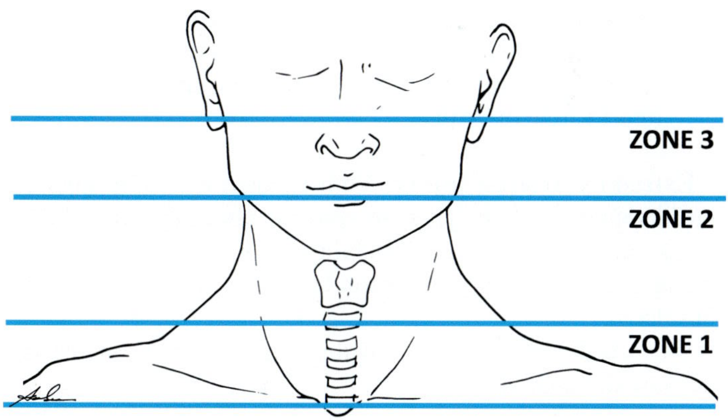

Fig. 19.4 Zones of neck. (Illustration by © Sara B. Edwards, MD MS FACS Visceral Anatomy LLC)

- Operative approach.
  - Zone I: comprises clavicle to cricoid, contains innominate vessels, origin of common carotid, subclavian and vertebral vessels; difficult to access. Exposure via sternotomy, endovascular approach recommended.
  - Zone II: comprises cricoid to angle of mandible, contains carotid and vertebral vessels, jugular veins; exposure via standard anterior sternocleidomastoid incision from base of skull to sternal notch. Sternotomy or endovascular balloon occlusion may be necessary for proximal control.
  - Zone III: comprises angle of mandible to base of skull, contains distal carotid and vertebral arteries, difficult to access. May require mandible subluxation or mandibulotomy. Endovascular approach recommended.
  - Contraindications to endovascular intervention include inability to safely pass a guidewire beyond injury, uncontrolled hemorrhage, airway compromise, concomitant aerodigestive injuries, and infected wounds.
  - Small injuries: primary repair.
  - Large or destructive injuries: patch angioplasty, resection and primary anastomosis, interposition graft or external carotid artery transposition.
  - Damage control: consideration should be given to shunting in the unstable patient. Ligation has been described without residual ischemic sequelae, predicated upon presence of intact Circle of Willis.

Extremity arterial injury: With isolated extremity injuries, consideration should be given to systemic anticoagulation. In the setting of hemodynamic instability and severe physiologic derangement, temporary intravascular shunts should strongly be considered.

Subclavian artery injury: challenging to access, increasing endovascular approach.

- Management:
  - Open approach: Right-sided injury—sternotomy with supraclavicular extension, left-sided injury—high thoracotomy (3–4 interspace). Due to the time-consuming and

morbid nature of these approaches, endovascular balloon occlusion should be strongly considered.
  - Small injuries: primary repair.
  - Large or destructive injuries: patch angioplasty, interposition graft
  - Stenting has been shown to be feasible for repair of these injuries [52].

Axillary Artery

- Management.
  - Open approach: infraclavicular incision that extends laterally into the deltopectoral groove, again, endovascular occlusion should be considered for proximal control.
  - Small injuries: primary repair.
  - Large or destructive injuries: patch angioplasty, interposition graft.
  - Stenting has been shown to be feasible for repair of these injuries [52].

Brachial artery: Due to its proximity to the humerus, supracondylar humerus fractures can be associated with intimal injury and subsequent thrombosis of the brachial artery or arterial transection. This may not be readily apparent due to extensive collateralization in the area.

- Management.
  - Open approach: longitudinal incision in the groove between biceps and triceps, avoid injury to the median nerve. Distal control can be obtained in the antecubital fossa via a curvilinear incision. The biceps tendon obscures the artery and often needs to be divided.
  - Small injuries: primary repair.
  - Large or destructive injuries: resection, mobilization and primary anastomosis may be performed, interposition graft may be necessary.

  - In the setting of injury distal to the radial/ulnar bifurcation, the decision to proceed with a complex revascularization or ligation depends on the presence of an intact palmar arch and adequate extremity perfusion.

Lower Extremity

Femoral arterial injury: Most commonly injured in penetrating mechanism

- Management.
  - Exposure: vertical incision over femoral triangle allowing easy proximal or distal extension. An oblique incision superior to the inguinal ligament allows retroperitoneal exposure of the iliac vessels.
  - Small injuries: repair primarily. If <50% circumference after debridement to clean edges, patch angioplasty.
  - <2 cm segmental defects adequate dissection may allow sufficient mobilization for primary tension-free repair.
  - Long defects, autologous (from contralateral extremity) or synthetic conduit may be utilized.
  - With concomitant complex orthopedic injuries or hemorrhagic shock, a vascular shunt should be placed. Orthopedic manipulation should then occur, followed by definitive repair if the patient's physiologic status permits. Early reperfusion is associated with improved neurologic outcomes [53].
  - Four compartment fasciotomies should be liberally performed.

Popliteal artery is the most commonly injured vessel following blunt mechanism; generally intimal disruption followed by thrombosis after posterior knee dislocation or tibial plateau fractures. Failure of timely revascularize leads to very high amputation rate in young trauma patients without well-developed arterial collaterals [54]. For penetrating injuries to the popliteal fossa, injury to the popliteal artery and vein must be ruled out. AV fistulas are not uncommon after missed injury and can be limb-threatening.

- Exposure: medial incision above knee to obtain proximal control with extension distally for distal control (which may require division of the medial head of the gastrocnemius). Care should be taken to preserve saphenous vein and deep veins.
- Management: Care should be taken to thoroughly evaluate the internal surface of the artery following blunt trauma, as the zone of injury and intimal disruption may propagate further than suggested on initial assessment.
  - Interposition graft with contralateral saphenous vein or synthetic conduit most commonly performed.

Shank Vessels

- *Tibioperoneal trunk* exposed through an incision along medial edge of tibia with division of medial head of gastrocnemius. The deep posterior compartment of the leg is entered, attachments of soleus and tibia are taken down.
- *Anterior tibial artery* exposure best obtained through anterolateral incision two fingerbreaths lateral to the anterior edge of the tibia. This is carried past the fascia between the tibialis anterior and extensor hallucis longus muscle.
- In the setting of hemodynamic instability or significant physiologic derangement, ligation of a single shank vessel should be considered instead of pursuing timely repair.

Venous Trauma

Most venous injuries can be ligated in setting of damage control, but improved outcomes have been demonstrated if attempts are made at venous injury repair [55].

IVC injury rare [56] but associated with 66% mortality rate [57].

Infrarenal IVC

- Exposure: right-sided medial visceral rotation.
- Management.
  - Low pressure system, trial gentle pressure, and application of topical hemostatic agent.
  - Small injury (<50% of circumference) repair transversely with lateral venorrhaphy [58], if larger or will cause narrowing, patch angioplasty should be performed.
  - Damage control: Ligation of infra-renal IVC is acceptable [59] but is associated with lower extremity edema and venous insufficiency, consider 4 compartment fasciotomies [60].

Suprarenal IVC

- Exposure: right-sided medial visceral rotation with Kocher maneuver to expose a space above the renal veins to allow for vascular control.
- Management: repair primarily, patch or shunt. Ligation of the suprarenal IVC should not be performed.

Retro/Suprahepatic Caval

- Exposure: divide all hepatic ligaments and completely mobilize liver.
- Management: Large bore chest tubes (36-40Fr) can be utilized as atriocaval shunts [61] or total hepatic isolation can be performed.

Portal Venous Injuries: Rare

- Management.
  - Control with Pringle maneuver followed by dissection of portal structures in combination with reduction of arterial

inflow with REBOA or aortic cross clamping can facilitate identification of focal injury.
  - Portal vein injuries should ideally be repaired or reconstructed, however after confirmation of a patent hepatic artery to decrease the likelihood of acute hepatic necrosis, the portal vein can be ligated.

Mesenteric Venous Injuries: Rare

Ligation of SMV highly morbid due to resultant visceral ischemia. Reconstruction is recommended.

Iliac Venous Injury

- Management.
  - Control with sponge-stick compression.
  - Small injuries: repair primarily.
  - Larger injuries: Interposition grafts or vein patches.
  - Damage control: Ligation is well tolerated [62]. Postoperative elevation and compression as well as monitoring for the development of compartment syndrome is critical.

Extremity Vein Injury

- Management: attempt repair, restoration of venous outflow may improve limb outcomes.
- Damage control: liberal use of shunts. Ligation is appropriate for patients in extremis.

Questions and Answers

1. 24 year old F sp. GSW to pelvis and chest. She has a L tube thoracostomy in the emergency department which drains 800c

of blood, and a positive abdominal FAST exam. In operating room the left iliac vein is 75% disrupted. Her pH is 6.9, temperature is 32 degrees F, and she has received 18PRBC/18FFP as well as platelets and TXA. The best option for management of the iliac vein injury is:
   (A) Interposition repair with synthetic graft
   (B) Interposition repair with biologic graft
   (C) Shunting with a size-matched hollow-bore tube
   (D) Ligation with lower extremity compression and elevation
2. 48 year old M sp. motorcycle collision arrives to the ED hypotensive with obvious pelvic deformity. He does not respond to resuscitation with blood products and his abdominal FAST exam is negative. While awaiting the IR team to mobilize, his SBP drops from 92/58 to 68/42, and REBOA is performed. In what Zone is the balloon inflated?
   (a) Zone 1
   (b) Zone 2
   (c) Zone 3
   (d) Zone 4
3. 19 year old M sp. GSW to right popliteal fossa. Entry and exit wounds are visible along with absence of right pedal pulses and signals. What is the next step?
   (a) CTA
   (b) Arterial and venous duplex
   (c) Operating room for an on-table angiogram and surgical intervention
   (d) Start anti-coagulation with q1hour vascular checks in ICU

Answers: 1 (D), 2(c), 3 (c)

References

1. Roberts DJ, Ball CG, Feliciano DV, et al. History of the innovation of damage control for Management of Trauma Patients: 1902–2016. Ann Surg. 2017;265(5):1034–44.
2. Frykberg ER. Advances in the diagnosis and treatment of extremity vascular trauma. Surg Clin North Am. 1995;75(2):207–23.

3. Mills WJ, Barei DP, McNair P. The value of the ankle-brachial index for diagnosing arterial injury after knee dislocation: a prospective study. J Trauma. 2004;56(6):1261–5.
4. Lynch K, Johansen K. Can Doppler pressure measurement replace "exclusion" arteriography in the diagnosis of occult extremity arterial trauma? Ann Surg. 1991;214(6):737–41.
5. Inaba K, Branco BC, Reddy S, et al. Prospective evaluation of multidetector computed tomography for extremity vascular trauma. J Trauma. 2011;70(4):808–15.
6. Rhee PM, Acosta J, Bridgeman A, Wang D, Jordan M, Rich N. Survival after emergency department thoracotomy: review of published data from the past 25 years. J Am Coll Surg. 2000;190(3):288–98.
7. Assar AN, Zarins CK. Endovascular proximal control of ruptured abdominal aortic aneurysms: the internal aortic clamp. J Cardiovasc Surg. 2009;50(3):381–5.
8. White JM, Cannon JW, Stannard A, Markov NP, Spencer JR, Rasmussen TE. Endovascular balloon occlusion of the aorta is superior to resuscitative thoracotomy with aortic clamping in a porcine model of hemorrhagic shock. Surgery. 2011;150(3):400–9.
9. Moore LJ, Brenner M, Kozar RA, et al. Implementation of resuscitative endovascular balloon occlusion of the aorta as an alternative to resuscitative thoracotomy for noncompressible truncal hemorrhage. J Trauma Acute Care Surg. 2015;79(4):523–30; discussion 530–522
10. Romagnoli AN, Teeter W, Wasicek P, et al. No wire? No problem: resuscitative endovascular balloon occlusion of the aorta can be performed effectively and more rapidly with a wire-free device. J Trauma Acute Care Surg. 2018;85(5):894–8.
11. Brenner M, Inaba K, Aiolfi A, et al. Resuscitative endovascular balloon occlusion of the aorta and resuscitative thoracotomy in select patients with hemorrhagic shock: early results from the American Association for the Surgery of Trauma's aortic occlusion in resuscitation for trauma and acute care surgery registry. J Am Coll Surg. 2018;226(5):730–40.
12. Stannard A, Eliason JL, Rasmussen TE. Resuscitative endovascular balloon occlusion of the aorta (REBOA) as an adjunct for hemorrhagic shock. J Trauma. 2011;71(6):1869–72.
13. Brenner M, Hoehn M, Pasley J, Dubose J, Stein D, Scalea T. Basic endovascular skills for trauma course: bridging the gap between endovascular techniques and the acute care surgeon. J Trauma Acute Care Surg. 2014;77(2):286–91.
14. Arthurs ZM, Starnes BW, Sohn VY, Singh N, Martin MJ, Andersen CA. Functional and survival outcomes in traumatic blunt thoracic aortic injuries: an analysis of the National Trauma Databank. J Vasc Surg. 2009;49(4):988–94.
15. Smith RS, Chang FC. Traumatic rupture of the aorta: still a lethal injury. Am J Surg. 1986;152(6):660–3.

16. Clancy TV, Gary Maxwell J, Covington DL, Brinker CC, Blackman D. A statewide analysis of level I and II trauma centers for patients with major injuries. J Trauma. 2001;51(2):346–51.
17. Richens D, Field M, Neale M, Oakley C. The mechanism of injury in blunt traumatic rupture of the aorta. Eur J Cardiothorac Surg. 2002;21(2):288–93.
18. Parmley LF, Mattingly TW, Manion WC, Jahnke EJ Jr. Nonpenetrating traumatic injury of the aorta. Circulation. 1958;17(6):1086–101.
19. Teixeira PG, Inaba K, Barmparas G, et al. Blunt thoracic aortic injuries: an autopsy study. J Trauma. 2011;70(1):197–202.
20. O'Conor CE. Diagnosing traumatic rupture of the thoracic aorta in the emergency department. Emerg Med J. 2004;21(4):414–9.
21. Woodring JH. The normal mediastinum in blunt traumatic rupture of the thoracic aorta and brachiocephalic arteries. J Emerg Med. 1990;8(4):467–76.
22. Mirvis SE, Bidwell JK, Buddemeyer EU, et al. Value of chest radiography in excluding traumatic aortic rupture. Radiology. 1987;163(2):487–93.
23. Gavant ML, Menke PG, Fabian T, Flick PA, Graney MJ, Gold RE. Blunt traumatic aortic rupture: detection with helical CT of the chest. Radiology. 1995;197(1):125–33.
24. Wicky S, Capasso P, Meuli R, Fischer A, von Segesser L, Schnyder P. Spiral CT aortography: an efficient technique for the diagnosis of traumatic aortic injury. Eur Radiol. 1998;8(5):828–33.
25. Bruckner BA, DiBardino DJ, Cumbie TC, et al. Critical evaluation of chest computed tomography scans for blunt descending thoracic aortic injury. Ann Thorac Surg. 2006;81(4):1339–46.
26. Azizzadeh A, Keyhani K, Miller CC 3rd, Coogan SM, Safi HJ, Estrera AL. Blunt traumatic aortic injury: initial experience with endovascular repair. J Vasc Surg. 2009;49(6):1403–8.
27. Lee WA, Matsumura JS, Mitchell RS, et al. Endovascular repair of traumatic thoracic aortic injury: clinical practice guidelines of the Society for Vascular Surgery. J Vasc Surg. 2011;53(1):187–92.
28. Fabian TC, Davis KA, Gavant ML, et al. Prospective study of blunt aortic injury: helical CT is diagnostic and antihypertensive therapy reduces rupture. Ann Surg. 1998;227(5):666–76; discussion 676–667
29. Shalhub S, Starnes BW, Tran NT, et al. Blunt abdominal aortic injury. J Vasc Surg. 2012;55(5):1277–85.
30. Osgood MJ, Heck JM, Rellinger EJ, et al. Natural history of grade I-II blunt traumatic aortic injury. J Vasc Surg. 2014;59(2):334–41.
31. DuBose JJ, Leake SS, Brenner M, et al. Contemporary management and outcomes of blunt thoracic aortic injury: a multicenter retrospective study. J Trauma Acute Care Surg. 2015;78(2):360–9.
32. Brenner M, Teeter W, Hadud M, et al. Long-term outcomes of thoracic endovascular aortic repair: a single institution's 11-year experience. J Trauma Acute Care Surg. 2017;82(4):687–93.

33. Demetriades D, Velmahos GC, Scalea TM, et al. Blunt traumatic thoracic aortic injuries: early or delayed repair--results of an American Association for the Surgery of Trauma prospective study. J Trauma. 2009;66(4):967–73.
34. Daly K, Ho C, Persson D, Gay S. Traumatic retroperitoneal injuries: review of multidetector CT findings. Radiographics. 2008;28:1571–90
35. Starnes BW, Lundgren RS, Gunn M, et al. A new classification scheme for treating blunt aortic injury. J Vasc Surg. 2012;55(1):47–54.
36. Shalhub S, Starnes BW, Brenner ML, et al. Blunt abdominal aortic injury: a Western trauma association multicenter study. J Trauma Acute Care Surg. 2014;77(6):879–85; discussion 885.
37. Starnes BW, Arthurs ZM. Endovascular management of vascular trauma. Perspect Vasc Surg Endovasc Ther. 2006;18(2):114–29.
38. DuBose J, Inaba K, Barmparas G, et al. Bilateral internal iliac artery ligation as a damage control approach in massive retroperitoneal bleeding after pelvic fracture. J Trauma. 2010;69(6):1507–14.
39. Asensio JA, Petrone P, Kimbrell B, Kuncir E. Lessons learned in the management of thirteen celiac axis injuries. South Med J. 2005;98(4):462–6.
40. Graham JM, Mattox KL, Beall AC, DeBakey ME. Injuries to the visceral arteries. Surgery. 1978;84(6):835–9.
41. Feliciano DV. Abdominal vascular injuries. Surg Clin North Am. 1988;68(4):741–55.
42. Fullen WD, Hunt J, Altemeier WA. The clinical spectrum of penetrating injury to the superior mesenteric arterial circulation. J Trauma. 1972;12(8):656–64.
43. Reilly PM, Rotondo MF, Carpenter JP, Sherr SA, Schwab CW. Temporary vascular continuity during damage control: intraluminal shunting for proximal superior mesenteric artery injury. J Trauma. 1995;39(4):757–60.
44. Demetriades D, Asensio JA, Velmahos G, Thal E. Complex problems in penetrating neck trauma. Surg Clin North Am. 1996;76(4):661–83.
45. Lee TS, Ducic Y, Gordin E, Stroman D. Management of carotid artery trauma. Craniomaxillofac Trauma Reconstr. 2014;7(3):175–89.
46. Beliaev AM, Barber PA, Marshall RJ, Civil I. Denver screening protocol for blunt cerebrovascular injury reduces the use of multi-detector computed tomography angiography. ANZ J Surg. 2014;84(6):429–32.
47. Biffl WL, Cothren CC, Moore EE, et al. Western trauma association critical decisions in trauma: screening for and treatment of blunt cerebrovascular injuries. J Trauma. 2009;67(6):1150–3.
48. Biffl WL, Moore EE, Offner PJ, Brega KE, Franciose RJ, Burch JM. Blunt carotid arterial injuries: implications of a new grading scale. J Trauma. 1999;47(5):845–53.
49. Biffl WL, Ray CE, Moore EE, et al. Treatment-related outcomes from blunt cerebrovascular injuries: importance of routine follow-up arteriography. Ann Surg. 2002;235(5):699–706; discussion 706–697

50. Fabian TC, Patton JH, Croce MA, Minard G, Kudsk KA, Pritchard FE. Blunt carotid injury. Importance of early diagnosis and anticoagulant therapy. Ann Surg. 1996;223(5):513–22; discussion 522–515
51. Jarvik J, Philips G, Schwab C, Schwartz J, Grossman R. Penetrating neck trauma: sensitivity of clinical examination and cost- effectiveness of angiography. AJNR Am J Neuroradiol. 1995;16:647–54.
52. Xenos ES, Freeman M, Stevens S, Cassada D, Pacanowski J, Goldman M. Covered stents for injuries of subclavian and axillary arteries. J Vasc Surg. 2003;38(3):451–4.
53. Burkhardt GE, Gifford SM, Propper B, et al. The impact of ischemic intervals on neuromuscular recovery in a porcine (sus scrofa) survival model of extremity vascular injury. J Vasc Surg. 2011;53(1):165–73.
54. Steele HL, Singh A. Vascular injury after occult knee dislocation presenting as compartment syndrome. J Emerg Med. 2012;42(3):271–4.
55. Hudorovic N. Wartime major venous vessel injuries. Interact Cardiovasc Thorac Surg. 2008;7(1):158–60.
56. Buckman RF, Pathak AS, Badellino MM, Bradley KM. Injuries of the inferior vena cava. Surg Clin North Am. 2001;81(6):1431–47.
57. Rosengart MR, Smith DR, Melton SM, May AK, Rue LW. Prognostic factors in patients with inferior vena cava injuries. Am Surg. 1999;65(9):849–55; discussion 855–846
58. Carr JA, Kralovich KA, Patton JH, Horst HM. Primary venorrhaphy for traumatic inferior vena cava injuries. Am Surg. 2001;67(3):207–13; discussion 213–204
59. Huerta S, Bui TD, Nguyen TH, Banimahd FN, Porral D, Dolich MO. Predictors of mortality and management of patients with traumatic inferior vena cava injuries. Am Surg. 2006;72(4):290–6.
60. Mullins RJ, Lucas CE, Ledgerwood AM. The natural history following venous ligation for civilian injuries. J Trauma. 1980;20(9):737–43.
61. Burch JM, Feliciano DV, Mattox KL. The atriocaval shunt. Facts and fiction. Ann Surg. 1988;207(5):555–68.
62. Timberlake GA, O'Connell RC, Kerstein MD. Venous injury: to repair or ligate, the dilemma. J Vasc Surg. 1986;4(6):553–8.

20 Techniques of Vascular Access and Endovascular Surgery

Sharon Kiang, Hans Keenan Boggs, and Roger Tomihama

Vascular Access [1, 2]

1 French = 0.33 mm.

Vascular access: initial step for endovascular intervention

- The common femoral artery (preferably from the right) is by far the most common location, with axillary/brachial (usually from the left) being second.
- Anterograde access = in direction of blood flow.
- Retrograde access = against direction of blood flow.
- Can be done via percutaneous route or open cutdown.

S. Kiang (✉)
Department of Vascular Surgery, Loma Linda University Medical Center, Loma Linda, CA, USA
e-mail: Skiang@llu.edu

H. K. Boggs
Department of Surgery, Loma Linda University Medical Center, Loma Linda, CA, USA
e-mail: HAboggs@llu.edu

R. Tomihama
Department of Interventional Radiology, Loma Linda University Medical Center, Loma Linda, CA, USA
e-mail: RTomihama@llu.edu

A. Murga et al. (eds.), *The Vascular Surgery In-Training Examination Review (VSITE)*,
https://doi.org/10.1007/978-3-031-24121-5_20

Arterial vs. Venous Access

- Generally similar in theory and technique; important caveats:
- Lower pressure in venous system.
  - Easier hemostasis → decreased bleeding complications.
  - Less radial force against the vessel wall keeping it open → harder access.
- Veins are capacitance vessels and can be large; however, they do not stretch and can be prone to tear from a large device.
- A syringe may need to be used with venous access.
  - Vacuum generated can confirm entry.
  - Avoids inadvertent air embolism.

Identifying Point of Access

1. Manual Palpation.
   (a) Typically involves having two fingers on pulse—one proximal and one distal.
   (b) With vessel oriented in a straight line, access needle inserted between two fingers.
   (c) Appropriate if pulse is readily palpable and necessary landmarks are easy to identify.
2. Radiographic guidance (used as adjunct to ultrasound guidance).
   (a) Typically fluoroscopy, used to visualize the bony landmarks mentioned above.
   (b) Optimal access is again at the CFA overlying the medial 1/3 of the femoral head.
   (c) Useful in pulseless or hostile groin; but largely replaced by ultrasound for initial access.
   (d) Provides only 2-dimensions of guidance.
3. Ultrasound (US) guidance (preferred method).
   (a) Allows direct visualization of the vascular structures (specifically visualizing the bifurcation of the SFA and profunda in order to access proximally see Fig. 20.1).
   (b) Allows for small corrections in angle and approach.

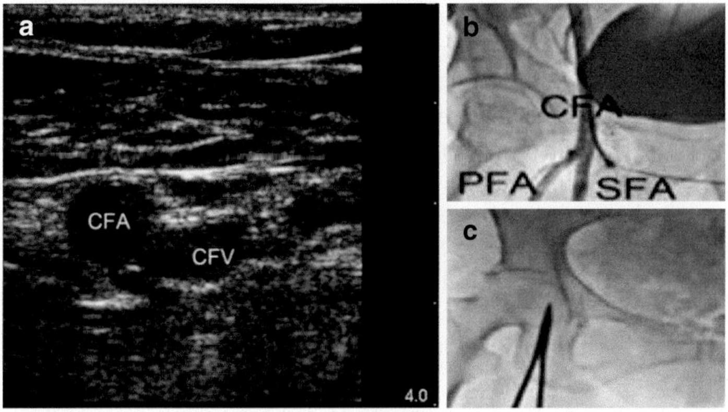

Fig. 20.1 (**a**) Femoral vessels. (Taken from Handbook of Endovascular Peripheral Interventions. Ch 1 p 20). (**b**) Angiography demonstrating sheath placement within common femoral artery. (**c**) Access point for femoral artery over femoral head. (Taken from Handbook of Endovascular Peripheral Interventions. Ch 1. p 5)

Seldinger Technique: Universal Means for Percutaneous Access

1. Access vessel with needle, typically under US guidance.
2. Hold access with guidewire.
3. Position sheath or other catheter into vessel lumen over guidewire.
4. Remove the guidewire.

When Choosing a Site for Percutaneous Access, Must Consider

1. Appropriateness for the procedure.
   (a) Vessels must be appropriately sized for the devices/catheters to be used.
   (b) Chosen location must permit catheterization of the vessels of interest.

   (c) Possible interventions to follow primary diagnostic procedure should be considered.
2. Ability for hemostasis.
   (a) Access site must be able to be readily sealed.
   (b) Hemostasis is generally achieved through manual compression.
   (c) In common femoral region, vessels lie *anterior to the medial 1/3* of the femoral head, against which they can be compressed; similarly, the brachial artery against the humerus.
   (d) Unsatisfactory compression may result in hematoma or pseudoaneurysm.
   (e) Closure devices: a variety of devices exist.
      - Cannot be used in areas of significant calcification.
      - Limited use in smaller diameter vessels.
      - Not intended for use in access sizes >8 French, except for Perclose technique.
3. Ability to convert open.
   (a) May be required in situations where access is lost or there is failure of hemostasis.
   (b) This is facilitated by ready accessibility.
4. Ensuring minimal injury to downstream tissue.
   (a) Blood flow to distal tissues may be affected by indwelling catheters.
      - Thrombosis may occur with sluggish flow.
   (b) Rarely an issue in diagnostic angiography given relatively small diameters of diagnostic catheters.
   (c) Cannulation of smaller vessels risks dissection and occlusion of flow.
   (d) Anticoagulation, typically heparin, is frequently used in peripheral interventions to reduce thrombogenicity.

Potential Points of Access [1]

CFA: The typical first choice for vascular access in most diagnostic and therapeutic procedures

- 5–8 cm long on average
- Can permit devices up to 26 French.
- Lateral to medial: Femoral nerve; CFA; CFV (recall *NAVEL* mnemonic).
- Ideal location for access of CFA is where it crosses the medial border of the femoral head, between inguinal ligament and the CFA bifurcation; see Fig. 20.1b, c.
- Can palpate anterior superior iliac spine and pubic tubercle (landmarks of inguinal ligament) to identify superior-most border of safe access.
- The crossing of the inguinal ligament can be visualized on ultrasound by seeing the CFA "dive" underneath the ligament.
- Anterograde access too close to CFA bifurcation can make selective catheterization of superficial femoral artery (SFA) difficult due to angle of entry.

Popliteal Artery: continuation of SFA at exit of Hunter's canal in distal medial thigh, travels behind knee

- Access medially either above/below knee, or posteriorly from prone.
- Not commonly used diagnostically.
- Retrograde access helpful for to cross and reenter SFA occlusion.
- Hemostasis can be difficult: fatty space, little to compress against.

Tibial Arteries: anterior, posterior, peroneal arteries

- Some utility as adjunctive access in recanalizing severe tibial disease.
- Commonly accessed using micropuncture.
- Typically requires smaller sheaths and wires.
- Easiest to access at dorsalis pedis as it is relatively superficial, easy hemostasis.
- Posterior tibial also superficial and compressible.
- Peroneal generally too deep for access.

Axillary Artery

- Cannulate at intramuscular groove between the triceps and coracobrachialis.
- Can compress against humerus.
- Bleeding into axillary sheath can cause compartment syndrome involving the median nerve.
- Open cutdown is related to lower complication rates compared to percutaneous access.
- Minimal caliber change to brachial artery.

Brachial Artery

- Sole vascular supply to the distal upper extremity.
- Palpable over the olecranon process.
- Use ultrasound and micropuncture; must delineate bifurcation to achieve access at largest portion.
- Similar risk for compartment syndrome of median nerve from hematoma.
- Open cutdown is related to lower complication rates compared to percutaneous access.
- 6 French sheaths are safe in most; can accommodate up to 7–8 Fr.

Radial Artery

- Readily palpable over distal radius; can be accessed without ultrasound but almost always ultrasound-guided.
- Compressible against radius.
- Accommodates 4–6 French sheath, facilitating a 0.014″ or 0.018″ platform.
- Most patients will be ulnar dominant: vessel trauma may have minimal downstream effect.
- Modified Allen's test can be used to identify patients with incomplete palmar arches who may be at risk of hand ischemia

in case of flow limitation of the radial artery.
- Antispasmodic drugs (e.g. calcium-channel blocker) may need to be infused in order to prevent reactive spasm and thrombosis.

Common Femoral Vein
- Most common access for diagnostic procedures of the vena cava and branches.
- Medial to CFA.
- Can similarly be compressed against medial femoral head.

Popliteal Vein: Both paired veins on each side of popliteal artery can be used for access.

Saphenous Veins: Greater and Smaller

- Both will generally accommodate 6 French sheath.
- Smaller saphenous often used as access in thrombolysis of femoral deep vein thrombosis.

Cephalic/Basilic Vein
- Sometimes used for dialysis or vein mapping though mapping usually done with US.

Internal Jugular Vein
- Lateral to carotid artery; recommended to always use US to avoid injury.
- Access between sternal and clavicular heads of the sternocleidomastoid.
- Optimal access for vena cava filter removal.

Access Technique [1]

Access Needles

- Single-wall puncture needles.
  - Almost universally used for vascular access.

  - 18-gauge needle permits passage of a 0.035-in. guide wire
  - 21-gauge needle permits 0.018-in. guide wire
- Double-wall puncture needles.
  - Blunt tip, hollow with inner beveled stylet.
  - Historically inserted through-and-through with removal of stylet and gradual withdrawal of the needle until blood returns.
  - Causes unnecessary vessel trauma and is avoided in standard femoral cannulation.
  - Still used in translumbar aortic cannulation of endoleaks in order to avoid piercing endograft once aneurysm sac is accessed.
- **Positive control of the wire must be maintained at all times in order to prevent loss of the wire or inadvertent removal.**

Micropuncture Needle Technique

- 21-gauge needle inserted at a 30–45 degree angle ideally under US guidance.
- Once in vessel, 0.018″ floppy tip guidewire is inserted, with or without fluoroscopic confirmation, and needle is removed.
- 4 French introducer sheath is placed over the wire.
- Inner cannula of sheath and 0.018″ wire is removed; 0.035″ wire is placed through sheath.
- Larger and longer sheath can be placed for definitive access.

Standard Needle Technique: most helpful to avoid the less supportive 0.018″ guidewire in (1) scarred tissue, (2) deep vessels, (3) accessing Dacron grafts

- Similar to micropuncture technique but avoids initial 4 French sheath.
- 18-gauge needle to access artery; 0.035″ guidewire placed through needle; 5–6 French sheath placed.

Techniques for Catheterization [1, 2]

Guidewires: maintains arterial access and acts rail for placement of further sheaths, catheters, and devices

- J-tipped; angled; straight wires.
- Standard entry wire = 0.035″ J-tipped moveable core steel guidewire; intended for atraumatic passage through iliacs.
  - Fluoroscopy can confirm safe wire placement.
  - It is critical that hydrophilic-coated wires are <u>not</u> used as entry wires; coating can be sheared and embolize from use with entry needles.
- Once with sheath access, a wide variety of guidewires can be utilized for catheter placement.
- Two general size categories, by transverse diameter (in inches):
  - Larger, 0.035″/0.038″.
  - Smaller, 0.014″/0.018″.
  - Other sizes are usually device-specific and uncommonly used in vascular surgery.
  - Larger gauge wires have more "<u>trackability</u>"—ability of a device to pass over the wire under tortuous configurations.
- Lengths are typically 120–360 cm; longer wires are usually "exchange length" wires for use with very long catheters or when introducing devices far from site of access.
- <u>Stiffness versus Flexibility:</u> stiff wires provide more support for catheters/devices but pose higher risk for vessel trauma.
  - Stiffness determined by.
    - outer spring coil,
    - core wire (mandrel),
  - Steel core = very stiff.
  - Nitinol core = very flexible.

- Coatings can be added to wires to reduce friction and increase trackability.
  - Hydrophilic coating attracts water—e.g. Polyurethane.
    Creates gel-like surface on wire; increased lubricity.
    Can reduce tactile feedback and increase risk of subintimal dissection or vessel perforation.
  - Hydrophobic coating repels water—e.g. Teflon/PTFE.
    Creates wax-like surface; decreased lubricity.
    Can increase tactile feedback.
- Wires should be cleaned with heparin/saline routinely between manipulations; wipe towards the body to minimize displacement of the wire.
- Wire Tips.
  - Effect "steerability"—ability to direct the intraluminal tip via manipulation of the extra-anatomic portion.
  - Soft, floppy tips protect against vessel trauma but difficult to make turns, cannulate side branches.
  - Stiffer, slightly angled tips can allow for better maneuvering through tortuous vessels and side branch cannulation.
  - J-tip wires are ideal for cannulating, for sheath exchange—reduced risk of vessel trauma or inadvertent cannulation of a side branch.

Sheaths—maintain vascular access and act as entry for all further wires, catheters, devices, etc.

- Allows for rapid exchange, minimizing trauma to the arteriotomy.
- Come in an array of lengths (5–100 cm) and internal diameter (typically 4–11 F).
- Diameter measured in French size; 1F = 0.013″ = 0.33 mm.
- Standard diagnostic sheath = 10 cm; catheter length variable.
  - Smaller sheaths for shorter working distances.
  - Longer sheaths for remote work.
- Side ports permit aspiration; hemostatic valve maintains hemostasis.
- Braided sheaths can prevent kinking in dense tissue.

Diagnostic Catheters—vehicles for delivery of contrast to a site of interest; vary in size, length, and tip

- Similar to wires, may have coating to reduce friction, increase trackability.
- Can be braided to increase torque responsiveness and reduce kinking.
- Caliber measured as <u>outer</u> diameter; thus, a 5F catheter may fit in a 5F sheath.
- Range between 2–6 F; 2–3 F are microcatheters—primarily used for embolization coil delivery.
- Two main types: Non-Selective and Selective.
  - Non-Selective: for large volume contrast, usually under power injection, into a large vessel (e.g. aortography, vena cavography).

    Catheter tips usually take circular shape without guidewire support.

    Have multiple terminal side holes—reduce "jet-effect"; allow for dispersal of contrast.
  - Selective: shape allows for engagement of a branch vessel orifice for either contrast administration or guidewire passage.

    Generally have only an end hole—risk of vessel trauma from fluid jet with high pressure contrast.

    Single-curved—for cannulating side branches with <45 degree take off (e.g. Kumpe).

    Double-curved—angled up to 90 degrees; for more acute take offs.

    Reverse-curved—usually 180 degree curve with flared tip; for steep take offs.
  - Crossing Catheters: low profile, still, tapered tip for crossing stenotic or occluded vessels.
  - Guiding Catheters: function similarly to long sheaths but with different tip shapes; constant diameter throughout, allowing for smaller instruments to be passed through.

Achieving Hemostasis

- Manual compression: effective for the majority, especially in smaller punctures (4–8F).
  - Complete occlusion may result in thrombosis.
  - Insufficient pressure → hematoma, pseudoaneurysm.
  - 5–20 min of compression—dependent on anticoagulation, size of puncture, blood pressure, etc.
  - Mandated bed rest in addition, ~6 h.
- Closure Devices: a range of proprietary devices exist—extravascular plugs, suture-based.
  - Can increase the risk of groin infection and limb ischemia.
  - Decreased time to hemostasis; reduced mandatory bedrest.
  - Limited by puncture size.
  - No clear evidence of superiority over manual compression.

Complications

- Access site = most common site of complication after percutaneous diagnostic endovascular procedure.
- Risk increased with obesity, access vessel disease, use of large sheaths, and in patients on anticoagulation.
- Risk may be reduced with imaging guidance.
- Bedrest and keeping the leg extended for 4 h after a 4–5 Fr arteriotomy is recommended; add 2+ h for >6 Fr.
- Common complications include.
  - Clinically significant hematoma (3%).
  - Thrombosis (2%).
  - Bleeding (1%).
  - Traumatic arteriovenous fistula (0.9%).
  - Pseudoaneurysm (0.6%).

    Most are asymptomatic and will spontaneously resolve.

    If persisting, symptomatic, or enlarging → can treat most with percutaneous thrombin injection.
  - Specific to CFA/CFV access:

    Too cephalad relative to the femoral head → retroperitoneal hematoma.

    Too caudad → inadequate compression.

- Catheters and Guidewires may injure the vessel wall, resulting in dissection, perforation, or embolization.
  - Can be mitigated through: (1) appropriate selection of instruments, (2) fluoroscopic guidance.
  - Catheters should not be excessively larger than the occupied vessel.
- Systemic Complications.
  - Anticoagulation: failure of hemostasis, bleeding, HITT.
    0.2% incidence of Heparin-Induced Thrombocytopenia (HIT)
    - Can lead to thrombosis and cardiovascular collapse.
    - Remove all sources of heparin and switch agents (e.g. Argatroban).
  - Contrast: allergic reaction, renal injury.
    Routinely use lowest dose possible.
    Facilitate by diluting contrast, titrating by real-time visualization, and selective catheterization.
    CO_2 contrast can be a useful adjunct below the diaphragm.
  - Radiation: burns, fibrosis; "As low as reasonably achievable" (ALARA).

Questions and Answers

1. You are preparing for a diagnostic angiogram with possible angioplasty in a 76-year-old woman with new-onset rest pain in her right lower extremity. You prepare for micropuncture access. What is the correct needle and wire combination below?
   (a) 21 Gauge; 0.018 inches
   (b) 14 Gauge; 4 French
   (c) 24 Gauge; 6 French
   (d) 18 Gauge; 0.035 inches

2. A 67-year-old man is in the PACU, 1 h postoperatively from angioplasty and stenting of his left SFA. Vascular access was achieved percutaneously from the right groin. He becomes hypotensive. POC hemoglobin in 6.5. He has distal pulses but his abdomen is tender in the RLQ and appears slightly distended. Blood transfusion is initiated. What is the likely technical error that preceded this complication?
   (a) Choice of percutaneous access over open cutdown
   (b) Poor wire control
   (c) Access above the inguinal ligament
   (d) Inappropriate sheath sizing
3. Which of the following is NOT an appropriate option for management of percutaneous common femoral artery access after the completion of a procedure?
   (a) Manual compression with bedrest
   (b) Suture-based closure device
   (c) Extravascular plug-based closure device
   (d) Bedrest alone

Answers: 1 (a), 2 (c) 3 (d)

References

1. Sidawy AN, Perler BA. Rutherford's vascular surgery and endovascular therapy, volumes 1 and 2. 9th ed. Philadelphia, PA: Elsevier; 2018. p. 747–60.
2. Moore WS. Vascular and endovascular surgery: a comprehensive review. 7th ed. Philadelphia, PA: Elsevier; 1986. p. 303–24.

21 Vascular Grafts

Isabella J. Kuo and Shelley Maithel

Autogenous Vein Graft

- Graft of choice for infrainguinal revascularization.
- Common used veins:
  - Great saphenous vein (GSV): primary patency 85% at 1 year, 75% at 5 years [1, 2].
  - Small saphenous vein (SSV): difficult because harvest requires prone position, primary patency 68% at 1 year, 54% at 5 years [3].
  - Arm vein: often requires composite construction, mostly often cephalic vein or cephalic and basilic vein composite; primary patency 70% at 1 year, 55% at 5 years [4, 5].
  - Femoral vein: used if larger caliber needed (i.e. aorta in setting of aortic graft infection or mesenteric reconstruction, central venous bypass, creation of arteriovenous fistula via local transposition), excellent long-term primary patency but more complications [6, 7].

    Incision 5 cm below inguinal crease down to level of knee with dissection performed medial to sartorius proximally and lateral to sartorius distally.

I. J. Kuo (✉) · S. Maithel
University of California Irvine, Orange, CA, USA
e-mail: ijkuo@hs.uci.edu; smaithel@hs.uci.edu

A. Murga et al. (eds.), *The Vascular Surgery In-Training Examination Review (VSITE)*,
https://doi.org/10.1007/978-3-031-24121-5_21

- Advantages: easily accessible, removal typically inconsequential, low risk of infection.
- Disadvantages: limited availability, potential for size mismatch.
- Surgical technique.
  - Pre-operative vein mapping: minimum diameter of 2 mm–3 mm.
  - Dissection: atraumatic, "no-touch" technique to reduce endothelial damage during harvest with ligation of branches away from the wall to avoid luminal narrowing.
    - Endoscopic GSV harvest has fewer wound complications but lower patency.
  - Distention of the vein to maximum pressure of 100–150 mm Hg.
    - Assess for leaks.
    - Identify diameter of vein.
    - Identify adventitial bands.
  - Irrigation solution: buffered crystalloid solution.
  - Pharmacologic adjuncts.
    - Unfractionated heparin ranging from 4–10 U/mL.
    - Papaverine 120 mg/L.
- Graft configuration.
  - Reversed vein grafts.
    - Maintains antegrade flow through intact valves.
    - Potential size mismatch with artery and vein at both proximal and distal anastomotic sites.
  - Nonreversed vein grafts.
    - Requires valve lysis.
    - Avoids potential size mismatch of artery and vein.
  - In situ vein grafts.
    - Surgical technique: mobilization of proximal and distal vein segments, removal of valves near arterial anastomosis, interrupting venous side branches.

Arterial Autografts

- Superficial femoral artery grafts.
  - Create conduit by performing eversion endarterectomy.
  - High incidence of rupture when used in infected fields
- Hypogastric artery grafts.
  - Conduit of choice for renovascular reconstruction in pediatric population.
- Superficial temporal artery: extracranial-intracranial bypass.

Biologic Grafts

- Allograft (same species graft—cryopreserved vein and human umbilical vein) versus xenograft (different species—typically bovine).
- Cryopreserved vein allografts.
  - Expensive compared to other grafts.
  - Can use cryopreserved GSV, femoral vein, femoral artery, aorta.
  - Increased rate of aneurysmal degeneration and thrombosis from late rejection.
  - Use in infected fields when no autogenous grafts are available.
  - Poor primary patency.
    - 1 year patency for infrainguinal reconstruction: cryopreserved GSV ~30% [8].
    - Better when using femoral vein, typically when use for portal or superior mesenteric vein reconstructions.
  - Human umbilical vein allograft.
    - No longer being manufactured.
  - Bovine.
    - Bovine carotid artery or mesenteric vein graft.
    - Compliant and soft.
    - Requires rinsing prior to use.

Synthetic Grafts

- Ideal vascular prosthetic graft properties: Impermeable, thromboresistant, compliant, resistant to infection, readily available, cost-effective, easy to implant.
- Dacron grafts.
  - Collagen-coated polyester graft.
  - Knitted, woven (less porosity/bleeding but reduced compliance), or reinforced by external rings.
  - Higher risk of dilation than other grafts.
  - Primary used as tube graft in aortic aneurysmal disease or bifurcated form in aortic occlusive disease (5 year patency 86%) [9].
- Expanded Polytetrafluoroethylene (ePTFE) grafts.
  - Paste-extruded fiber, which delivers better tensile stretch and less shrinkage compared to non-expanded PTFE.
  - Ringed or non-ringed.
  - Heparin bonded is default graft (propaten): better long term patency in infrainguinal bypass, not shown in dialysis access [10, 11].
  - Primary patency in infrainguinal heparin bonded ePTFE bypass: 60–65% versus 85% for autogenous vein bypass [12, 13].
  - Amenable to catheter thrombectomy.

Bioengineered Grafts

- Isolated vessels: intact blood vessels isolated from animals or humans that are then treated with chemical decellularization and then fixation of remaining collagen, connective tissue proteins, and cells with glutaraldehyde to reduce antigenicity.
  - Primary patency rates from phase II human trials: 63% at 6 months, 28% at 1 year.

    Loss of primary patency often due to in situ thrombosis.

  - Examples: Bovine carotid artery graft (Artegraft), Bovine mesenteric vein (Procol), Cryopreserved human saphenous vein (CryoVein).
- Tissue-Engineered Vascular Grafts: cellular-based vascular conduits designed to have synthetic components degrade over time and replaced by autogenous material, creating a blood vessel.
  - Examples: Omniflow, Humacyte, Lifeline (Cytograft), Allogenic sheet-based (Cytograft).

Nonaortic Stent Grafts

- Background
  - Balloon angioplasty had technical failure due to elastic recoil, vasospasm, plaque rupture, or dissection.
  - Stenting introduced to improve results of angioplasty; however, placement of stent itself causes remodeling of the vessel due to intimal damage.
- Two categories of stents.
  - Self-expanding and balloon expanding (Table 21.1).
    Can be covered (PTFE) or uncovered.

Table 21.1 Characteristics of self-expanding and balloon expanding stents

Characteristic	Self-expanding	Balloon expanding
Material	Nitinol	Stainless steel
Radial force	Low	High
Flexibility	High	Low
Requires delivery sheath	No	Yes
Radiopacity	Variable	High
Oversizing recommended	Yes	No
Treats lesions with variable diameter	Yes	No
Resistant to external compression	Yes	No

Aortic Stent Grafts

- Principles of aortic repair involve following the instructions for use (IFU) in order to decrease rate complications including endoleak, device failure, migration, conversion to open, and aneurysm rupture.
- Thoracic aorta.
  - Standard thoracic endovascular aneurysm repair: 2 cm of landing zone.

    10–20% oversizing in relation to the native aortic diameter
    - Too much oversize → device infolding, gutter formation, endoleak, accelerated aneurysmal degeneration.
    - Undersized → device migration, endoleaks.
  - May need combination of extra-anatomic bypass with elective coverage of left subclavian artery.
- Abdominal aortic grafts.
  - Modular bifurcated covered self-expanding graft with either Dacron or PTFE fabric.

    Important to insert and deploy main body of graft with contralateral gate in anterolateral position for ease of subsequent retrograde cannulation.
- Advanced endovascular grafts [14].
  - Fenestrated grafts (see Fig. 21.1).

    Inadequate or short neck/landing zone but target vessels original from normal aorta.

    Fenestrations/scallops with radiopaque markers to facilitate accurate positioning over branch arteries → alignment stents used to prevent vessel occlusion/stenosis.
  - Branched endovascular repair (see Fig. 21.1).

    Inadequate or short neck/landing zone and target vessels originate from aneurysmal aorta.

    Fenestrated branches: based on reinforced fenestration, bridged by balloon-expandable covered stents (connects fenestration to target vessel).

    Directional branches: based on pre-sewn cuff.

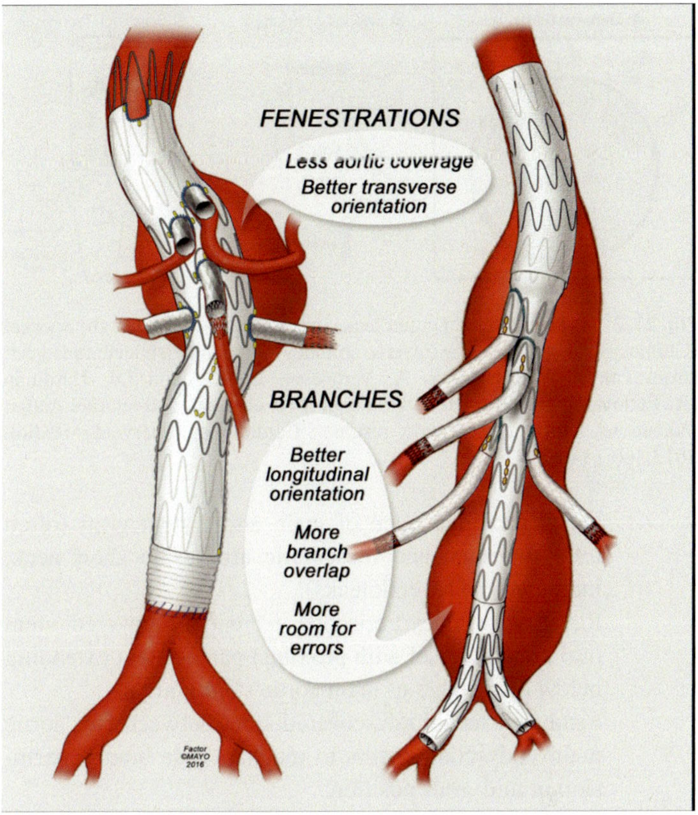

Fig. 21.1 [15] Fenestrated versus branches aortic graft (from Oderich GS, Ribeiro M, Reis de Souza L, Hofer J, Wigham J, Cha S. Endovascular repair of thoracoabdominal aortic aneurysms using fenestrated and branched endografts. The Journal of thoracic and cardiovascular surgery. 2017;153 (2):S32–S41.e7)

– Parallel graft technique (see Fig. 21.2).

  When stent grafts deployed alongside each other.

  • Typically use only two stent grafts to avoid "gutter" endoleaks.

  Chimney/Snorkel technique: placement of covered stent into branch vessel with proximal part of stent extending

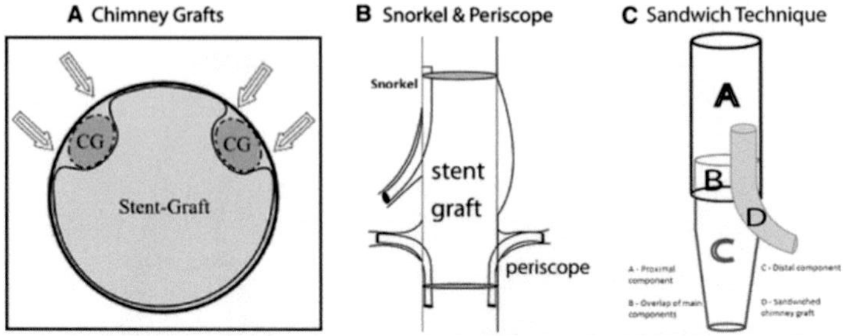

Fig. 21.2 [16] (**a**) Potential gutter leaks in Chimney grafts (CG). (**b**) Snorkel (Chimney) versus Periscope (reverse chimney). (**c**) Sandwich technique graft (from Patel RP, Katsargyris A, Verhoeven ELG, Adam DJ, Hardman JA. Endovascular aortic aneurysm repair with chimney and snorkel grafts: indications, techniques and results. Cardiovasc Intervent Radiol. 2013;36(6):1443–51)

above proximal edge of main aortic stent graft (often used for renal and mesenteric arteries in short neck, increase type IA endoleaks).

Reverse chimney/Periscope technique: covered stent into branch vessel with proximal part of stent extending below distal edge of main aortic stent graft.

Sandwich technique: covered stent between two aortic main body components to maintain side branch perfusion in mid-graft position.

Can be used as bailout maneuver if inadvertent coverage of vessel.

Questions and Answers

1. The best conduit for lower extremity bypass is:
   (a) ePTFE.
   (b) Great saphenous vein.
   (c) Femoral vein.
   (d) Cryopreserved vein.

2. The following are all TRUE of cryopreserved vein EXCEPT:
   (a) More expensive than other conduits.
   (b) Good for use in infected field.
   (c) Patency rate is better than saphenous vein.
   (d) High rate of aneurysmal degeneration.
3. The following is a property of balloon expandable stent.
   (a) High flexibility.
   (b) High radial force.
   (c) Can treat lesions of variable diameter.
   (d) Can resist external compression.

Answers: 1 (b), 2 (c), 3 (b)

References

1. Shah DM, Darling RC 3rd, Chang BB, Fitzgerald KM, Paty PS, Leather RP. Long-term results of in situ saphenous vein bypass. Analysis of 2058 cases. Ann Surg. 1995;222(4):438–46; discussion 46–8
2. Taylor LM Jr, Edwards JM, Porter JM. Present status of reversed vein bypass grafting: five-year results of a modern series. J Vasc Surg. 1990;11(2):193–205.
3. Nierlich P, Metzger P, Enzmann FK, Aspalter M, Dabernig W, Hitzl W, et al. The small saphenous vein: an underestimated source for autologous distal vein bypass. Eur J Vasc Endovasc Surg. 2019;58(4):556–63.
4. Holzenbein TJ, Pomposelli FB Jr, Miller A, Contreras MA, Gibbons GW, Campbell DR, et al. Results of a policy with arm veins used as the first alternative to an unavailable ipsilateral greater saphenous vein for infrainguinal bypass. J Vasc Surg. 1996;23(1):130–40.
5. Faries PL, Arora S, Pomposelli FB Jr, Pulling MC, Smakowski P, Rohan DI, et al. The use of arm vein in lower-extremity revascularization: results of 520 procedures performed in eight years. J Vasc Surg. 2000;31(1 Pt 1):50–9.
6. Jackson MR, Ali AT, Bell C, Modrall JG, Welborn MB 3rd, Scoggins E, et al. Aortofemoral bypass in young patients with premature atherosclerosis: is superficial femoral vein superior to Dacron? J Vasc Surg. 2004;40(1):17–23.
7. McKeever SC, Escobar GA, Moursi MM, Ali AT, Smeds MR. Management of noninfected prosthetic aortic bypass failures using femoral vein. J Vasc Surg. 2016;63(3):642–5.

8. Guevara-Noriega KA, Lucar-Lopez GA, Pomar JL. Cryopreserved allografts for treatment of chronic limb-threatening ischemia in patients without autologous saphenous veins. Ann Vasc Surg. 2019;60:379–87.
9. Sachwani GR, Hans SS, Khoury MD, King TF, Mitsuya M, Rizk YS, et al. Results of iliac stenting and aortofemoral grafting for iliac artery occlusions. J Vasc Surg. 2013;57(4):1030–7.
10. Samson RH, Morales R, Showalter DP, Lepore MR Jr, Nair DG. Heparin-bonded expanded polytetrafluoroethylene femoropopliteal bypass grafts outperform expanded polytetrafluoroethylene grafts without heparin in a long-term comparison. J Vasc Surg. 2016;64(3):638–47.
11. Zea N, Menard G, Le L, Luo Q, Bazan HA, Sternbergh WC 3rd, et al. Heparin-bonded polytetrafluorethylene does not improve hemodialysis arteriovenous graft function. Ann Vasc Surg. 2016;30:28–33.
12. Park KM, Kim YW, Yang SS, Kim DI. Comparisons between prosthetic vascular graft and saphenous vein graft in femoro-popliteal bypass. Ann Surg Treat Res. 2014;87(1):35–40.
13. Ambler GK, Twine CP. Graft type for femoro-popliteal bypass surgery. Cochrane Database Syst Rev. 2018;2:Cd001487.
14. Kansagra K, Kang J, Taon MC, Ganguli S, Gandhi R, Vatakencherry G, et al. Advanced endografting techniques: snorkels, chimneys, periscopes, fenestrations, and branched endografts. Cardiovasc Diagn Ther. 2018;8(Suppl 1):S175–s83.
15. Oderich GS, Ribeiro M, Reis de Souza L, Hofer J, Wigham J, Cha S. Endovascular repair of thoracoabdominal aortic aneurysms using fenestrated and branched endografts. J Thorac Cardiovasc Surg. 2017;153(2):S32–S41.e7.
16. Patel RP, Katsargyris A, Verhoeven ELG, Adam DJ, Hardman JA. Endovascular aortic aneurysm repair with chimney and snorkel grafts: indications, techniques and results. Cardiovasc Intervent Radiol. 2013;36(6):1443–51.

22 Lymphatic Disease

Andrew Son and Thomas F. O'Donnell Jr.

Pathophysiology

In 2004, Adamson and colleagues revealed that the effect of capillary oncotic pressure on transvascular fluid exchange is significantly less than predicted from the original Ernest Henry Starling model that was originally described in 1896 that later became known as the widely referenced "Starling Principle" [1, 2]. This new discovery led to a revision of the principle by Levick and Michel based upon evidence that capillaries push fluid into the interstitial space along their entire length, not just at the arteriolar-capillary junction [3]. As noted by Mortimer and Rockson, the expected reabsorption of interstitial fluid via the venules simply does not occur; rather, interstitial fluid returns into the circulation only via the lymphatic system [4].

A. Son (✉)
Department of Surgery, Division of Vascular Surgery, Loma Linda University School of Medicine, Coleman Pavilion, Loma Linda, CA, USA
e-mail: anson@llu.edu

T. F. O'Donnell Jr.
Tufts University School of Medicine, The Cardiovascular Center at Tufts Medical Center, Boston, MA, USA
e-mail: todonnell@tuftsmedicalcenter.org

A. Murga et al. (eds.), *The Vascular Surgery In-Training Examination Review (VSITE)*,
https://doi.org/10.1007/978-3-031-24121-5_22

- Impairment of lymphatic flow causing accumulation of protein-rich interstitial fluid in body regions. This can be due to high-input impairment (i.e. venous edema), low-output impairment (i.e. lymphatic channel obstruction), an imbalance of lymphatic fluid production and absorption, or a combination of the above.
- Etiology: Primary versus secondary.
- Primary Lymphedema: Inheritable causes; typically subclassified by age of onset.
- Secondary Lymphedema: Filariasis (i.e. Wuchereria Bancrofti infection); post-surgery or radiation therapy, pretibial myxedema from thyrotoxicosis, malignancy.
  - Lipedema: Lymphedema secondary to lipedema typically occurs in lipedema's advanced stages, as pressure from fat accumulation compromises lymphatic transport (lipo-lymphedema). Since, among other things, the lymphatics are responsible for clearing lipids and fatty acids, compromised lymphatic flow can result in additional congestion of fat (adipocyte hypertrophy), including hands and feet.
  - Risk factors for developing lymphedema: Obesity/higher BMI, lower education, age > 55, hypertension, post-surgical infection.

Complications

- Infection (i.e. Cellulitis): 25% of patients with lymphedema will have at least one episode of cellulitis or related skin infection in the affected limb [5].
- Malnutrition and immunodeficiency.
- Malignancy: Kaposi's sarcoma, squamous cell carcinoma, melanoma, malignant lymphoma, lymphangiosarcoma (Stewart-Treves Syndrome)—purple nodules over areas of chronic lymphedema (should biopsy nodule and obtain CT chest to look for lung metastasis if suspicion arises).

Classification and Staging

- Primary lymphedema classification (many instances are associated with genetic disorders) based on age of onset:
  - Congenital Lymphedema (onset before age 2): Klinefelter syndrome, Trisomy 21, Noonan syndrome (PTPN11 gene mutation), Milroy disease, Meige disease, lymphedema-distichiasis syndrome, hypotrichosis-lymphedema-telangiectasia syndrome, HGF and MET mutations (can be silent, then unmasked after trauma).
  - Lymphedema Praecox (aka Meige disease, onset between ages 2–35)—most common type of primary lymphedema (77–94% of all primary cases); has predilection for adolescent females and involvement of the left leg [6].
  - Lymphedema Tarda (onset after age 35).

Based on Clinical Severity

The Staging System (see Table 22.1) is based solely on subjective symptoms, making it prone to substantial observer bias (similar to CEAP classification for venous disease) [7].

Table 22.1 Staging System for lymphedema. (Reproduced with permission from Vascular and Endovascular Surgery A Comprehensive Review 9th ed. Chapter 56)

	Fibrosis	Pitting	Elevation	Skin
Stage 0 (latent or sub-clinical condition)	None	None	No effect	No change
Stage 1 (early protein rich fluid accumulation)	None or minimal	May be present with pressure	Reduces edema	No change
Stage 2 (initial fibrosis development)	Moderate	May be present	Minimal to no reduction	Early changes
Stage 3 (marked fibrosis)	Substantial	None to minimal	No reduction	Marked trophic changes

Clinical Presentation and Symptoms

- Edema.
- Skin Changes: Hyperkeratosis, Peau d' orange, lichenification, lymphorrhea, chylorrhea, yellow nail syndrome.
- Stemmer's Sign: Positive when unable to tent the skin when pinching the base of the second or third digit on the affected limb.
- Buffalo Hump: Edema on the dorsum of the foot of the affected limb (see Fig. 22.1).

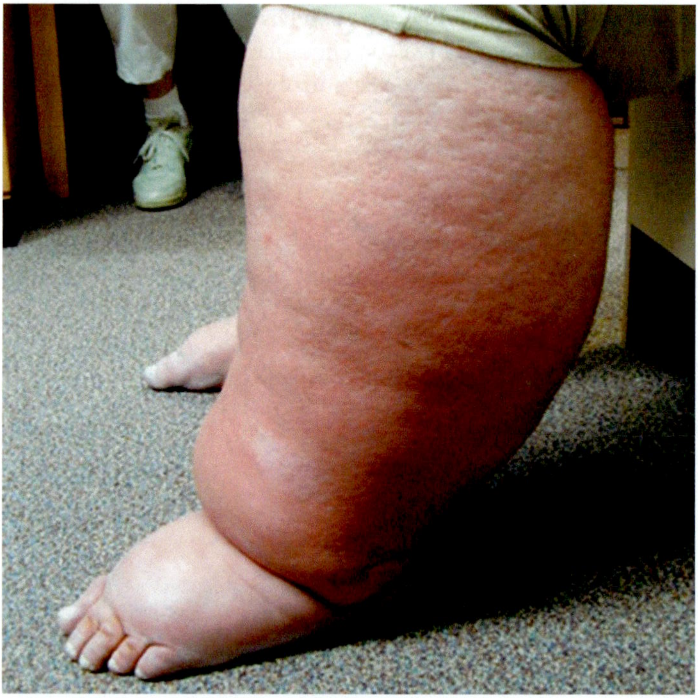

Fig. 22.1 Buffalo Hump. (Reproduced with permission from Vascular and Endovascular Surgery A Comprehensive Review ninth ed. Ch 56)

Diagnosis

- Thorough history and physical and rule out other causes of limb swelling: Venous insufficiency, lipedema, hereditary angioedema, allergic reactions, congenital heart failure, chronic steroid use, concomitant vascular malformations [8].
- Physical Exam: Observation of aforementioned signs.
- Imaging: Lymphoscintigraphy (first choice gold standard, see Fig. 22.2), CT, MRI (characteristic honeycomb appearance of edema in epifascial compartments), direct-contrast lymphangiography (rarely used anymore because of lymphangitis complication) [9].

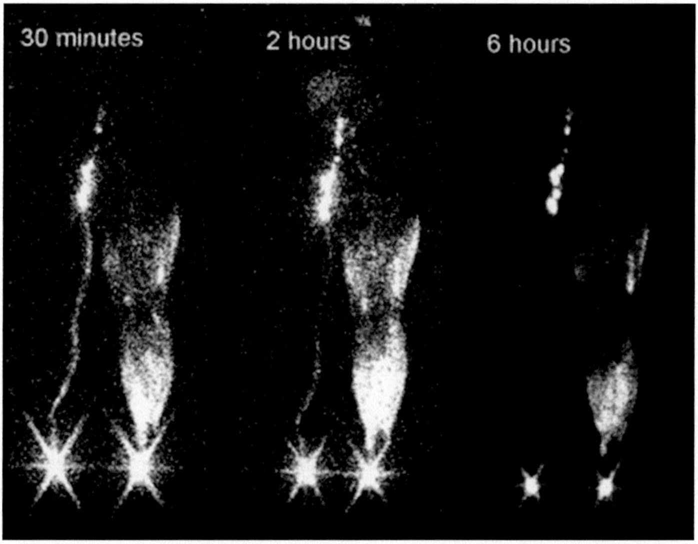

Fig. 22.2 Lymphoscintigraphy showing left leg lymphedema. (Reproduced with permission from Vascular and Endovascular Surgery A Comprehensive Review ninth ed. Ch 56)

Treatment

Treatment rates for lymphedema are variable, with highest treatments rates being lymphedema secondary to breast cancer and lowest treatment rates being related to non-cancer etiologies [10]. Also, efficacy of treatment (especially surgical) is suboptimal.

Non-operative Treatment: The main stay of therapy for both early and advanced stage lymphedema

1. Main components include: Manual lymphatic drainage/physiotherapy, compression bandages and garments, pneumatic compression devices, limb elevation.
2. Complex decongestive therapy (CDT): First line treatment for stage II and III lymphedema (performed in the acute phase).
   (a) Consists of 4 components in 2 phases:
      - Manual lymphatic drainage: Multi-layer wrapping and investment with specialized physical therapist (no strong evidence yet to support this).
      - Compression bandaging: Elastic wrapping.
      - Compression garments: Properly fitting, graduated elastic compression.
      - Compression devices: Sequential pneumatic compression.

   (b) Two phases: Initial (reductive) phase—focus on reducing size of affected body region and proper skin care along with CDT; maintenance phase—follows initial phase and emphasizes maintaining phase 1 progress life-long. Pneumatic compression devices play a role for home therapy [11, 12].
3. Pharmacological: Diuretics (not recommended anymore), Coumarin (used in the past for anti-inflammatory properties, but no longer). Early antibiotic treatments for minor infections since it can spread rapidly (Penicillin based).
4. Preventative: Creams to prevent skin breakdown and infection, self-hygiene, clothing precautions/compression garments, limb elevation, watching fluid balance, exercise, avoiding trauma.

Surgical/Operative Treatment

1. Offered as a last resort if conservative treatment is unsuccessful. Several operations are divided into:
   (a) Physiologic:
      - Microsurgical lymphovenous anastomosis creation to improve lymphatic drainage—plagued by low patency rates.
      - Vascularized lymph node transfer (VLNT)—theorized to help redirect lymphatic flow and stimulate lymphangiogenesis.
      - Autologous lymphatic grafting: Mostly for treatment of secondary lymphedema as a result of local lymphatic obstruction/trauma.

   (b) Reductive.
      - Liposuction.
      - Resection: Segmental removal of skin and subcutaneous tissue down to fascia; best done in a staged fashion.
      - Coverage with split-thickness skin grafting (STSG), less frequently performed and reserved for massive stage III lymphedema where the skin is severely damaged.

Review Questions

1. A 50-year-old female presents to your office with a history of progressively worsening swelling in her right leg that started 10 years ago. She states it has gotten significantly worse in the last 2 years and has noticed her skin on the affected leg becoming thick. She denies any previous surgeries, trauma, or radiation treatment. What is the best classification of her condition?
   (a) Secondary lymphedema.
   (b) Congenital lymphedema.
   (c) Lymphedema Praecox.
   (d) Lymphedema Tarda.
   (e) Meige disease.

2. A 70-year-old female presents to your office as a referral for chronic left arm swelling as a result of a modified radical mastectomy done 20 years ago. She has been wearing compression sleeves, but her swelling has been debilitating and she no longer really has full functional use of her arm. On exam, you notice a dark purple nodule on the lateral aspect of her edematous arm. What is the next best step?
   (a) Reassurance of the nodule and recommend follow-up in 6 months.
   (b) Recommend topical moisturizers as the nodule is likely a result of chronic irritation from compression sleeves.
   (c) Referral to a dermatologist and geneticist to evaluate for neurofibromatosis.
   (d) Increase the compression gradient on her sleeves and refer her to a specialized physical therapist.
   (e) Recommend biopsy of the nodule and a CT scan of the chest to evaluate for metastasis.
3. Which one of the following is NOT considered a routine integral part of non-operative treatment for chronic lymphedema?
   (a) Diuretics such as furosemide.
   (b) Manual lymphatic drainage.
   (c) Compression garments.
   (d) Sequential pneumatic compression.
   (e) Proper preventive measures such as good hygiene and limb elevation.

Answers: 1 (d), 2 (e), 3 (a)

References

1. Starling EH. On the absorption of fluids from the connective tissue spaces. J Physiol. 1896;19(4):312–26.
2. Adamson A, Lenz J, Zhang X, Adamson G, Weinbaum S, Curry F. Oncotic pressures opposing filtration across non-fenestrated rat microvessels. J Physiol. 2004;557(Pt 3):889–907.
3. Levick J, Michel C. Microvascular fluid exchange and the revised Starling principle. Cardiovasc Res. 2010;87(2):198–210.

4. Mortimer P, Rockson S. New developments in clinical aspects of lymphatic disease. J Clin Invest. 2014;124(3):915–21.
5. Badger C, Seers K, Preston N, Mortimer P. Antibiotics / anti-inflammatories for reducing acute inflammatory episodes in lymphoedema of the limbs. Cochrane Database Syst Rev. 2004;2:CD003143.
6. Kinmoth J, Taylor G, Tracy G, Marsh J. Primary lymphoedema: clinical and lymphangiographic studies of a series of 107 patients in which the lower limbs were affected. Br J Surg. 1957;45(189):1–9.
7. The International Lymphoedema Framework. Best practice for the management of lymphoedema. In: Compression therapy: a position document compression bandaging. 2nd ed; 2012. Available from: http://www.lympho.org/mod_turbolead/upload//file/Resources/Compression%20bandaging%20-%20final.pdf
8. Gloviczki P. Handbook of venous disorders: guidelines of the American venous forum. 4th ed. Boca Raton, FL: CRC Press; 2017.
9. O'Donnell TF, Sevick EM, Rasmussen J. New diagnostic modalities in the evaluation of lymphedema. J Vasc Surg Venous Lymphat Disord. 2017;5:261–73.
10. Son A, O'Donnell TF Jr, Izhakoff J, Gaebler JA, Niecko T, Iafrati MA. Lymphedema-associated comorbidities and treatment gap. J Vasc Surg Venous Lymphat Disord. 2019;7(5):724–30.
11. Richmand DM, O'Donnell TF, Zelikovski A. Sequential pneumatic compression for lymphedema: a controlled trial. Arch Surg. 1985;120:1116–9.
12. Pappas C, O'Donnell TF. The long-term results of compression treatment for lymphedema. J Vasc Surg. 1992;16:555–64.

23 Vascular Malformations

Tyler Miskin, Sharon Kiang,
and Roger Tomihama

Definition and Classification

- Introduction
  - Vascular malformations and tumors comprise a wide, heterogeneous spectrum of lesions that involve all parts of the body and can cause significant morbidity and even mortality in both adults and children.
  - Vascular lesions represent the most common cause of pediatric soft-tissue masses.
  - The International Society for the Study of Vascular Anomalies (ISSVA) classifies lesions into broad categories consisting of tumors and malformations [1].

T. Miskin · R. Tomihama (✉)
Vascular and Interventional Radiology, Department of Radiology, Loma Linda University Medical Center, Loma Linda, CA, USA
e-mail: tmiskin@llu.edu; RTomihama@llu.edu

S. Kiang
Division of Vascular Surgery, Institutional Review Board (IRB) Committee, Vascular Non-Invasive Laboratory, Va Loma Linda Healthcare System, Loma Linda, CA, USA

Department of Surgery, Division of Vascular Surgery, Center of Excellence for Surgical Research, Loma Linda Surgery, Loma Linda University|School of Medicine, Loma Linda, CA, USA
e-mail: skiang@llu.edu

A. Murga et al. (eds.), *The Vascular Surgery In-Training Examination Review (VSITE)*,
https://doi.org/10.1007/978-3-031-24121-5_23

  - Correct diagnosis and classification of a vascular anomaly are crucial as treatment strategy depends on the type of malformation.
- Diagnosis.
  - Diagnosis of vascular malformations and tumors is often achieved with the clinical history and physical examination.
  - An informal bedside ultrasound exam.
    - Useful in confirming the diagnosis.
    - Determining the degree of vascularity.
    - Providing preprocedural target planning for future intervention.
  - Cross-sectional imaging (CT or MRI) usually provides the information required for treatment planning.
    - Depth and extent of the lesion.
    - Relationship to adjacent sensitive structures.
  - Magnetic resonance imaging.
    - Conventional MRI with gadolinium contrast.
      - Helpful in confirming the diagnosis of low flow vascular malformations (i.e. lymphatic or venous).
      - Evaluating the extent and depth of lesions and their relationship to adjacent structures.
    - Conventional and time-resolved MR angiography is useful for the evaluation of high flow vascular malformations.

Benign Vascular Tumors

- Infantile hemangioma.
  - Most common vascular tumor of infancy [2].
  - Clinical findings.
    - Proliferative phase: Rapidly growing, strawberry-like, pulsatile, warm lesion. It begins in the first few weeks of life and may proliferate for up to 1 year (see Fig. 23.1).
    - Involuting phase: Dark grayish-red mass that regresses by 10 years of age.
    - Common locations: face and neck > trunk > extremities [3].
    - Female-to-male ratio, 4:1.

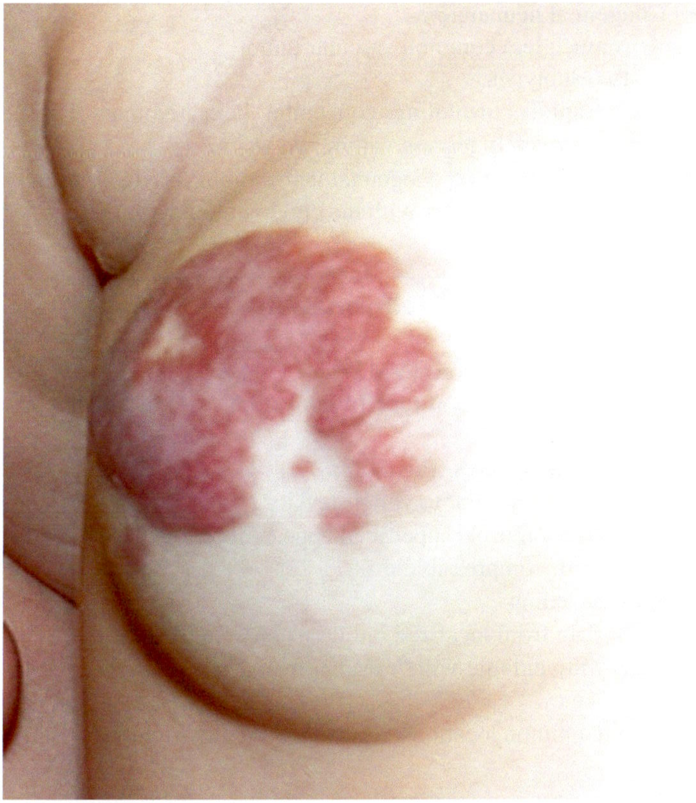

Fig. 23.1 Infantile hemangioma in a 12-month-old infant which demonstrates a superficial lobulated mass in the right chest wall with its strawberry-like appearance. (Reprinted with permission from [9])

- Treatment.

  Usually, no treatment is required due to spontaneous involution.

  However, treatment with propranolol may be used.

  - If the hemangioma is symptomatic.
  - This occurs in regions where there is a possible secondary loss of function or lifetime aesthetic impairment.

- Congenital hemangioma.
  - A much less common vascular tumor.
  - Two subtypes.
    - Rapidly involuting congenital hemangiomas (RICH) completely regress within two years.
    - Noninvoluting congenital hemangiomas (NICH) usually continue to grow with the child without regression.

Low Flow Vascular Malformations

- Venous malformations (VM).
  - The most common type of congenital vascular malformation [4].
  - Clinical Features (Fig. 23.2).
    - Can be similar to varicose veins.
    - Bluish/purple superficial appearance.
    - Soft, compressible mass.
    - Swelling.
    - Pain from localized intravascular coagulation.
    - May enlarge with Valsalva maneuver, puberty, or pregnancy.
    - Common locations: head and neck = extremities > trunk.

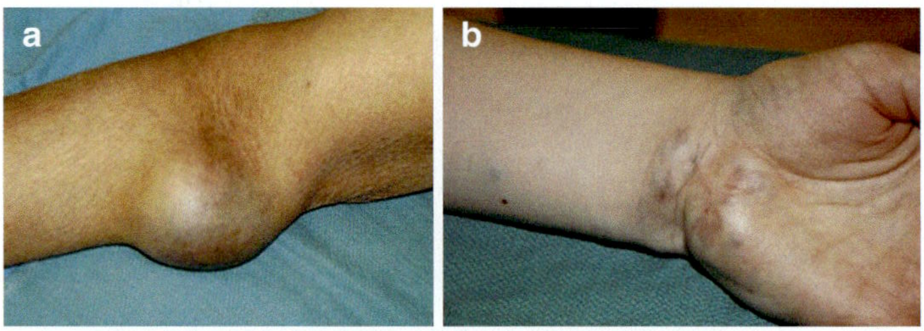

Fig. 23.2 Clinical appearance of venous malformations. (**a**) Protuberant subcutaneous VM near the elbow resulting in a mild "blue tinge" on examination. (**b**) Superficially visible component of a much deeper and diffusely infiltrative VM involving the entire elbow, forearm, and wrist. (Reprinted with permission from [10])

Many forms.
- Well-defined or diffuse.
- Focal or infiltrative.
- Superficial or deep.

– Imaging findings.

X-rays.
- Phleboliths formed from thrombosis and calcification are pathognomonic.

MRI (Fig. 23.3).
- Septated lobulated mass.
- No mass effect on surrounding structures.
- Calcifications (phleboliths).
- Infiltrative tissue planes.
- Possible surrounding edema.
- Slow gradual enhancement on delayed images.

– Treatment.

Indications for treatment [4].
- Pain.
- Functional impairment.
- Cosmetic implications.

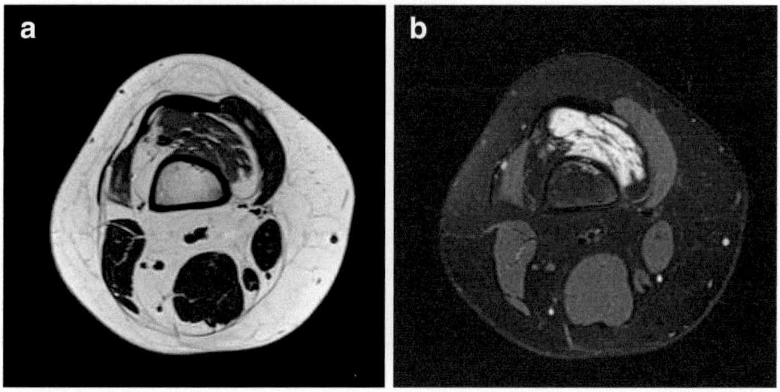

Fig. 23.3 MRI of a thigh venous malformation in a 17-year-old teenager. (**a**) Axial T1-weighted image shows a poorly defined, partially infiltrating hypointense mass in the anterior to the femur bone. (**b**) Axial T2-weighted image shows the well-defined exophytic hyperintense fluid intensity mass in the left chest wall

- Recurrent thrombosis.
- VMs in vital areas or in areas with the chance of future complications.
- VMs that result in significantly adverse hemodynamic states.

Lesions of the extremities.

- Compression stockings to minimize symptoms of swelling and thrombophlebitis.

The majority of venous malformations are primarily treated via sclerotherapy.

- Percutaneous sclerotherapy injection (Fig. 23.4).
- Agents include.
  - Absolute ethanol.
  - Sodium tetradecyl sulfate (STS).
  - Bleomycin.

Other treatment options include.

- Surgical resection.

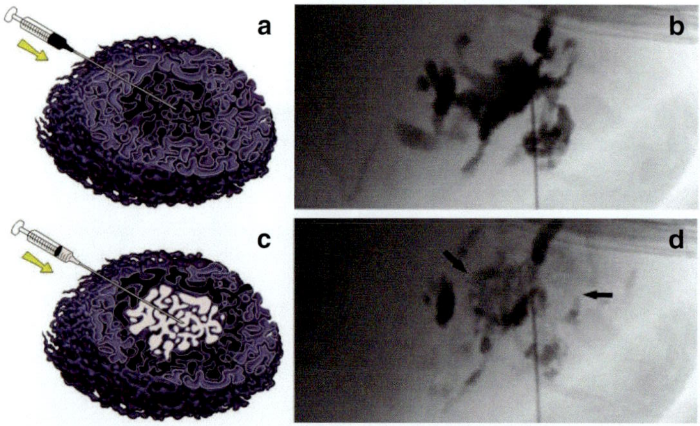

Fig. 23.4 Conventional sclerotherapy technique. (**a**) Contrast is administered into the lesion during the fluoroscopy to demonstrate volume and distribution within the lesion. (**b**) While under close fluoroscopic observation, radiolucent sclerosant is slowly administered through the same site displacing the contrast peripherally within the lesion. (**c** and **d**) Reprinted with permission from [10])

    - Nd-YAG laser photocoagulation.
    - Thermal ablation.
- Lymphatic malformations (LM).
  - Consist of chyle-filled cysts that result from sequestered lymphatic sacs that fail to communicate with peripheral draining channels.
  - Two types.

    Microcystic: cysts <2 cm.

    Macrocystic: cysts >2 cm.

    Mixed: cysts of varying sizes.
  - Clinical features.

    The majority are clinically apparent within the first 2 years of life [5].

    Vary in size from small to massive.

    Lesions are rubbery and usually non-compressible.

    Common locations: neck and axillary region.

    Symptoms relate to the mass-effect on surrounding structures resulting in a wide variety of presentations based on the location of the LM.
  - Imaging findings (Fig. 23.5).

    On MRI, simple LMs can appear as lobulated masses that have the signal characteristics of water (decreased signal intensity on T1-weighted images and increased signal intensity on T2-weighted and STIR images).

    Other findings.
    - Sometimes can have fluid-fluid levels.
    - Macrocystic lesions have rim and septal enhancement.
    - Microcystic lesions have no significant to slight diffuse enhancement.
  - Treatment.

    Macrocystic LMs are primarily treated via sclerotherapy.
    - Doxycycline.
    - Bleomycin.
    - Absolute ethanol.
    - Sodium tetradecyl sulfate (STS).

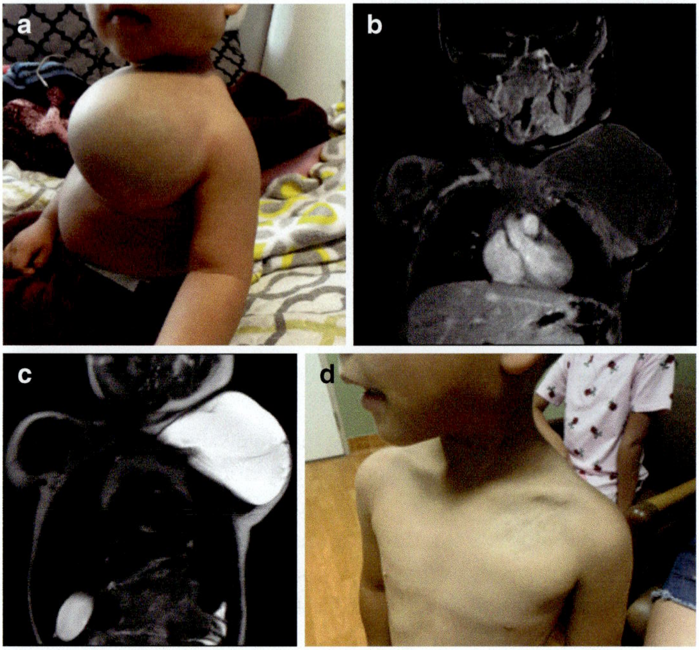

Fig. 23.5 Lymphatic malformation in a 17-month-old child. (**a**) Photograph shows a protuberant mass in the left chest wall. (**b**) Coronal T1-weighted image shows the well-defined exophytic hypointense mass in the left chest wall. (**c**) Coronal T2-weighted image shows the well-defined exophytic hyperintense fluid intensity mass in the left chest wall. (**d**) Photograph shows interval resolution of the lymphatic malformation after several sessions of percutaneous sclerotherapy

- OK-432 (picibanil).

Microcystic malformations.

- Are more difficult to treat.
- Treatment options include.
  - Surgical resection.
  - Intralesional infiltration with bleomycin.
  - Nd-YAG laser photocoagulation.
  - Thermal ablation.

High Flow Vascular Malformations

- Arteriovenous malformations.
  - Clinical Features.
    - Enlarging, red, warm, pulsatile mass with a thrill.
    - Pain.
    - Ulceration and bleeding.
    - Shunt-related cardiac overload.
    - Individual lesions may progress from a quiescent to a more aggressive lesion.
  - Imaging findings.
    - MRI findings (Fig. 23.6).

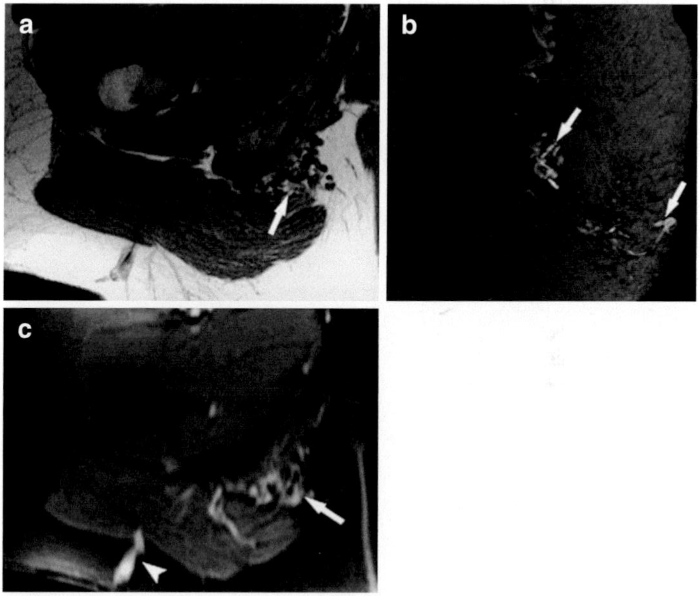

Fig. 23.6 MRI of a high flow arteriovenous malformation (AVM). (**a**) Axial T1-weighted sequence shows numerous tortuous vascular spaces with flow voids (arrow) within an AVM of the ischial region with a characteristic lack of discernible "mass." (**b**) Axial T2-weighted sequence reveals mixture of focal high signal intensity owing to turbulent or abnormal flow (arrows). (**c**) Gadolinium-enhanced fat-saturated sequence reveals hyperintensity with the arteriovenous nidus (arrow) and within venous drainage (arrowhead). (Reprinted with permission from [11])

  - No well-defined mass.
  - Enlarged feeding arteries and draining veins.
  - The early enhancement of enlarged feeding arteries and nidus with shunting to draining veins.
  - Vessels without signal on non-contrast images ("MRI flow voids").
  - Infiltrative tissue planes.

  Angiographic images (Fig. 23.7).
  - Enlarged tortuous feeding arterial feeding vessels.
  - Complex vascular nidus.
  - Enlarged tortuous early draining venous vessels.

– Treatment.

  Indications for treatment.
  - Significant mass.
  - Pain.
  - Bleeding.
  - Ischemia.
  - Growth disturbance.
  - High-output cardiac state.
  - Cosmetically disfiguring lesions where there can be psychosocial repercussions.

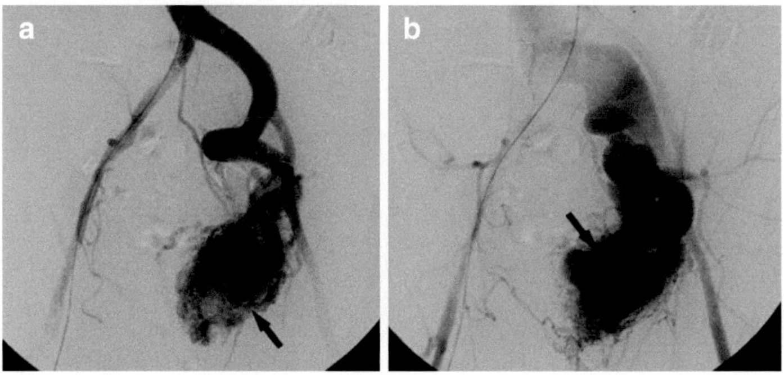

Fig. 23.7 Angiography of high flow AVM. (**a**) Early arterial phase pelvic arteriogram reveals a markedly enlarged internal iliac arterial distribution leading to a hypervascular nidus (arrow). (**b**) Late arterial phase image shows the full extent of the nidus with grossly enlarged internal iliac draining veins (arrow). (Reprinted with permission from [11])

Treatment options.

- There are a variety of approaches to treating these lesions.
  - Arterial based embolization.
  - Venous based embolization.
  - Direct puncture nidus embolization.
  - Surgery.
  - Systemic medical therapy (i.e. Sirolimus).
- Pre-intervention diagnostic angiography is helpful first to assess feeding vessel characteristics, nidus, and draining pathways.
- The goal of treatment is to eliminate the nidus, which is a low-pressure area that will stimulate collateral recruitment and recurrence if it is not eliminated.
- Elimination of the nidus is performed by superselective embolization making sure immediately adjacent vessels are treated.
- Arterial, direct puncture, or venous access may be used individually or in combination to ensure the successful embolization of the nidus (Fig. 23.8).
- Embolic agents.
  - Many options available and dependent on lesion characteristics and operator preference.
  - Embolic particles (i.e. polyvinyl alcohol (PVA) particles).
  - Coils.
  - Plugs.
  - Liquid embolic (i.e. ethylene vinyl alcohol copolymer or n-butyl-2-cyanoacrylate) [6].
  - Sclerosants (i.e. absolute ethanol).

Vascular Malformation Syndromes

- Klippel-Trenaunay Syndrome.
  - A vascular malformation syndrome that exhibits complex low-flow vascular malformations of an extremity.
  - Clinical features (three classic findings) [7].

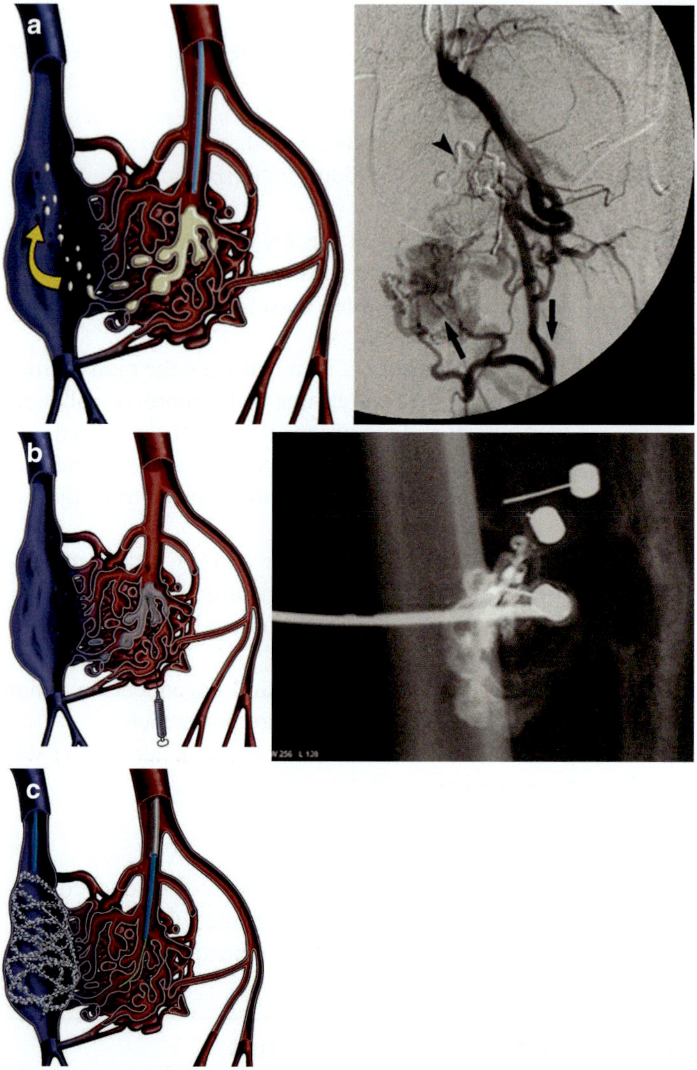

Fig. 23.8 Treatment options of high flow AVMs. (**a**) A superselective catheter site close to the nidus of an AVM should be chosen for embolosclerotherapy to be maximally effective. (**b**) Direct percutaneous needle puncture into the nidus for administration of sclerosant that allows for maximal endothelial-cidal effect of the agent and protection against nontarget embolization. (**c**) Venous embolization of AVM nidus can reduce total flow within the lesion allowing greater effectiveness of transarterial sclerosant. This technique also may serve as the most definitive AVM closure technique during multitechnique therapy. (Reprinted with permission from [11])

    Capillary malformations or patchy port wine stains covering a large area of the affected limb.

    Congenital varicose veins or venous malformations characterized by abnormally dilated blood vessels called lateral megaveins that develop on the lateral aspect of the affected limb.

    Bone and soft-tissue hypertrophy resulting from overgrowth.

  - Treatment.

    Ultrasound of the affected extremity is first performed to assess the status of the normal deep venous system. Alternatively, venography can be performed.

    Treatment is usually conservative and consists of compression therapy with support stockings.

    Sclerotherapy, and laser or radiofrequency ablation may also be employed to treat symptomatic varicose veins and swelling.

- Parkes Weber Syndrome.
  - A rare syndrome characterized by a combination of capillary and high flow arteriovenous malformations typically affecting one limb, most commonly the leg [7].
  - RASA1 mutation [8].
  - Clinical features.

    Capillary malformations, "port-wine stains."

    Arteriovenous malformations.

    Hypertrophy of the bone and soft tissue of the affected limb.

    Recurrent hemorrhage.

    High-output heart failure.

    Pain.

  - Treatment.

    Patients are treated on a symptomatic basis in much the same way as arteriovenous malformations.

Study Questions and Answers

1. A 2-week-old child is noted to have a warm, raised, red cutaneous lesion developed on the malar region of the child's face two days after birth. Since its appearance, the lesion has enlarged in size but is painless. Ultrasound demonstrates a well defined mass with prominent vascularity. What treatment should be offered?
   (A) Surgical excision
   (B) Conservative management
   (C) Sclerotherapy
   (D) Endovascular embolization
2. A 17 year-old male presents with asymmetric enlargement of the right leg and with multiple varices throughout the limb presents to your clinic complaining of a particularly painful varix on the lateral aspect of the thigh. The patient states his lower extremities have had this appearance for several years and has no history of trauma or malignancy. Ultrasound demonstrates numerous tortuous blood vessels with low, continuous velocity and no deep venous thrombosis. What is the most likely diagnosis?
   (A) Klippel-Trénaunay syndrome.
   (B) May-Thurner syndrome.
   (C) Parkes-Weber syndrome.
   (D) Maffucci Syndrome.
3. A 34-year-female presents to the emergency department with gross hematuria. Contrast enhanced CT of the abdomen and pelvis demonstrates a numerous vessels involving the lower pole of the right kidney. Sonographic examination reveals complex vessels in the lower pole of the right kidney with high velocity, pulsatile waveforms. When treating these lesions, what structure(s) should be targeted for treatment?
   (A) The inflow arterial branches.
   (B) The outflow venous branches.
   (C) The arterial inflow and venous outflow branches.
   (D) The nidus.

Answers: 1 (B), 2 (A), 3 (D)

References

1. ISSVA Classification of Vascular Anomalies ©2018 International Society for the Study of Vascular Anomalies Available at "issva.org/classification" Accessed December 12, 2019, https://www.issva.org/UserFiles/file/ISSVA Classification-2018.pdf.
2. Laffan EE, Ngan B-Y, Navarro OM. Pediatric soft-tissue tumors and pseudotumors: MR imaging features with pathologic correlation: part 2. Tumors of fibroblastic/myofibroblastic, so-called fibrohistiocytic, muscular, lymphomatous, neurogenic, hair matrix, and uncertain origin. Radiographics. 2009;29:e36.
3. Zheng JW, Zhang L, Zhou Q, et al. A practical guide to treatment of infantile hemangiomas of the head and neck. Int J Clin Exp Med. 2013;6:851–60.
4. Behravesh S, Yakes W, Gupta N, et al. Venous malformations: clinical diagnosis and treatment. Cardiovasc Diagn Ther. 2016;6:557–69.
5. de Serres LM, Sie KC, Richardson MA. Lymphatic malformations of the head and neck. A proposal for staging. Arch Otolaryngol Head Neck Surg. 1995;121:577–82.
6. Numan F, Omeroglu A, Kara B, et al. Embolization of peripheral vascular malformations with ethylene vinyl alcohol copolymer (onyx). J Vasc Interv Radiol. 2004;15:939–46.
7. Nozaki T, Nosaka S, Miyazaki O, et al. Syndromes associated with vascular tumors and malformations: a pictorial review. Radiographics. 2013;33:175–95.
8. Revencu N, Boon LM, Mulliken JB, et al. Parkes weber syndrome, vein of Galen aneurysmal malformation, and other fast-flow vascular anomalies are caused by RASA1 mutations. Hum Mutat. 2008;29:959–65.
9. Flors L, Leiva-Salinas C, Maged IM, et al. MR imaging of soft-tissue vascular malformations: diagnosis, classification, and therapy follow-up. Radiographics. 2011;31:1321–40; discussion 1340–1
10. Legiehn GM, Heran MKS. Venous malformations: classification, development, diagnosis, and interventional radiologic management. Radiol Clin N Am. 2008;46:545–97, vi.
11. Legiehn GM, Heran MKS. Classification, diagnosis, and interventional radiologic management of vascular malformations. Orthop Clin North Am. 2006;37:435–74, vii–viii.

24 Complications of Vascular Surgery

Christian Ochoa
and Miguel Francisco Manzur

Diagnosis and Management of Complications of Vascular Therapy

1. Pseudoaneurysms (PSA)
   (a) Most commonly develop after angiographic procedures when access site arteriotomy has not adequately sealed after sheath removal
   (b) Blood spreads into the surrounding soft tissue which leads to compressed thrombus along with the soft tissue to pseudocapsule formation
   (c) Etiology—inability to adequately compress access site vessel or closure device failure after sheath removed
      - Seen with superficial femoral artery, low common femoral artery, or external iliac artery puncture that is not compressible by the femoral head
   (d) Risk factors—female sex, increasing age, concomitant venous puncture, hypertension, severely calcified vessels,

C. Ochoa (✉)
Vascular Surgery, Keck Medical Center of USC, Los Angeles, CA, USA
e-mail: Christian.ochoa@med.usc.edu

M. F. Manzur
Vascular Surgery, LAC+USC/Keck Medical Center of USC, Los Angeles, CA, USA
e-mail: miguel.manzur@med.usc.edu

A. Murga et al. (eds.), *The Vascular Surgery In-Training Examination Review (VSITE)*,
https://doi.org/10.1007/978-3-031-24121-5_24

large access sheath size (>6 French (Fr)), use of anticoagulation at time of access or immediately afterwards [1]

(e) Physical exam—severe groin pain, ecchymosis, pulsatile groin mass, systolic bruit
   - Can present from 24 h after procedure to 7–10 days afterward

(f) Diagnosis
   - Arterial Duplex—pulsatile echolucent sac, swirling flow pattern, "to- and-fro" pattern, able to evaluate size, neck diameter and length (Fig. 24.1)

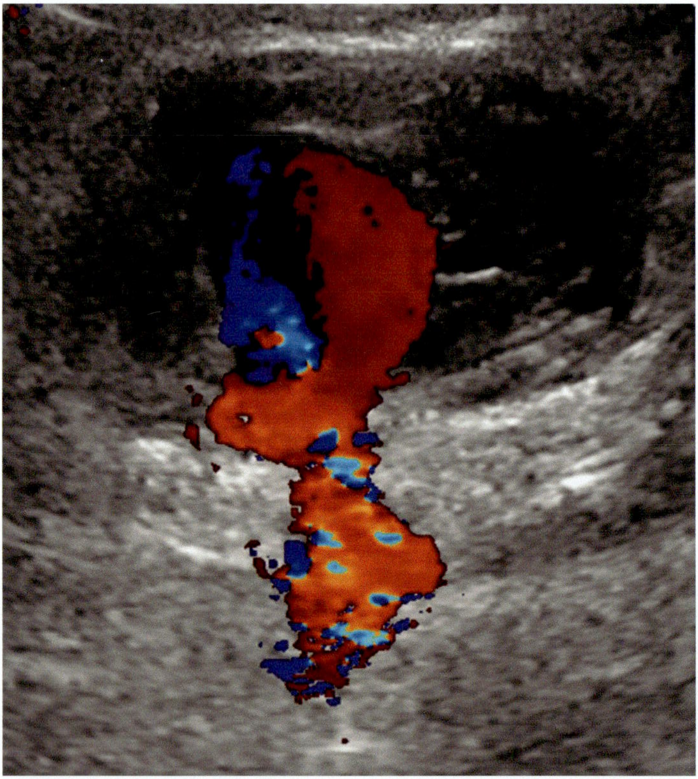

Fig. 24.1 Arterial duplex demonstrating "to-and-fro" mosaic pattern

- Computed tomography (CT) angiogram—concern for high arterial puncture and retroperitoneal extension, evaluate size and neck diameter, and additional injury sites

(g) Management
- Observation
  - Small PSAs that are less than <2 cm [2]
- Treatment—>2 cm or on anticoagulation/antiplatelet therapy
  - Ultrasound-guided thrombin (1000 IU/mL) injection (found to be more successful than compression method, >90% successful) [3, 4]

    Use thrombin to convert fibrinogen to fibrin—form clot and ultimately thrombosis of PSA

    Bedrest post-procedure and then repeat duplex examination in 24 h.

    Complications—distal embolization/local thrombosis (wide necks >1 cm), anaphylaxis (Bovine preparations)
  - Ultrasound-guided compression—cycles of 10–20 min of compression

    Success ~70% [3]
    - More likely to fail if patient on anticoagulation, large size of PSA, patient discomfort, or obese
  - Surgical Management

    Indications: Larger PSAs/active hemorrhage, wide neck, failed compression/thrombin injection, ischemic necrosis of the overlying skin, compression neuropathy of the femoral nerve

    Options—endovascular (covered stent) vs. direct open surgical repair (primary repair vs. patch repair)

2. Anastomotic Aneurysm

(a) Complicate 1–4% of arterial anastomoses, mean of 6 years following graft implantation (shorter timespan if infection) [5–7]

(b) Most common is the femoral artery (0.5–24%) [8]
(c) Pathogenesis—suture line disruption leading to the egress of blood and formation of false aneurysm [9]
  - Local factors [9]
    - Arterial wall degeneration—progression of atherosclerosis, attenuated arterial wall (decreased elastic fibers in media and replacement with fibrous connective tissue)
    - Suture line disruption—loss of tensile strength of suture. Monofilament polypropylene (Prolene) has inherent resistance to infection and maintains tensile strength but will fray and fracture with handling of suture
    - Graft failure—can fray with handling, recommended to incorporate greater margin of graft into anastomosis
    - Infection/Inflammation—seen with early postoperative anastomotic aneurysms. Associated with hematomas, lymphoceles, and smoldering infections
    - Technical errors—lack of good arterial bites, graft tension, poor suture handling
    - Mechanical stress—compliance mismatch, the greater the diameter and angle (end-to-side) the greater the tension/turbulence on the suture line, end to end has less anastomotic turbulence
  - Systemic factors—Smoking, hypertension, hyperlipidemia effects vessel wall integrity. Acquired vasculitis (Bechets, Takayasu's) [9]
(d) Diagnosis—seen on routine surveillance or imaging of unrelated clinical issues. Most likely present as asymptomatic pulsatile mass but can also present as acute thrombosis, embolization or cause local compression (vein, nerves) [7, 10]
  - Imaging—CT (Fig. 24.2) or Magnetic resonance imaging (MRI), if suspect infection, erythrocyte sedimentation rate (ESR), C-reactive protein (CRP), and tagged white blood cell (WBC) scan may aid in narrowing the diagnosis

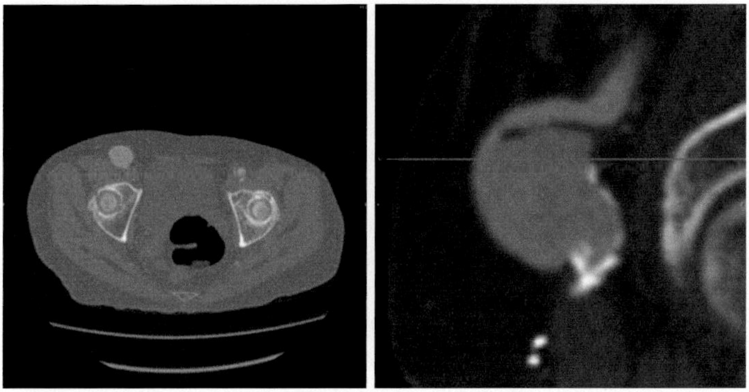

Fig. 24.2 CT scan demonstrating right common femoral anastomotic aneurysm that had developed after Aortobifemoral bypass

- Need to evaluate other anastomoses—synchronous anastomotic aneurysms in 36%

(e) Treatment—for open repair need to maintain principles of proximal and distal control along with control of other collateral branches, may need to employ balloon occlusion in hostile/scarred fields

- Femoral—may need proximal control of the external iliac artery via a suprainguinal incision and retroperitoneal exposure [7]
  - Infectious—extra-anatomic reconstruction (i.e. obturator bypass) and debridement
  - Non-infectious—interposition graft replacement (end to end, if need to preserve retrograde pelvic circulation do end to side)
- Aortic—pre-operative imaging critical for planning for proximal clamp placement (supraceliac or suprarenal), proximity to visceral branches [9, 11, 12]
  - Open repair—if infectious etiology then will need graft excision with in situ aortic replacement or extra-anatomic bypass, if not then can do replacement with tube graft with potential visceral bypass
  - Endovascular repair—tubular, bifurcated, or fenestrated/branched, chimney techniques. Need to

ensure adequate proximal seal for fixation and exclusion

- Iliac—usually near the distal anastomosis at the iliac bifurcation [9]
  - Open repair—ureter protection, may need to make separate bypass to the internal iliac artery
  - Endovascular repair—may need to either cover and coil the internal iliac artery to ensure exclusion but if need to preserve can use commercially available branched iliac endograft or separate bypass [13, 14]
- Carotid—rule out infection in setting of patient's with history of patch angioplasty using prosthetic patch material [15, 16]
  - Open—resect the aneurysm and interposition graft or repair with patch angioplasty. Suspect infection—reconstruction with saphenous vein. Carotid artery ligation if fail reconstruction but associated with high incidence of ipsilateral stroke and with an associated 30–50% mortality [17]
  - Endovascular—employed to avoid difficult dissection and risk of cranial nerve injury [16]

3. Aortoenteric Fistula/Erosion
   (a) Communication between the aorta and the gastrointestinal (GI) tract
   (b) Primary aortoenteric (AE) fistula—Native aorta and GI tract, most commonly seen associated with aneurysmal disease, but can be seen with foreign bodies, tumors, infection, peptic ulcer disease, and post-radiated fields [9, 18].
      - Commonly seen in the third and fourth portion of the duodenum
      - Pulsatile pressure from the aneurysmal aorta leads to local compression and ischemia leading to erosion and fistula [9]
   (c) Secondary AE fistula—Reconstructed aorta and GI tract, more common and related to prior vascular surgery, usually 2–6 years afterwards [19]

- Can be seen in distal duodenum/proximal jejunum but can be seen anywhere there is bowel in contact with the prosthetic material or its suture line.
- Mechanism related to infection, pulsatile pressure and technical error (graft inoculation, delayed bowel injury) [9]
  - Limit bowel contact—retroperitoneal approach, close aneurysm sac, interpose omentum between graft and bowel
- Seen with endovascular repair—persistent endoleak, erosion of stent graft through the aorta, multiple rounds of coiling, infection at time of graft placement [20]

(d) Diagnosis—most commonly present with GI bleed but can present with abdominal pain, pulsatile abdominal mass, fever/sepsis [21]

- "Herald bleed"—minor bleed that is self-limited or can be recurring and can be followed by massive exsanguination
- Secondary AE fistula can also present with occult peripheral abscess, graft limb thrombosis, groin fistula or femoral pseudoaneurysm
- CT scan—will see perigraft fluid and soft tissue thickening, gas, extravasation of contrast from aorta into the bowel
- Endoscopy—can be used to exclude other sources of bleeding, only try to do in patients who are hemodynamically stable. May see graft, ulcer, adherent clot, pulsatile mass [9]

(e) Treatment

- Unstable—central venous access, volume resuscitation, intravenous antibiotics
  - Midline laparotomy, proximal control (infrarenal or supraceliac, or balloon control), and distal control
  - Dissect off bowel, control spillage, primary repair or resect bowel (higher incidence of recurrence with primary repair), and place tissue in between repair and aorta [22].

  - Repair of aorta: If no infection attempt repair with either prosthetic graft, cadaveric artery, or femoral vein. If infected debride the retroperitoneum and either perform in situ autogenous aortic graft replacement or oversow and cover the aortic stump with omentum, then do extra-anatomic bypass.
- Stable—try to perform the extra-anatomic bypass first, reduces clamp time and preserves pelvic circulation and allows the limbs to be perfused
  - Primary AE Fistula

    Mild Contamination—in situ replacement of aorta with local debridement and long term intravenous (IV) antibiotics

    Gross contamination—extra-anatomic bypass, aneurysm resection and omentoplasty of aortic stump, retroperitoneal debridement
  - Secondary AE Fistula—goal is to remove all infected synthetic material [9]

    Graft excision without replacement—graft originally placed for occlusive disease or chronically occluded. If end-to side do patch repair after removed

    In-site aortic graft replacement—cryopreserved allografts, antibiotic (Rifampin) soaked synthetic grafts or dacron coated with silver

    Neo-Aortoiliac System (NAIS) Procedure—using autologous tissue, no aortic stump, inexpensive but labor intensive (harvesting femoral vein) [23]

    Extra-anatomic bypass—axillobifemoral bypass; however, if contamination spreads into the femoral arteries may need to do bilateral axillo-unifemoral bypasses down to the superficial femoral or profunda arteries [9].

    Endovascular repair—allows rapid control of hemorrhage but only temporizing until definitive repair [24, 25]

      Majority of patients die from septic complications or recurrent hemorrhage
  - In all cases—long term IV antibiotics (6 weeks) and long-term surveillance

4. Aortocaval Fistula
   (a) Seen with rupture or erosion of an atherosclerotic, inflammatory, or mycotic aortic or iliac aneurysm into the inferior vena cava (IVC), iliac vein, or retro-aortic left renal vein [26]
   (b) If large arteriovenous fistula (AVF) get increase in preload leading to cardiomegaly and, if left untreated can lead to high-output congestive heart failure (CHF)
   (c) Diagnosis—Can present with aortic pulsation with associated epigastric thrill or bruit, lower extremity venous hypertension, abdominal or back pain, or cardiac decompensation from CHF
       - Imaging
         - Duplex ultrasound—visualize the AVF, color mosaic, diminished or reversal of flow in the distal artery, high velocity flow in the distal vein
         - CT angiography
   (d) Treatment
       - Endovascular repair—feasible option that may be limited by anatomic constraints (neck length, aortic neck angulation, access vessels), may need additional stent or IVC filter to prevent pulmonary embolization on the venous side [27–30]
       - Open repair—Obtain control of aorta and IVC, open aorta and ligate the connection to the IVC from inside the aorta [9]. Be mindful of open IVC and risk of embolism of thrombus or air.
5. Graft Infections
   (a) Incidence low, 0.2–5% of open operations and influenced by implant site (femoral, subcutaneous tunnel) and indication (emergent) [31]
   (b) Early (<4 months)—caused by virulent hospital acquired bacteria and can present with sepsis and wound infection. Seen with extra-anatomical grafts [9, 32]

(c) Late (>4 months)—colonization by low virulence organisms such as *Staphylococcus epidermidis*. Seen most commonly with grafts in anatomical positions (aortic) [9]

(d) Sources—contamination (during implantation, surgical wound, hematogenous/lymphatic sources), bacteremia (hematogenous from separate source), contiguous infectious process (diverticulitis, infected lymphocele), mechanical erosion (skin, GI or GU tract), immunodeficiency (autoimmune, drugs, diabetes mellitus, malnutrition, malignancy) [9]

(e) Bacteriology
  - Early—Most common *Staphylococcus aureus*, however, gram negative bacteria such as *Escherichia coli* or *Pseudomonas aeruginosa* more virulent because of destructive endotoxins [33]
  - Late—*S. epidermidis*. Usually lack signs of systemic sepsis [34]

(f) Diagnosis [9]
  - Can present asymptomatic, smoldering fevers, or the following presenting signs/symptoms
    - Aortic grafts—sepsis, ileus, GI bleed
    - Extra-anatomic grafts—cellulitis, draining sinus tract, anastomotic pseudoaneurysm
  - Imaging—start with CT scan with IV contrast—will have loss of normal tissue planes in the retroperitoneum or in the subcutaneous tissues, false aneurysms, gas present >2 months after implantation

(g) Treatment
  - Goals of treatment—eradicate infectious source and maintain sufficient arterial perfusion
  - Aortic—total graft excision, retroperitoneal debridement and revascularization via extra-anatomic routes. Close aortic stump in two layers and buttress with omentum
    - No revascularization needed—excise graft only in those whose initial indication for surgery was claudication or low risk for limb ischemia

    - Revascularization needed
      Urgent—do excision in conjunction with revascularization
      Non-urgent—axillofemoral bypass prior to excision of aortic graft or in situ replacement [35, 36]
        - In situ replacement—NAIS procedure, rifampin soaked dacron, cryopreserved aorta [37–40]
  - Peripheral
    - No revascularization needed—excise graft in those whose initial indication for surgery was claudication or low risk for limb ischemia
    - Revascularization needed
      Excise graft and utilize greater saphenous vein to reconstruct or femoral vein for large diameter arterial reconstruction or perform extra-anatomic bypass (obturator bypass) [41]
  - Parenteral antibiotics based on perigraft/graft culture results for 4–6 weeks
  - Post-operative imaging at 1 year for surveillance
  - If area of graft exposed or has been preserved or replaced with new in situ graft plan for soft tissue coverage
    - Aorta—pedicled omentum
    - Peripheral—sartorius muscle flap in the groin, other options include gracilis, rectus femoris or rectus abdominis flaps [42]

6. Colon Ischemia after aortic surgery
   (a) Associated with ligation of inferior mesentery artery (IMA), no revascularization of the internal iliac arteries, iliofemoral disease, superior mesenteric artery (SMA) stenosis, retractor injury, previous colonic resection [43]
   (b) Postoperative diarrhea, melena, or hematochezia warrants further investigation via flexible sigmoidoscopy or colonoscopy [43]
   (c) Aggressively resuscitate, start on IV broad spectrum antibiotics

   (d) Non-operative therapy—Limited to mucosa and no systemic instability
   (e) Operative therapy—full thickness ischemia, organ failure, exploration laparotomy, and bowel resection
7. Tracheoinnominate Fistula [44]
   (a) Sentinel bleed followed by massive hemoptysis, seen 3–4 weeks after tracheostomy creation, earlier bleeding (48 h) associated with anterior jugular or inferior thyroid veins
   (b) Tracheostomy tube and cuff can place pressure on the anterior tracheal wall. Avoided if tracheostomy placed above the third tracheal ring, between the second and third ring, and cuff pressure kept below 25 mmHg.
   (c) If no longer requiring ventilation change tube to cuff-less or down size and decannulate
   (d) Stable patient
      - CT angiography to visualize anatomic relationships and if indeed a fistulous tract has formed and then OR if the tract exists
      - High index of suspicion—take to OR and perform flexible or rigid bronchoscopy
   (e) Unstable patient/Hemorrhaging
      - First try to overinflate the tracheostomy cuff, if unsuccessful, extend the tracheostomy incision to allow finger pressure anteriorly to compress the innominate artery. Secure airway with oral endotracheal tube. Transport to OR.
   (f) Operative management—median sternotomy, divide the thymus and mobilize the innominate vein. Proximal and distal control on the innominate artery. Resect and over sow with 4-0 prolene suture in two layers.
      - Ligate the innominate artery proximally at its origin and distally just proximal to bifurcation of the right common carotid the right subclavian artery.
      - Debride the tracheal injury and repaired with 4-0 PDS suture and buttress the repair with sternocleidomastoid or strap muscle flap
      - Bronchoscopy at the end to remove all blood from the distal airways

    - Alternative is endovascular repair but only for bridge to definitive therapy depending on the status of the patient

8. Chylous Ascites/Chylothorax
   (a) Chylous Ascites—very rare after abdominal aortic reconstruction
      - Progressive abdominal pain, dyspnea, nausea/decreased oral intake
      - Diagnosis—CT scan and paracentesis for confirmation of chyle (+sudan stain) [9, 45]
      - Treatment—mild/moderate case restrict diet to medium chain triglyceride diet, if severe, complete bowel rest and parenteral nutrition [45, 46]
         – No resolution—operative exploration and closure/ligation of lymphatic injury
   (b) Chylothorax—very rare after cardiothoracic surgery, seen more in children with congenital vascular anomalies [47]
      - Diagnosis—pleural effusion seen on chest X-ray or CT scan. Thoracentesis confirms the fluid
      - Treatment—drainage first and foremost with tube thoracostomy [48, 49]
         – Similar approach to treatment as with above for chylous ascites
         – Surgical ligation of thoracic duct if high output fistula (>1 L/24 h) or if remains >200 mL/24 h after 1 week

           Video-assisted thoracoscopic surgery (VATS) is the preferred approach

Questions

1. Which modality of non-surgical treatment for arterial iatrogenic access pseudoaneurysms has been found to be the most successful for inducing thrombosis?
   (a) Observation
   (b) Ultrasound guided compression
   (c) Ultrasound guided thrombin injection
   (d) Fem-stop

2. What diet has been shown to help reduce the production of chylous ascites in mild cases?
   (a) High fatty diet
   (b) Medium chain triglyceride diet
   (c) Carbohydrate controlled diet
   (d) Low residue diet
3. Which bacteria have been implicated in late graft infections?
   (a) *S. aureus*
   (b) *P. aeruginosa*
   (c) *E. faecalis*
   (d) *S. epidermidis*

Answer: 1 (c), 2 (b), 3 (d)

References

1. Kresowik TF, Khoury MD, Miller BV, Winniford MD, Shamma AR, Sharp WJ, Blecha MB, Corson JD. A prospective study of the incidence and natural history of femoral vascular complications after percutaneous transluminal coronary angioplasty. J Vasc Surg. 1991;13(2):328.
2. Toursarkissian B, Allen BT, Petrinec D, Thompson RW, Rubin BG, Reilly JM, Anderson CB, Flye MW, Sicard GA. Spontaneous closure of selected iatrogenic pseudoaneurysms and arteriovenous fistulae. J Vasc Surg. 1997;25(5):803.
3. Lönn L, Olmarker A, Geterud K, Risberg B. Prospective randomized study comparing ultrasound-guided thrombin injection to compression in the treatment of femoral pseudoaneurysms. J Endovasc Ther. 2004;11(5):570.
4. Khoury M, Rebecca A, Greene K, Rama K, Colaiuta E, Flynn L, Berg R. Duplex scanning-guided thrombin injection for the treatment of iatrogenic pseudoaneurysms. J Vasc Surg. 2002;35(3):517.
5. Abou-Zamzam AM Jr, Ballard JL. Management of sterile para-anastomotic aneurysms of the aorta. Semin Vasc Surg. 2001;14(4):282–91.
6. Youkey JR, Clagett GP, Rich NM, Brigham RA, Orecchia PM, Salander JM. Femoral anastomotic false aneurysms. An 11-year experience analyzed with a case control study. Ann Surg. 1984;199(6):703–9.
7. Dennis JW, Littooy FN, Greisler HP, Baker WH, Anastomotic pseudoaneurysms. A continuing late complication of vascular reconstructive procedures. Arch Surg. 1986;121(3):314–7.

8. Szilagyi DE, Elliott JP Jr, Smith RF, Reddy DJ, McPharlin M. A thirty-year survey of the reconstructive surgical treatment of aortoiliac occlusive disease. J Vasc Surg. 1986;3(3):421–36.
9. Sidawy A, Perler B. Rutherford's vascular surgery and endovascular therapy. 9th ed. Philadelphia, PA: Elsevier; 2019.
10. Demarche M, Waltregny D, Van Damme H, Limet R. Femoral anastomotic aneurysms: pathogenic factors, clinical presentations and treatment. A study of 142 cases. Cardiovasc Surg. 1999;7(3):315–22.
11. Van Herwaarden JA, Waasdorp EJ, Bendermacher BL, Van den Berg JC, Teijink JA, Moll FL. Endovascular repair of paraanastomotic aneurysms after previous open aortic prosthetic reconstruction. Ann Vasc Surg. 2004;18(3):280–6.
12. Wu Z, Xu L, Raithel D, Qu L. Endovascular repair of proximal para-anastomotic aneurysms after previous open abdominal aortic aneurysm reconstruction. Vascular. 2016;24(3):227–32.
13. Sanchez LA, Patel AV, Ohki T. Midterm experience with the endovascular treatment of isolated iliac aneurysms. J Vasc Surg. 1999;30(5):907–13.
14. Criado E, Marston WA, Ligush J, Mauro MA, Keagy BA. Endovascular repair of peripheral aneurysms, pseudoaneurysms, and arteriovenous fistulas. Ann Vasc Surg. 1997;11(3):256–63.
15. Zhou W, Lin PH, Bush RL. Carotid artery aneurysm: evolution of management over two decades. J Vasc Surg. 2006;43(3):493–6.
16. Borazjani BH, Wilson SE, Fujitani RM, Gordon I, Mueller M, Williams RA. Postoperative complications of carotid patching: pseudoaneurysm and infection. Ann Vasc Surg. 2003;17(2):156–61.
17. Branch CL Jr, Davis CH Jr. False aneurysm complicating carotid endarterectomy. Neurosurgery. 1986;19(3):421–5.
18. Saers SJ, Scheltinga MR. Primary aortoenteric fistula. Br J Surg. 2005;92:143.
19. Hallett JW Jr, Marsal DM, Petterson TM, Gray DT, Bower TC, Cherry KJ Jr, Gloviczki P, Pairolero PC. Graft-related complications after abdominal aortic aneurysm repair: reassurance from a 36-year population-based experience. J Vasc Surg. 1997;25:277.
20. Kahlberg A, Rinaldi E, Piffaretti G, Speziale F, Trimarchi S, Bonardelli S, Melissano G, Chlesa R. Results from the multicenter study on aortoenteric fistulization after stent grafting of the abdominal aorta (MAEFISTO). J Vasc Surg. 2016;64:313.
21. Ranasinghe W, Loa J, Allaf N, Lewis K, Sebastian MG. Primary aortoenteric fistulae: the challenges in diagnosis and review of treatment. Ann Vasc Surg. 2011;25:386.e1.
22. Rodrigues dos Santos C, Casaca R, Mendes de Almeida JC, Mendes-Pedro L. Enteric repair in aortoduodenal fistulas: a forgotten but often lethal player. Ann Vasc Surg. 2014;28:756.
23. Chung J, Clagett GP. Neoaortoiliac system (NAIS) procedure for the treatment of the infected aortic graft. Semin Vasc Surg. 2011;24:220.

24. Antoniou GA, Koustsia S, Antonious SA, Georgiakakis A, Lazarides MK, Giannoukas AD. Outcome after endovascular stent graft repair of aortoenteric fistula: a systematic review. J Vasc Surg. 2009;49:782.
25. Kakkos SK, Antoniadis PN, Klonaris CN, Papazoglou KO, Giannoukas AD, Matsagkas MI, Kotsis T, Dervisis K, Gerasimidis T, Tsolakis IA, Lipais CD. Open or endovascular repair of aortoenteric fistulas? A multicentre comparative study. Eur J Vasc Endovasc Surg. 2011;41:625.
26. Brewster DG, et al. Aortocaval and iliac arteriovenous fistulas: recognition and treatment. J Vasc Surg. 1991;13:258–65.
27. Parodi JC. Endovascular repair of aortic aneurysms, arteriovenous fistulas and false aneurysms. World J Surg. 1996;20:655–63.
28. Lau LL, O'reilly MJ, Johnston LC, Lee B. Endovascular stent-graft repair of primary aortocaval fistula with an abdominal aortoiliac aneurysm. J Vasc Surg. 2001;33:425–8.
29. Umscheid T, Stelter WJ. Endovascular treatment of an aortic aneurysm ruptured into the inferior vena cava. J Endovasc Ther. 2000;7:31–5.
30. Kwon SH, Oh JH, Park SJ, Park HC. Endovascular repair of a spontaneous right common iliac artery—inferior vena cava fistula due to infrarenal aortoiliac aneurysm. Vasc Endovasc Surg. 2008;42:279–83.
31. Bandyk DF. Vascular graft infections: epidemiology, microbiology, pathogenesis, and prevention. In: Bernhard VM, Towne JB, editors. Complications in vascular surgery. St Louis: Quality Medical; 1991. p. 223.
32. Szilagyi DE, Smith RF, Elliott JP, Vrandecic MP. Infection in arterial reconstruction with synthetic grafts. Ann Surg. 1972;176:321.
33. Nasim A, Thompson MM, Naylor AR, Bell PR, London NJ. The impact of MRSA on vascular surgery. Eur J Vasc Endovasc Surg. 2001;22:211.
34. Bergamini TM, et al. Identification of Staphylococcus epidermidis vascular graft infections: a comparison of culture techniques. J Vasc Surg. 1989;9:665.
35. Reilly LM, Stoney RJ, Goldstone J, Ehrenfeld WK. Improved management of aortic graft infection: the influence of operation sequence and staging. J Vasc Surg. 1987;5:421.
36. Seeger JM, et al. Long-term outcome after treatment of aortic graft infection with staged extra-anatomic bypass and aortic graft removal. J Vasc Surg. 2000;32:451.
37. Clagett GP, Valentine RJ, Hagino RT. Autogenous aortoiliac/femoral reconstruction from superficial femoral-popliteal veins: feasibility and durability. J Vasc Surg. 1997;25:255–66.
38. Batt M, et al. In situ revascularization with silver coated polyester grafts to treat aortic infection: early and midterm results. J Vasc Surg. 2003;38:983.
39. Oderich GS, Bower TC, Hofer J, Kalra M, Duncan AA, Wilson JW, Cha S, Gloviczki P. In situ rifampin-soaked grafts with omental coverage and

antibiotic suppression are durable with low reinfection rates in patients with aortic graft enteric erosion or fistula. J Vasc Surg. 2011;53:99.
40. Bisdas T, Bredt M, Pichlmaier M, Aper T, Wilhemi M, Bisdas S, Haverich A, Teebken OE. Eight-year experience with cryopreserved arterial homografts for the in situ reconstruction of abdominal aortic infections. J Vasc Surg. 2010;52:323.
41. Seeger JM, Wheeler JR, Gregory RT, Snyder SO, Gayle RG. Autogenous graft replacement of infected prosthetic grafts in the femoral position. Surgery. 1983;93:39.
42. Armstrong PA, Back MR, Bandyk DF, Johnson BL, Shames ML. Selective application of sartorius muscle flaps and aggressive staged surgical debridement can influence long-term outcomes of complex prosthetic graft infections. J Vasc Surg. 2007;46:71.
43. Menegaux F, Tresallet C, Kieffer E, Bodin L, Thabut D, Rouby J-J. Aggressive management of nonocclusive ischemic colitis following aortic reconstruction. Arch Surg. 2006;141:678–82.
44. Ailawadi G. Technique for managing tracheo-innominate artery fistula. J Op Techs Thorac Cardiovasc Surg. 2009;9:66–72.
45. Ablan CJ, Littooy FN, Freeark RJ. Postoperative chylous ascites: diagnosis and treatment. Arch Surg. 1990;125:270.
46. Weninger M, D'Haese JG, Angele MK, Kleespies A, Werner J, Hartwig W. Treatment options for chylous ascites after major abdominal surgery: a systematic review. Am J Surg. 2016;211:206.
47. Kostiainen S, Meurala H, Mattila S, Appelqvist P. Chylothorax: clinical experience in nine cases. Scand J Thorac Cardiovasc Surg. 1983;17:79–83.
48. Cerfolio RJ, Allen MS, Deschamps C, Trastek VF, Pairolero PC. Postoperative chylothorax. J Thorac Cardiovasc Surg. 1996;112:1361–5.
49. Hirata N, Ueno T, Amemiya A, Shigemura N, Akashi A, Kido T. Advantage of earlier thoracoscopic clipping of thoracic duct for post-operation chylothorax following thoracic aneurysm surgery. J Thorac Cardiovasc Surg. 2003;51:378–80.

25 Amputations

Cassra N. Arbabi and Allen Murga

Amputations

Primary objective of an amputation:

- Eliminate infected, necrotic, malignant, and/or painful tissue
- Achieve adequate wound healing
- Maximize functional potential (prosthesis, ambulation)

Major Amputation—Above the ankle

Minor Amputation—Below the ankle

Primary Amputation—performed without an attempt at limb salvage

Secondary Amputation—performed after a failed attempt at limb salvage

Traumatic Amputation—limb loss secondary to trauma, often due to a mangled extremity or failed attempt to salvage the limb

C. N. Arbabi
Department of Vascular Surgery, Cedars-Sinai Medical Center, Beverly Hills, CA, USA

A. Murga (✉)
Department of Vascular Surgery, Loma Linda University, Loma Linda, CA, USA
e-mail: amurga@llu.edu

A. Murga et al. (eds.), *The Vascular Surgery In-Training Examination Review (VSITE)*,
https://doi.org/10.1007/978-3-031-24121-5_25

Most common indications for amputation [1]:

- Infectious—wet gangrene, necrotizing soft tissue infection (NSTI), osteomyelitis
- Ischemic—dry gangrene secondary to chronic limb threatening ischemia (CLTI), acute limb ischemia (non-salvageable limb)
- Traumatic—mangled extremity, vascular injury not amenable to repair or failed repair
- Malignancy—tumor not amenable to limb salvage operation

Risk factor:

- Diabetes Mellitus (DM)
  - Diabetics—8× greater risk of amputation than those without DM [2]
    DM → Neuropathy → wounds/ulcers (i.e. mal perforans) → diabetic foot infection (DFI) and/or diabetic foot osteomyelitis (DFO)
    DM → Increased risk of infection
    DM → Increased prevalence of atherosclerosis → PAD
- Peripheral arterial disease (PAD)
- Smoking

Risk factors for mortality:

- DNR status
- Congestive heart failure (CHF)
- Age >80
- Dependent living status
- Coronary artery disease
- Chronic obstructive pulmonary disease
- End-stage renal disease
- AKA has 2× the mortality risk compared to BKA [3]

Determination of amputation level—multifactorial, determined by:

- Extent/level of tissue loss
- Presence/severity of infection
- Revascularization status
- Healing potential
- Patient characteristics (functional status, age, comorbidities)

Imaging and adjunctive studies:

- Ankle-Brachial Index (ABI)
- Toe Pressures and Toe-Brachial Index (TBI)
  - More reliable than ABI in patients with diabetes and noncompressible tibial vessels
  - Normal TBI $\geq$0.7
  - Absolute Toe Pressure >30 mmHg predictive of wound healing
- Transcutaneous oxygen pressure measurement ($TCPO_2$)
  - Levels $\geq$30 mmHg are predictive of wound healing
  - Limitations—unreliable in the setting of edema, inflammation, overlying soft tissue necrosis, or infection
- Skin Perfusion Pressure (SPP)
- Arterial Duplex Ultrasound
- Computerized Tomography Angiography (CTA)/Magnetic Resonance Angiography (MRA)
- Conventional angiography

Sepsis or septic shock secondary to wet:

- Requires source control leading to a guillotine amputation followed by formalization
- A two-stage approach results in higher primary healing rates and decreased risk of more proximal amputation [4, 5]

Predictors of poor functional outcomes after major amputation:

- Dementia
- End stage renal disease (ESRD)
- Advanced coronary artery disease (CAD)
- Poor pre-operative functional status [6]
- Preoperative non-ambulatory status highest odds ratio (OR 9.5) of poor postoperative functional outcome [6]

Types of Amputation

Major Amputation:

- Above ankle amputations
  - Overall 30-day mortality approximately 5–8%
  - Nearly 20% in very high risk patients [3, 7]
- Below knee amputation:
  - Palpable popliteal pulse strongly predictive of wound healing in a BKA
  - Most common major lower extremity amputation performed
  - Five Types of Flaps
    - Posterior flap (preferred technique if healthy tissue exists) (see Fig. 25.1)
    - Sagittal flap
    - Skew flap
    - Fish-mouth flap
    - Medial flap
  - Requires 10–40% more than baseline energy expenditure to ambulate with a prosthesis (depending on length of the stump) [8]
  - 15–25% BKA to AKA revision [9–11]
  - 20–30% of BKAs fail to heal properly
  - Overall survival following BKA → 70% and 35% at 1 and 5 years, respectively
    - Significantly worse in patients with DM and ESRD [9, 12].

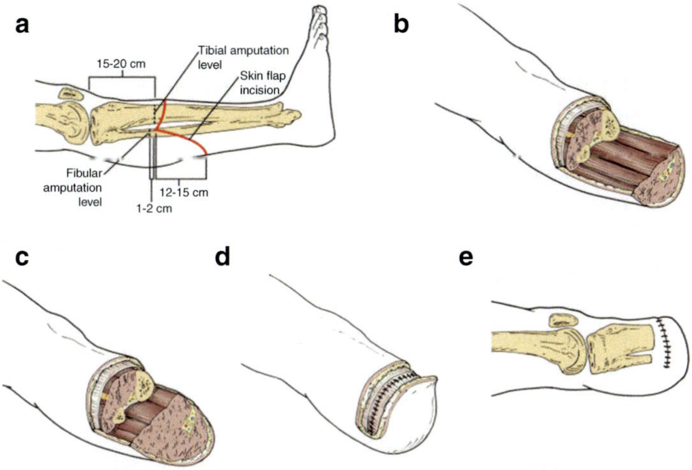

Fig. 25.1 Below the knee amputation. (**a**) Placement of incisions. (**b**) Posterior flap after bone resection. (**c**) Soleus muscle is trimmed to create flap. (**d**) Suturing of fascia. (**e**) Final skin incision. (Taken from Rutherford's Vascular Surgery and Endovascular Therapy 9th Ed. Ch. 112)

- Above Knee Amputation (AKA):
  - Palpable femoral pulse strongly predictive of wound healing in an AKA
  - Higher mortality risk (2×) compared to BKA
  - Superior wound healing compared to BKA
  - Requires two-thirds more than baseline energy expenditure to ambulate with a prosthesis [8]
- Through Knee Amputation (TKA):
  - Reserved for patients with good rehab potential
  - Preserves more limb length
  - Less energy expenditure during ambulation compared to AKA
  - Migration or nonunion of patella in 3% [9]
  - Reamputation at a higher level in 10–15% of patients after TKA [9]
- Hip Disarticulation:
  - Very high morbidity
  - Requires 80% more than baseline energy expenditure to ambulate with a prosthesis [8]
  - Very low ambulation rates

Minor Amputation: At or below the ankle

- Approximately 25% of toe amputations fail to heal and require additional amputation at a higher level
- 40% will require BKA [13, 14]
- Toe Amputations:
  - Includes partial digit and total digital amputations
  - For treatment of wounds limited to middle/distal phalanx
- Ray Amputation**:**
  - Includes toe and metatarsal head
  - For treatment of wounds involving all or part of the metatarsal head

    Mal-perforans ulcers
  - Higher morbidity compared to toe amputation
  - Recurrent ulceration in nearly 2/3 of patients following 1st ray amputation
  - Nearly 20% reamputation rate after 1st ray
- Transmetatarsal Amputation (TMA): (see Fig. 25.2)
  - Lesions involving >3 metatarsal heads
  - Lesions involving the 1st metatarsal head + any number of additional metatarsal heads
  - Lesions involving the entire forefoot
  - Risk of revision or re-amputation 20–40%
  - Approximately 1/3 of TMAs will eventually require major amputation [15]
- Midfoot Amputation: Lis Franc, Chopart, Syme (see Fig. 25.3) [16]
  - Rarely performed due to significant failure rate, high rate of revision to BKA
  - Inferior wound healing and functional outcomes compared to BKA
  - **Lis Franc:** tarsometatarsal disarticulation + Achilles or gastrocnemius tendon lengthening and reimplantation of the tibialis anterior and peroneus brevis
  - **Chopart:** disarticulation through the transtarsal joints of the talonavicular and calcaneocuboid joints combined
  - **Syme:** Ankle disarticulation

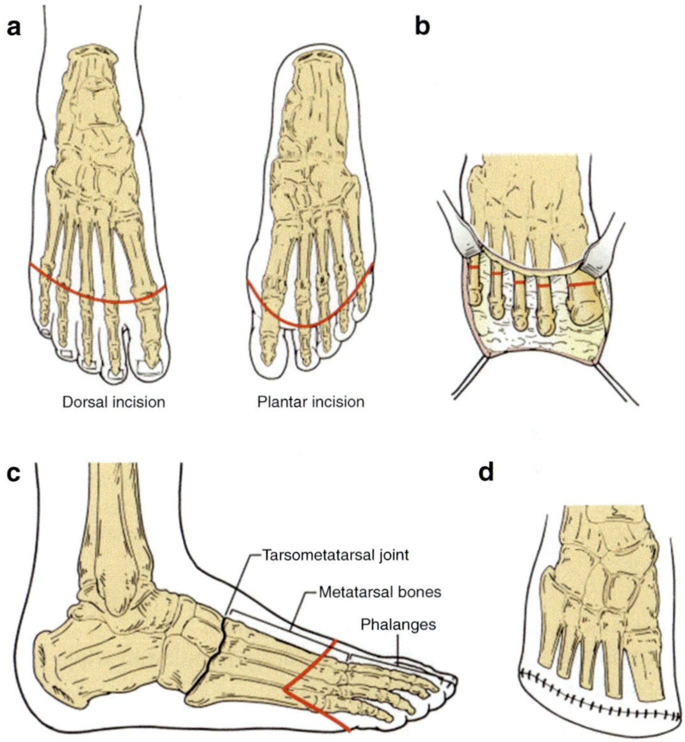

Fig. 25.2 Transmetatarsal amputation. (**a**) Marking of dorsal and plantar incision. (**b**) Bone transection. (**c**) Lateral view. (**d**) Skin closure. (Taken from Rutherford's Vascular Surgery and Endovascular Therapy 9th Ed. Ch. 112)

Cryo-Amputation

- A physiologic amputation which prevents the systemic spread of infectious organisms, toxic metabolites, inflammatory cytokines, and myoglobin
- Reserved for patients too high risk for surgery
- Temporizing measure
- Allows time for resuscitation of the patient and correction of metabolic derangements

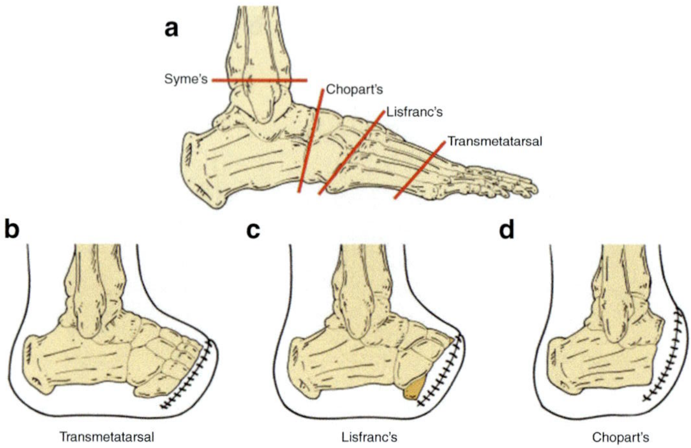

Fig. 25.3 Levels of foot amputations. (**a**) Level of bone transection for each respective amputation. (**b–d**) Skin incision closure for each respective foot amputation. (*Taken from Rutherford's Vascular Surgery and Endovascular Therapy 9th Ed. Ch. 112*)

- Second stage: formalization of amputation
- Improves mortality in frail and elderly population when compared to surgical amputation [17]

Complications

- General Complications:
  - Nonhealing stump
  - Wound infection
  - Osteomyelitis
  - Pressure ulcers (boney prominences)
  - Bleeding
- Local Stump complications occur in approximately 10% of patients after BKA [18]
- Myocardial infarction most common cause of death after lower extremity amputation in patients with PAD

Phantom Limb Syndrome

- The sensation that an amputated limb is still attached
- A majority will experience non-painful symptoms
- Phantom Limb pain—presence of burning, aching, and/or shooting pain in the amputated limb
- Diagnosis of exclusion—must rule out other causes of pain such as infection, neuroma, ischemia, necrosis

Contracture

- Can occur at the hip or knee joint leading to inability to ambulate
- More likely to develop in elderly with dementia
- Postoperative knee immobilizer can help prevent contracture
- Physical and occupational therapy

Questions

1. A 60-year-old male with poorly controlled diabetes presents to the ED with left foot wet gangrene involving the entire forefoot. He is febrile, tachycardic with a blood pressure 85/40. He is awake, alert but in mild distress. He has a palpable dorsalis pedis and posterior tibial pulse. X-ray shows soft tissue gas tracking to the level of the ankle. After adequate resuscitation and initiation of broad spectrum antibiotics, what is the next step in management of this patient?
   (a) Open guillotine amputation above the ankle followed by formal BKA after sepsis has resolved
   (b) Formal BKA
   (c) Primary transmetatarsal amputation
   (d) Hyperbaric oxygen therapy
   (e) Local wound debridement

2. What is the most common cause of death after major amputation in patients with PAD?
   (a) Sepsis
   (b) Myocardial infarction
   (c) Pulmonary Embolism
   (d) Stroke
3. Transcutaneous oxygen pressure ($TCPO_2$) measurement can be a useful adjunctive test to help determine amputation levels. All of the following will decrease the accuracy of $TCPO_2$, *except?*
   (a) Pitting edema
   (b) Inflammation
   (c) Overlying skin necrosis
   (d) Infection
   (e) Presence of peripheral artery disease

Answer: 1 (a), 2 (b), 3 (e)

References

1. The Global Lower Extremity Amputation Study Group. Epidemiology of lower extremity amputation in centres in Europe, North America and East Asia. Br J Surg. 2000;87:328.
2. Li Y, Burrows NR, Gregg EW, et al. Declining rates of hospitalization for nontraumatic lower extremity amputation in the diabetic population aged 40 years or older: U.S., 1988-2008. Diabetes Care. 2012;35:273.
3. Jolissaint JS, Shah SK, Martin MC, et al. Risk prediction of 30-day mortality after lower extremity major amputation. J Vasc Surg. 2019;70(6):1868–76.
4. Fisher DF Jr, Clagett GP, Fry RE, et al. One-stage versus two-stage amputation for wet gangrene of the lower extremity: a randomized study. J Vasc Surg. 1988;8(4):428–33.
5. McIntyre KE Jr, Bailey SA, Malone JM, et al. Guillotine amputation in the treatment of nonsalvageable lower-extremity infections. Arch Surg. 1984;119(4):450–3.
6. Taylor SM, Kalbaugh CA, Blackhurst DW, et al. Preoperative clinical factors predict postoperative functional outcomes after major lower limb amputation: an analysis of 553 consecutive patients. J Vasc Surg. 2005;42(2):227–35.

7. Gabel J, Jabo B, Patel S, et al. Descriptive analysis of patients going major lower extremity amputation in the Vascular Quality Initiative. Ann Vasc Surg. 2018;47:75–82.
8. Malone JM, Anderson GG, Lalka SG, et al. Prospective comparison of noninvasive techniques for amputation level selection. Am J Surg. 1987;154(2):179–84.
9. Eidt JF, Kalapatapu VR. Lower extremity amputation: techniques and results. Rutherford's vascular surgery. 8th ed. Philadelphia: Elsevier Saunders; 2014. p. 1848–66.
10. Nehler MR, Coll JR, Hiatt WR, et al. Functional outcome in a contemporary series of major lower extremity amputations. J Vasc Surg. 2003;38(1):7–14.
11. Abou-Zamzam AM Jr, Teruya TH, Killeen JE, et al. Major lower extremity amputation in an academic vascular center. Ann Vasc Surg. 2003;17(1):86–90.
12. Aulivola B, Hile CN, Hamdan AD, et al. Major lower extremity amputation: outcome of a modern series. Arch Surg. 2004;139(4):395–9.
13. Izumi Y, Satterfield K, Lee S, et al. Risk of reamputation in diabetic patients stratified by limb and level of amputation: a 10 year observation. Diabetes Care. 2006;29(3):566–70.
14. Dillingham TR, Pezzin LE, Shore AD. Reamputation, mortality, and health care costs among persons with dysvascular lower limb amputations. Arch Phys Med Rehabil. 2005;86(3):480–6.
15. Iosue H, Rosenblum B. Transmetatarsal amputation: predictors of success and failure. Podiatry Today. 2017;30(8):42–7.
16. Brodsky JW, Saltzman CL. Amputations of the foot and ankle. Mann's surgery of the foot and ankle. 9th ed. Philadelphia: Elsevier Saunders; 2014. p. 1481–506.
17. Chen SL, Kuo IJ, Kabuty NK, et al. Physiologic cryoamputation in managing critically ill patients with septic, advanced acute limb ischemia. Ann Vasc Surg. 2017;42:50–5.
18. Belmont PJ, Davey S, Orr J, et al. Risk factors for 30-day postoperative complications and mortality after below-knee amputation study of 2,911 patients from the National Surgical Quality Improvement Program. J Am Coll Surg. 2011;213:370.

Portal Hypertension 26

Isabella J. Kuo and Shelley Maithel

Relevant Anatomy

- Portal venous system extends from intestinal capillaries to the hepatic sinusoids and carries blood from abdominal gastrointestinal tract, pancreas, spleen, and gallbladder to the liver
- Portal vein formed by union of superior mesenteric vein and splenic vein
  - Provides 2/3 of blood flow to liver but only 40% of oxygen
- Inferior mesenteric vein enters the splenic vein
- Left and right gastric veins and posterior superior pancreaticoduodenal vein drain directly into the portal vein
- Important embryonic connections between portal and systemic venous systems (Fig. 26.1)
  - Lower esophagus: Left gastric (portal) with hemiazygos/azygos (systemic)
  - Anal wall: Superior rectal (portal) with middle/inferior rectal (systemic)
  - Caput medusa: Paraumbilical vein (portal) with epigastric (systemic)

I. J. Kuo (✉) · S. Maithel
Surgery, University of California, Irvine, Orange, CA, USA
e-mail: ijkuo@hs.uci.edu; smaithel@hs.uci.edu

A. Murga et al. (eds.), *The Vascular Surgery In-Training Examination Review (VSITE)*,
https://doi.org/10.1007/978-3-031-24121-5_26

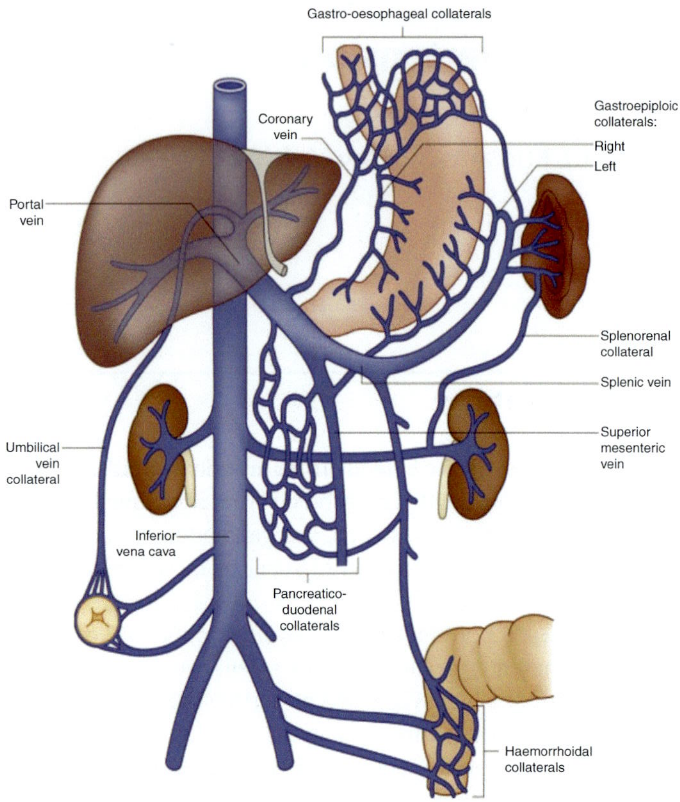

Fig. 26.1 Anatomy of portal venous system and diagram of collateral venous pathways between portal and systemic venous systems (from Allan P, Baxter G, Weston M. Clinical Ultrasound. Elsevier; 2011)

Causes

- Abnormal increase in pressure in veins that carry blood from visceral organs to the liver via portal venous system
- Pre-sinusoidal obstruction
  - Extrahepatic: Portal vein thrombosis (most common), pancreatitis, infectious such as omphalitis or appendicitis (most common in children to cause portal vein thrombosis)

  - Intrahepatic: Schistosomiasis (most common in developing countries), sarcoidosis
- Sinusoidal obstruction—most common
  - Cirrhosis, Wilson disease (hereditary disorder of copper metabolism so copper accumulates in hepatocytes)
- Post-sinusoidal obstruction
  - Budd Chiari syndrome (hepatic vein thrombosis), hepatic vein webs, congestive heart failure, constrictive pericarditis

Symptoms

- Ascites: >80% of patients, risk for spontaneous bacterial peritonitis (SBP)
- Varices: >30–50% of patients, risk for bleeding and rupture
  - Dilation and dysfunction of preexisting embryonic connections between portal and systemic systems such as left gastric (esophageal varices), short gastric veins into azygos venous system (esophageal, stomach varices)
- Hepatic encephalopathy: >30–40%
- Splenomegaly, Spider angiomas, palmar erythema, gynecomastia, asterixis

Diagnosis

- Portal venous pressure >15 or >10 mmHg above systemic venous pressure (corrected portal pressure)
  - Normal portal venous pressure is 5–10 mmHg
- Transhepatic percutaneous portal venography is necessary for evaluation of anatomy prior to surgical treatment
  - Determine hepatic vein wedge pressure

Child-Pugh Score

- Predicts operative risk of patients undergoing shunt surgery
- Scoring, see Table 26.1 [1]

Model for End-Stage Liver Disease (MELD) Score

- Originally created to predict survival of patients undergoing transjugular intrahepatic portosystemic shunts
- Now it used to rank priority of liver transplantation candidates
- Uses INR, creatinine, total bilirubin

Medical Management

- Ascites—spironolactone or furosemide
- Hepatic encephalopathy—lactulose (prevents ammonia absorption), neomycin (bad side effects: nephrotoxic, ototoxic)
- Varices
  - Nonselective beta-blockade (propranolol)—prevention of variceal bleeding
  - Endoscopic variceal band ligation—medium and large varices with high risk of bleeding

Table 26.1 Child-Pugh Score

Factor	**1 point**	**2 point**	**3 point**
Albumin (g/dL)	>3.5	2.8–3.5	<2.8
Bilirubin (mg/dL)	<2	2–3	>3
Encephalopathy	None	Mild-moderate (grade 1 or 2)	Severe (grade 3 or 4)
Ascites	None	Controlled with meds	Refractory
INR	<1.7	1.7–2.3	>2.3
	Class A	**Class B**	**Class C**
Total points	5–6	7–9	>10
1-year survival	100%	85%	45%

  - Endoscopic sclerotherapy—gastric varices
  - Vasopressin—active bleeding from varices
  - Somatostatin/octreotide—active bleeding from varices
  - Minnesota or Sengstaken-Blakemore tube—acute large hemorrhage from varices unresponsive to medical management; bridge to endoscopic or surgical management

Percutaneous Treatment

- Transjugular Intrahepatic Portosystemic Shunt (TIPS)
  - Allows antegrade flow from portal vein to the inferior vena cava (IVC) by creating connection between hepatic and portal vein
  - Indication: Child class B or C, refractory variceal bleeding or ascites
  - Contraindications: hepatic encephalopathy, sepsis, congestive heart failure, severe pulmonary hypertension [2]
  - Procedure, see Fig. 26.2 [3]
    - Catheter from the internal jugular vein into the right hepatic vein (best trajectory for portal vein, but middle and left vein can be used)
    - Needle is passed through liver parenchyma into portal vein target to create channel
    - Covered stent graft placed to establish channel from hepatic vein to portal vein
    - Repeat pressure measurements taken to confirm decrease in portosystemic gradient to <12 mmHg
  - Main complication is encephalopathy
- Balloon-occluded retrograde transvenous obliteration (BRTO)
  - Ideal for gastric varices for patients not candidate for TIPS due to encephalopathy
  - Used to occlude portosystemic collaterals between stomach and renal vein for gastric varices
    - Esophageal varices should be treated first
    - Portal vein must be patent

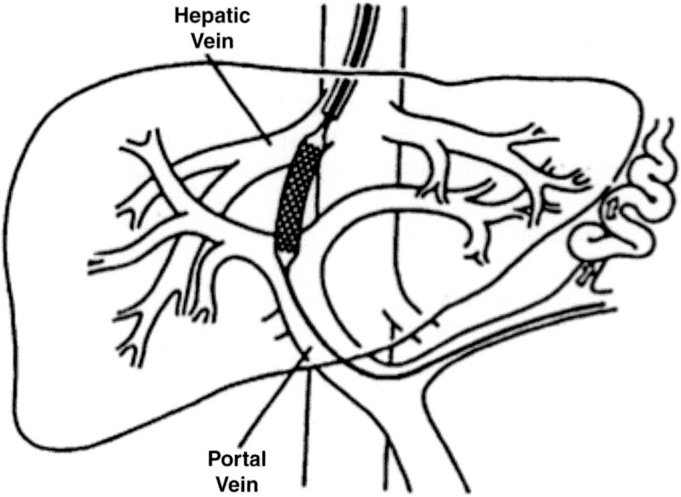

Fig. 26.2 Depiction of transjugular intrahepatic portosystemic shunt (TIPS) (from Waitches G, Leef J, Rosenblum J, Lipton MJ, Metz CE. Transjugular intrahepatic portosystemic shunts versus surgical shunts: quality assessment and outcome analysis. Academic radiology. 1996;3 Suppl 1:S62–5)

  - Occlusion balloon inserted from common femoral vein into outflow of gastrorenal shunt, resulting in occlusion of the tract so that a sclerosing agent can be injected into varices without reflux into systemic/portal system, see Fig. 26.3a [4]
  - Higher recurrence rate than TIPS can be used in combination with TIPS to facilitate flow toward the TIPS
- Balloon-occluded antegrade transvenous obliteration (BATO)—similar to BRTO but access via portal system into the gastric vein, see Fig. 26.3b [4]

Surgical Treatment

- Portacaval shunt
  - Midline or right subcostal incision, duodenum mobilized to expose IVC, dissection carried along IVC to level of first

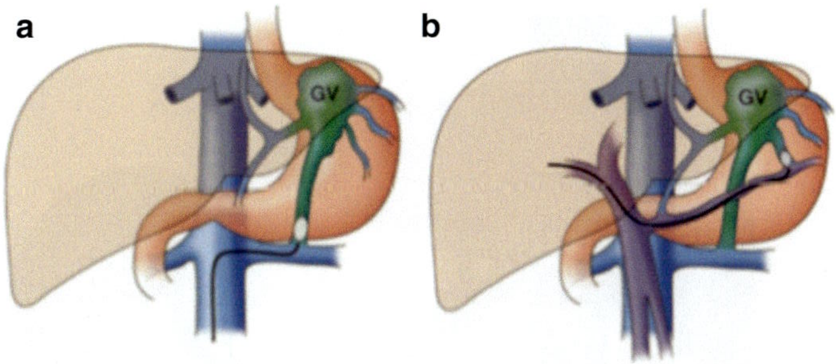

Fig. 26.3 (**a**) Illustration of balloon-occluded retrograde transvenous obliteration (BRTO) via transfemoral approach to approach the gastric varices (GV) from venous side. (**b**) Balloon-occluded antegrade transvenous obliteration (BATO) via portal venous system to obliterate the gastric varices (GV) (from Saad WE, Kitanosono T, Koizumi J. Balloon-occluded antegrade transvenous obliteration with or without balloon-occluded retrograde transvenous obliteration for the management of gastric varices: concept and technical applications. Techniques in vascular and interventional radiology. 2012;15 (3):203–25)

hepatic vein under liver, rotate bile duct and hepatic artery to expose portal vein, side to side or end to end anastomosis, need 50% reduction in portal venous pressure

- Mesocaval shunt—typically Dacron graft from SMV to IVC, rarely used due to massive lower extremity edema
- Distal splenorenal shunt (Fig. 26.4)
  - Must ligate left adrenal vein, left gonadal vein, inferior mesenteric vein, coronary vein, pancreatic branches of splenic vein
  - Can worsen ascites
- Nonsurgical shunt procedures
  - Splenectomy—best for isolated splenic vein thrombosis
  - Collateralization—omentopexy (produces collateral pathways by suturing omentum to peritoneum), transposition of spleen into thorax; not clinically proven
  - Ablation via periesophageal devascularization with partial transection (leaving only muscular layer) and oversewing of esophageal varices—acute hemorrhage in debilitated patient with both gastric and esophageal varices

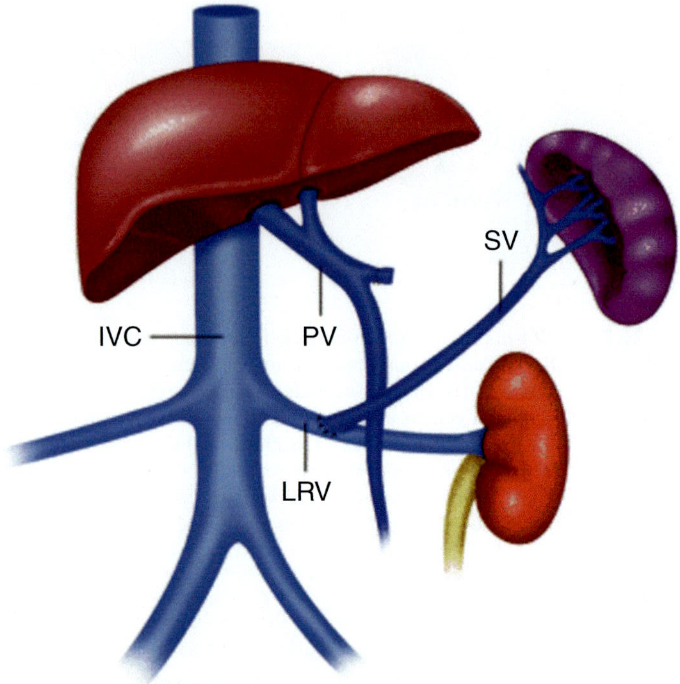

Fig. 26.4 Depiction of distal splenorenal shunt. *IVC* inferior vena cava, *PV* portal vein, *SV* splenic vein, *LRV* left renal vein (from Choudhury S.R. (2018) Portal Hypertension in Children. In: Pediatric Surgery. Springer, Singapore 8)

Questions

1. All of the following are components of the MELD score except:
   (a) INR
   (b) Creatinine
   (c) Hemoglobin
   (d) Bilirubin

2. The most common cause of sinusoidal portal hypertension is:
   (a) Cirrhosis
   (b) Schistosomiasis
   (c) Budd Chiari syndrome
   (d) Portal venous thrombosis
3. Which procedure is the best for isolated splenic vein thrombosis
   (a) Transjugular intrahepatic portovenous shunt (TIPS)
   (b) Splenectomy
   (c) Distal splenorenal shunt
   (d) Portocaval shunt

Answer: 1 (c), 2 (a), 3 (b)

References

1. Pugh RN, Murray-Lyon IM, Dawson JL, Pietroni MC, Williams R. Transection of the oesophagus for bleeding oesophageal varices. Br J Surg. 1973;60(8):646–9.
2. Boyer TD, Haskal ZJ. The role of transjugular intrahepatic portosystemic shunt in the management of portal hypertension. Hepatology. 2005;41(2):386–400.
3. Waitches G, Leef J, Rosenblum J, Lipton MJ, Metz CE. Transjugular intrahepatic portosystemic shunts versus surgical shunts: quality assessment and outcome analysis. Acad Radiol. 1996;3(Suppl 1):S62–5.
4. Saad WE, Kitanosono T, Koizumi J. Balloon-occluded antegrade transvenous obliteration with or without balloon-occluded retrograde transvenous obliteration for the management of gastric varices: concept and technical applications. Tech Vasc Interv Radiol. 2012;15(3):203–25.

Further Reading

Fischer JE, Gould JC. Fischer's Mastery of surgery. Philadelphia: Wolters Kluwer; 2019.

Moore WS. Vascular and endovascular surgery, a comprehensive review. Philadelphia: Elsevier; 2018.

Sidawy AN, Perler BA. Rutherford's vascular surgery and endovascular therapy, 2-Volume Set. Philadelphia: Saunders W.B.; 2018.

27 Miscellaneous

Seyed Saeed Pairawan,
B. S. Chloe Dominguez,
and Ahmed M. Abou-Zamzam Jr

Spine Exposures

- Numerous spinal pathologies require surgical intervention. Degenerative disc disease (DDD) is a major cause.
- Degenerative disc disease commonly affects the cervical and lumbar spine.
- Proteoglycan loss serves as a key event in degenerative disease of the intervertebral disc [1].
- Other pathologies include spondylosis, spondylolisthesis, and spinal stenosis.

S. S. Pairawan · B. S. Chloe Dominguez · A. M. Abou-Zamzam Jr (✉)
Division of Vascular Surgery, Loma Linda University Health,
CA, Loma Linda, USA
e-mail: Spairawan@llu.edu; cdominguez@students.llu.edu; AZamzam@llu.edu

A. Murga et al. (eds.), *The Vascular Surgery In-Training Examination Review (VSITE)*,
https://doi.org/10.1007/978-3-031-24121-5_27

Thoracic Spine Exposure

- The planned incision should always be confirmed following positioning in the operating room using C-arm fluoroscopy.
- Exposure of C7-T2 requires diagonal neck plus median sternotomy incision.
- T2 through T6 exposure is better approached through the right chest via a lateral approach. To approach the appropriate level, it requires an approach through the intercostal space usually 1–2 levels above the affected disc space. Partial removal of a rib in this access site can provide additional exposure and autologous bone for grafting.
- Lower thoracic spine can be accessed through a posterior, posterolateral, lateral, or an anterior approach.
- Lateral extra cavitary approach (LECA) has the advantage of providing a central view while allowing for posterior instrumentation through the same incision [2, 3].
- Anterior approach can be either transpleural or retropleural [4].
- Anterior thoracic approach is considered superior to posterior approach [5] because of:
  - Short-segment fixation.
  - Pain improvement.
  - Less bleeding.
  - Lower rate of wound infections.
  - Better wound healing.
- Anterior approach is favored when there is a presence of central calcified herniated discs and multilevel disease.
- Retropleural approach has less morbidity and potentially avoids lung-related injuries seen with transpleural approach, and the need for a chest tube.
- Thoracoscopic approach—offers more limited visualization, therefore only indicated for small, non-calcified herniated discs located between T4 and T11 in non-obese patient [3].
- Posterolateral approach is often preferred in non-calcified lateral and posterolateral disc herniations because the

complication risk is lower through this approach compared to transthoracic approach.

- Complications associated with anterior approach—lung injury, pneumothorax, chylothorax (left thoracic duct), spinal cord ischemia.
- LECA approach is prone to pulmonary complications such as pneumothoraxes and/or pleural effusions.
- Complications associated with thoracic spine approaches:
  - Overall, 20–30% complication rate. Anterior vs. non-anterior complication rate (26.8 vs. 9.6%) and mortality rate (0.7 vs. 0.2%).
  - Dural tear.
  - Neurological deterioration.
  - Intercostal neuralgia.
  - Lung-associated complications.
  - Incomplete disk resection.

Lumbar Spine Exposure

- Anterior abdominal approach is used for exposure of lower thoracic and entire lumbosacral spine. It can be approached in a transperitoneal or retroperitoneal manner [6].
- Retroperitoneal approach is preferred because of lower risk of postoperative ileus and lower rate of retrograde ejaculation. Additionally, there is minimal risk for the development of intraperitoneal adhesions.
- Most common incisions are vertical midline, vertical and oblique left paramedian, and lower abdominal transverse (mirroring Pfannenstiel for L4-5 and/or L5-S1). Incisions can be tailored according to disc level based on body habitus and intraoperative anterior-posterior and lateral lumbar X-ray.
- Exposure of the L1–L4 levels requires a left to right mobilization of the aorta with division of segmental lumbar arteries and veins.
- Exposures of the L4–L5 disc space require careful consideration of the relationships between the aortic bifurcation, iliac

vein confluence, and the disc space. The L4–L5 disc space may be exposed adjacent to the distal aorta above the left common iliac artery, between the left common iliac artery and vein, and (more rarely) below the left common iliac vein. Knowledge of the venous tributaries into the left common iliac vein (ascending lumbar vein and ilio-lumbar veins) is important. The median sacral vessels often need to be sacrificed to provide adequate exposure.

- L5-S1 disc space lies below the confluence of the iliac veins and aortic bifurcation, between the common iliac vessels and simply requires ligation of the median sacral vessels with minimal, if any, cephalad mobilization of the left common iliac vein.
- Vascular anatomic variations occur in 30% of cases including left sided IVC, double iliac veins, or large internal iliac vein [7]. Pelvic kidneys, fused renal ectopia, and other arterial variations may also occur and will be evident on cross-sectional imaging.
- Complications associated with anterior lumbar spine exposure:
  - Neurogenic—retrograde ejaculation, nerve injuries to lower extremity nerves.
  - Urologic—Ureteral injury.
  - Vascular—thrombosis or hemorrhage of arteries or veins.
  - Inflammatory—Pancreatitis, retroperitoneal fibrosis.
  - Intestinal—ileus, direct bowel injuries if peritoneum is violated.
  - Other—Rectus hematoma, wound infection, incisional hernia.

Complex Regional Pain Syndrome (CRPS)

- CRPS is a painful syndrome that develops secondary to a traumatic event.
  - Classification

    Classified into two types

CRPS type 1 also known as reflex sympathetic dystrophy.

CRPS type 2 previously known as causalgia.

- Clinical presentation

  Inciting events such as fractures are present in 36% of cases [8].

  Two phases occur

  - Acute phase with stigmata of inflammation including rubor, calor, tumor, and dolor. These symptoms typically appear distal to the area of insult and are accompanied by pain which is exacerbated by movement or temperature changes.
  - Chronic phase typically occurs after 6 months. Pain at rest is common in addition to muscular spasms. Patients may notice changes in their skin growth, hair growth, and muscle atrophy.

  Risk factors for development of CPRS:

  - Fracture-dislocation, intra-articular fractures and ankle fracture are predisposing factors for type 1 CRPS [9].
  - Female sex
  - High-energy injuries

- Diagnostic evaluation

  Diagnosis is guided by Budapest clinical criteria [10] including:

  - Presence of initiating noxious event with persisting pain, hyperalgesia, or allodynia where the pain is disproportionate to inciting event.
  - Patient reporting one symptom in three out of four categories: sensory (presence of allodynia or hyperesthesia), sudomotor (edema, sweating changes or asymmetry), vasomotor (changes in skin color or temperature asymmetry) or motor (changes in range of motion, weakness or change in skin, hair or nail). Persisting pain, hyperalgesia, or allodynia where the pain is disproportionate to inciting event.

  - Presence of at least one sign in two or more categories: sensory (hyperalgesia to pinpricking, or allodynia to touch and/or joint movement), sudomotor (presence of edema or sweating asymmetry), vasomotor (temperature or skin color asymmetry), or trophic (decreased ROM, weakness or trophic changes to skin, hair or nail).
  - Exclusion of other conditions explaining pain and dysfunction.

  There is no gold standard test for diagnosing CRPS.

  - Plain radiograph—may demonstrate non-specific bone demineralization.
  - MRI findings—bone-marrow edema, joint effusion, and/or uptake in the skin.
  - Serum osteoprotegerin, an osteoblastic marker suggesting increased bone turnover, demonstrated 74% sensitivity and 80% specificity [11] for CRPS.

– Nonsurgical treatment

  Patient education.

  Pharmacological agents

  - Non-steroidal anti-inflammatory drugs (NSAIDs)
  - Glucocorticoids
    – Prednisone, Methylprednisolone
  - Bisphosphonates
  - Calcitonin
  - Vitamin C
  - Vasoactive mediators
    – Clonidine
    – Phenoxybenzamine

  Physical therapy—first line therapy in CRPS.

– Sympathectomy

  Has demonstrated benefit in patients with CRPS.

  Can be performed in both thoracic and lumbar regions.

  Can be done endoscopically or open.

- Complications:
    - Lung-related injuries
    - Bleeding
    - Nerve injury including Horner's syndrome
    - Infection

Radiation and Radiation Safety

- Radiographic equipment
  - Sources: Intraoperative imaging
    - X-ray
    - C-arm and O-arm
    - Angiography
    - Fluoroscopy
  - Primary X-ray beam
    - Source of X-rays is the X-ray tube.
    - From this point, X-rays diverge into space.
    - Direct radiation is the most dangerous source of radiation for the surgeon [12].
    - X-ray tube is surrounded by lead-lined tube housing which absorbs some of the scattered rays.
    - The radiation that leaves the tube is called primary radiation, creating the radiation field.
    - Anatomic structures that have greater tissue density will absorb more radiation than less dense tissue.
  - Scatter Radiation
    - Travels out from the absorbing matter in all directions.
    - Less energy than the primary beam.
    - Primary form of exposure for operative staff [12].
- Allowable limits
  - International Commission on Radiological Protection (ICRP): maximum average of 20 mSv per year over a 5-year period with no exposure greater than 50 mSv in a single year.
  - Exposure to 1 Sv is associated with a 5% risk of developing cancer [13].

- Dose calculation
  - The average EVAR case was estimated to have a radiation effective dose of 12.4 mSv [14].
  - Dosages for both fluoroscopy time and kerma-area product during endovascular procedures do not exceed the International Atomic Energy Agency proposed trigger values for patients' follow-up for radiation-induced skin injuries [15].
  - Calculation of Peak Skin Dose: PSD (mGy) = 249 + 5.2*DAP Gy cm^2.
- Protective gear
  - Shielding: lead aprons, thyroid shields, lead gloves, lead skirts, and mobile shield screens.
  - Can reduce radiation exposure by 42–96.9% [12].
- Limiting exposure
  - Distance: The Inverse Square Law dictates that the radiation intensity is inversely proportional to the square of the distance ($1/d^2$), therefore radiation intensity decreases substantially with increasing distance from the radiation or scatter source.
  - When combined with appropriate shielding, scatter radiation may be reduced to 0.1% and 0.025% of the primary radiation at a distance of 3 and 6 ft. [16].
  - Dose reduction techniques such as shielding, pulsed imaging, lack of magnification, shuttering should be employed to attain "ALARA"—As Low As Reasonably Achievable.
- Radiation safety and occupational health issues
  - There has been an increased cancer risk identified in physicians routinely exposed to radiation—a cancer incidence of 29% in orthopedic surgeons exposed to medical radiation in the workplace compared to 4% in unexposed orthopedic surgeons [17].
  - The US population has seen a 600% increase in medical radiation since 1980, mostly from diagnostic procedures [18].

Frostbite

- Severe ischemic injury after sub-zero temperature exposure resulting in tissue necrosis and potential amputation.
- Both the temperature and duration of exposure impact prognosis.
- Other factors such as age, fat and muscle mass, health conditions, drug intake, and diabetes mellitus impact prognosis [19].
  - High fat and muscle mass act as good insulators.
  - Children and the elderly are more at risk.
  - Diabetes mellitus impairs the heat response against cold exposure.
- Symptoms include vasospasm, vasoconstriction, hemorrhage, and loss of blood supply to affected site resulting in ischemic injury [20].
- Pathophysiology includes increased blood viscosity, vasoconstriction of the capillaries and blood vessels, reduction in blood supply to the tissue, and shunting [19].
  - "Hunting response": after initial vasoconstriction upon cold exposure, there is vasodilation of affected blood supply for 5–10 min to protect from thermal injury [19].
  - If exposure is prolonged, vasoconstriction occurs to prevent further core cooling, creating an avascular and ischemic environment [19].
- Four grades of frostbite [21]:
  - Grade I: no cyanosis on the extremity, and little to no sequelae.
  - Grade II: cyanosis isolated to the distal phalanx. Predicts only soft tissue amputation and fingernail or toenail sequelae.
  - Grade III: intermediate and proximal phalangeal cyanosis. Predicts bone amputation of the digit and functional sequelae.
  - Grade IV: cyanosis over the carpal or tarsal bones. This predicts significant amputation of the limb with functional sequelae.

- Eighty-five percent of cases of frostbite are first degree frostbite
  - Digits of the lower limbs are the most common, followed by the hands, nose, and pinna of the ear [19].
- Diagnosis:
  - Tissue damage only becomes visible after 2–4 weeks, immediate evaluation is necessary to increase tissue salvage.
  - Imaging is critical in frostbite prognosis: radiography, digital subtraction angiography, SPECT/CT, and laser Doppler imaging.

    DSA to evaluate vascular perfusion and help monitor the effect of thrombolytic therapy.

    Fluorescence microangiography.

    Technetium-99m scintigraphy: visualizes microcirculation to establish candidacy for thrombolytic therapy [22].

    Single-photon emission computed tomography (SPECT).

    MRI.
- Treatment:
  - Field-management: changing wet clothing, warming, and warm water bath immersion.
  - Hospital care:

    Active and passive rewarming.

    Wound care: systemic antibiotics, non-steroidal anti-inflammatory drugs (NSAIDs).

    Thrombolytic therapy: aggressive management in the first 24 h has been shown to reduce damage [23].

    - Intra-arterial rTPA administration within the first 24 h can reduce digital amputation rates from 41 to 15% [19].
    - Intravenous Iloprost (prostacyclin PGI_2 analog): rate of amputation much lower in group receiving Iloprost than in other groups [24].

Pediatric Vascular Surgical Problems

- Pediatric vascular disease is very rare.
- Diseases are heterogeneous and involve multiple vascular territories.
- Complicated by issues related to small size, future growth, and vascular conduit availability [25].
- Diagnosis typically established with magnetic resonance angiography and ultrasound. Attempts are made to minimize radiation exposure with CT scans or conventional angiography.
- Indications for surgery: risk of expansion and rupture, potential thrombosis or embolization of aneurysmal thrombus, local soft tissue and nerve compression, and secondary hypertension in the case of aortic coarctation and renal artery lesions (stenoses or aneurysms).
- Individualized interventional technique, either surgical or endovascular, is necessary.

Abdominal Aortic Aneurysm in Pediatric Population

- Etiology: Developmental defects, infection, vasculitis, tuberous sclerosis, trauma, with infection after umbilical artery stump or cardiac catheterization being the most common cause [26].
  - Wiskott-Aldrich Syndrome [27]—rarely develop aortic aneurysms due to vasculitis but may require intervention due to slow progression.
- Effect of later growth must be considered when planning treatment and selecting the appropriate composition and diameter of graft.
- Correction should be deferred until child reaches 8–10 years [28] if risk of adverse outcomes is low.
- Children under 6 rarely have adequate autologous options for graft construction [29].
  - Benefit from cryopreserved arterial allografts.

- Technique:
  - Dacron or expanded polytetrafluoroethylene (ePTFE) can be used for revascularization, with Dacron favored [26].
  - Role of covered stents or stent-grafts is limited due to fixed size of stents and arterial access issues. This may be suitable as a bridge procedure in cases of critically ill children [29].

Blunt Thoracic Aortic Injury

- The rate of thoracic endovascular aortic repair (TEVAR) in the pediatric population is increasing steadily and shows no difference in risk of mortality with open thoracic aortic repair (OTAR) [30]. The size of the native aorta and the access vessels is a limiting factor.

Pediatric Non-aortic Arterial Aneurysms Are Rare, and Treatment Is Ill-Defined [31]

- Aneurysms in children have been described in many locations including the brachial [32], ulnar [33], femoral [34], and the external carotid arteries [35].
  - Saphenous vein grafts are commonly used during repair of these aneurysms.
- Most common factors are related to proximal juxta-aneurysmal stenoses, trauma, Kawasaki disease, Ehlers-Danlos type IV syndrome, and infection [31, 36, 37].
- Rheumatologist and geneticist consultation should be sought to help screen for associated conditions.

Pediatric Renal Arterial Occlusive Disease

- Most common cause of severe HTN in children over 1 year of age [38].
  - Etiology: Developmental renal artery stenosis is the most common cause [39], however renovascular hypertension (RVHT) is associated with many different diseases including Takayasu's arteritis, neurofibromatosis, and fibromuscular dysplasia.
  - Approach:

    Treat first with antihypertensives.

    Consider endovascular approaches in medically refractory patients. Percutaneous transluminal renal angioplasty (PTRA) is preferred treatment in children [25]. Stenting is controversial and should be used in select cases.

    Surgical correction only if angioplasty has failed.

Acute Arterial Occlusion: Medical Emergency Requiring Immediate Treatment

- Diagnosis and treatment is difficult due to frequent delay in diagnosis, technical difficulty accessing small-caliber vessels, and poor conduit for possible interposition grafting or bypass. Individualized surgical technique is necessary [25].
- Diagnosis: Careful pulse exam, hand-held Doppler, duplex ultrasonography.
- Etiology: Iatrogenic from vessel catheterization, idiopathic, traumatic, congenital [40].
- Technique: can be managed nonoperatively with anticoagulation although may require surgical repair.
  - Most surgical techniques can be used dependent upon patient and artery size, location and conduit availability.

Pediatric Chronic Arterial Occlusion

- Etiology: Iatrogenic (cardiac catheterizations), community trauma, vasculitis, congenital abnormality, or chronic embolism [25].
- Due to increased collateral circulation, occlusion is usually tolerated without significant symptoms and is rarely immediately limb-threatening [25].
- Treatment can be delayed until maturity if symptoms are minor or develop later.

Pediatric Vascular Access for Hemodialysis

- Frequently requires anesthesia and microscopic surgery.
- Kidney Disease Outcomes Quality Initiative (K-DOQI) guidelines recommend the placement of permanent access in dialysis patients aged 0–19 years who weigh >20 kg and are unlikely to receive a transplant within 1 year [41].
  - Peritoneal dialysis is more appropriate for children weighing less than 10 kg [25].

Vasculogenic Erectile Dysfunction

- Erectile dysfunction affects 18 million men in the US [42].
- Two categories—Psychogenic (20%) and Organic (80%). Organic includes vasculogenic, neurogenic and hormonal, with vasculogenic being the most prevalent.
  - Vasculogenic ED has two subtypes: Arterial insufficiency (AI) and Veno-Occlusive Disease (VOD) [43].
- Among men with diabetes, 51% also have ED [42].
- ED is independently associated with diabetes, lack of exercise, hyperlipidemia, obesity, and smoking [42, 44, 45].

- Endothelial dysfunction represents the probable link between vasculogenic ED, CAD, and PAD [44, 45].
- In patients with peripheral arterial disease, 86% of patients with severe ED also had bilateral internal pudendal artery stenosis, as opposed to those determined to have moderate ED, of which only 50% had bilateral stenosis [45].
- Therapy for ED:
  - Lifestyle modifications: lowering cardiovascular risk factors by improving diet, increasing exercise, and smoking cessation is the first line therapy.
  - Oral PDE-5 inhibitors (such as sildenafil and tadalafil) are effective for ED. These agents work by inducing relaxation through the prevention of degradation of cyclic guanosine monophosphate.
  - Patients with vasculogenic ED frequently require more invasive treatments.
- Endovascular treatment for refractory vasculogenic ED has increased in popularity, including angioplasty, or stenting for arterial insufficiency and embolization procedures for veno-occlusive dysfunction [44].
- Endovascular treatment:
  - VOD was successfully treated endovascularly in 59.5% of patients through embolization of the deep dorsal vein or the periprostatic venous plexus [44].

    Diagnosis: Duplex ultrasound, cavernosometry, and covernosography [44].
  - Arterial Insufficiency: treated with angioplasty or stenting of the internal pudendal, common iliac, and penile artery.

    Overall combined clinical success rate of endovascular AI therapy was 63.2% [44].

    Diagnosis: diagnostic angiography, duplex ultrasonography, pelvic computerized tomographic, magnetic resonance angiography [44].

Questions and Answers

1. An obese patient has a non-calcified lateral disc herniation involving T10. Which approach is preferred in this patient?
   (a) Posterior
   (b) Posterolateral
   (c) Anterior
   (d) Thoracoscopic
2. Exposure of the L4–L5 disc space requires careful consideration of following vascular structures except:
   (a) Aortic bifurcation
   (b) Segmental lumbar arteries and veins
   (c) Median sacral vessels
   (d) Left renal artery and vein
3. Which of the following is a common complication of using an anterior approach to access the upper thoracic spine?
   (a) Poor wound healing
   (b) Pancreatitis
   (c) Retrograde ejaculation
   (d) Lung injury
4. A woman comes to your clinic 1 year after a motorcycle accident where she fractured her right tibia. She has been seen by numerous other providers for constant pain in the right lower extremity. She reports that the pain has worsened from pain with movement to pain while resting. Upon examination of the right leg you notice mild right lower leg edema with skin thickening, asymmetry of skin color, and motor weakness. She most likely has:
   (a) Cellulitis
   (b) S1 radiculopathy
   (c) Complex regional pain syndrome
   (d) Chronic venous insufficiency
5. What is one of the criteria for diagnosing complex regional pain syndrome?
   (a) Symptoms greater than 1 year
   (b) Presence of initiating noxious event
   (c) Decreased peripheral pulses
   (d) Multiple joints affected

6. What is a risk factor for developing complex regional pain syndrome?
   (a) Past psychiatric diagnosis
   (b) Previous diagnosis with fibromyalgia
   (c) Fracture injury
   (d) Presence of a burn injury
7. Which type of radiation is most commonly experienced in the OR by the surgeon and surgical staff?
   (a) Direct
   (b) Scatter
8. When combined with appropriate shielding, at what distance can scatter radiation be decreased to 0.025% the dose of the primary radiation?
   (a) 2 feet
   (b) 10 feet
   (c) 6 feet
   (d) 1 foot
9. Maximum radiation exposure experienced over a single year should not exceed which?
   (a) 20 mSv
   (b) 5 mSv
   (c) 50 mSv
   (d) 35 mSv
10. You see a 60-year-old male in the ED who was found outside during a snowstorm. He is -complaining of pain in his bilateral feet. You examine his feet and see cyanosis over the intermediate and proximal phalanges. How do you grade his frostbite?
   (a) Grade 1
   (b) Grade 2
   (c) Grade 3
   (d) Grade 4
11. **Continued:** What is the best next step in management:
   (a) Fluorescence microangiography
   (b) Active and passive rewarming
   (c) NSAIDS
   (d) No intervention necessary

12. The Hunting response describes:
    - (a) Severe ischemic injury after sub-zero temperature exposure resulting in tissue necrosis and potential amputation.
    - (b) Vasodilation of affected blood supply for 5–10 min (after initial vasoconstriction) in order to protect from thermal injury.
    - (c) Immediate vasoconstriction to prevent further core cooling, creating an avascular and ischemic environment.
    - (d) Tissue damage being visible after 2–4 weeks.
13. What is the most common cause of pediatric abdominal aortic aneurysm?
    - (a) Infection after procedure
    - (b) Tuberous Sclerosis
    - (c) Wiskott-Aldrich Syndrome
    - (d) Developmental defect
14. What is the most appropriate catheter to place for dialysis in an infant weighing 9 kg with end-stage renal disease?
    - (a) Central Venous Catheter
    - (b) Peritoneal Dialysis catheter
    - (c) Arteriovenous graft
    - (d) Arteriovenous fistula
15. What is the most common cause of severe HTN in children over 1 year of age?
    - (a) Fibromuscular dysplasia
    - (b) Takayasu arteritis
    - (c) Congenital adrenal hyperplasia
    - (d) Developmental renal artery stenosis
16. What is the first line therapy for vasculogenic erectile dysfunction?
    - (a) Lifestyle modifications
    - (b) B-blocker
    - (c) Angioplasty
    - (d) Fibrates
17. What is the probable link between vasculogenic erectile dysfunction and coronary artery disease?
    - (a) Hyperhomocysteinemia
    - (b) Protein C deficiency

   (c) Endothelial dysfunction
   (d) Medication nonadherence
18. You suspect that your patient may have vasculogenic erectile dysfunction. What is the best next step?
   (a) Duplex ultrasonography
   (b) Lipid panel
   (c) Echocardiogram
   (d) Voiding cystourethrogram

Answers: 1 (b), 2 (d), 3 (d), 4 (c), 5 (a), 6 (c), 7 (b), 8 (c), 9 (c), 10 (c), 11 (b), 12 (b), 13 (a), 14 (b), 15 (d), 16 (a), 17 (c), 18 (a)

References

1. Roughley PJ. Biology of intervertebral disc aging and degeneration: involvement of the extracellular matrix. Spine (Phila Pa 1976). 2004;29(23):2691–9.
2. Foreman PM, et al. The lateral extracavitary approach to the thoracolumbar spine: a case series and systematic review. J Neurosurg Spine. 2016;24(4):570–9.
3. Bouthors C, Benzakour A, Court C. Surgical treatment of thoracic disc herniation: an overview. Int Orthop. 2019;43(4):807–16.
4. Berjano P, et al. Transthoracic lateral retropleural minimally invasive microdiscectomy for T9-T10 disc herniation. Eur Spine J. 2014;23(6):1376–8.
5. Gokaslan ZL, et al. Transthoracic vertebrectomy for metastatic spinal tumors. J Neurosurg. 1998;89(4):599–609.
6. Ikard RW. Methods and complications of anterior exposure of the thoracic and lumbar spine. Arch Surg. 2006;141(10):1025–34.
7. Harmon PH. A simplified surgical technic for anterior lumbar diskectomy and fusion; avoidance of complications; anatomy of the retroperitoneal veins. Clin Orthop Relat Res. 1964;37:130–44.
8. Goh EL, Chidambaram S, Ma D. Complex regional pain syndrome: a recent update. Burns Trauma. 2017;5:2.
9. Birklein F, et al. Complex regional pain syndrome - phenotypic characteristics and potential biomarkers. Nat Rev Neurol. 2018;14(5):272–84.
10. Harden NR, et al. Validation of proposed diagnostic criteria (the "Budapest Criteria") for Complex Regional Pain Syndrome. Pain. 2010;150(2):268–74.

11. Kramer HH, et al. Osteoprotegerin: a new biomarker for impaired bone metabolism in complex regional pain syndrome? Pain. 2014;155(5):889–95.
12. Narain AS, et al. Radiation exposure and reduction in the operating room: perspectives and future directions in spine surgery. World J Orthop. 2017;8(7):524–30.
13. Lin EC. Radiation risk from medical imaging. Mayo Clin Proc. 2010;85(12):1142–6; quiz 1146.
14. Walsh C, et al. Measurement and optimization of patient radiation doses in endovascular aneurysm repair. Eur J Vasc Endovasc Surg. 2012;43(5):534–9.
15. Kostova-Lefterova DD, et al. Patient doses in endovascular and hybrid revascularization of the lower extremities. Br J Radiol. 2018;91(1091):20180176.
16. Singer G. Occupational radiation exposure to the surgeon. J Am Acad Orthop Surg. 2005;13(1):69–76.
17. Mastrangelo G, et al. Increased cancer risk among surgeons in an orthopaedic hospital. Occup Med (Lond). 2005;55(6):498–500.
18. Linet MS, et al. Cancer risks associated with external radiation from diagnostic imaging procedures. CA Cancer J Clin. 2012;62(2):75–100.
19. Joshi K, et al. Frostbite: current status and advancements in therapeutics. J Therm Biol. 2020;93:102716.
20. Gonzaga T, et al. Use of intra-arterial thrombolytic therapy for acute treatment of frostbite in 62 patients with review of thrombolytic therapy in frostbite. J Burn Care Res. 2016;37(4):e323–34.
21. Carceller A, et al. Amputation risk factors in severely frostbitten patients. Int J Environ Res Public Health. 2019;16(8):1351.
22. Twomey JA, Peltier GL, Zera RT. An open-label study to evaluate the safety and efficacy of tissue plasminogen activator in treatment of severe frostbite. J Trauma. 2005;59(6):1350–4; discussion 1354–5.
23. Lindford A, et al. The evolution of the Helsinki frostbite management protocol. Burns. 2017;43(7):1455–63.
24. Cauchy E, Cheguillaume B, Chetaille E. A controlled trial of a prostacyclin and rt-PA in the treatment of severe frostbite. N Engl J Med. 2011;364(2):189–90.
25. Min SK, et al. Pediatric vascular surgery review with a 30-year-experience in a tertiary referral center. Vasc Specialist Int. 2017;33(2):47–54.
26. Eliason JL, et al. Surgical treatment of abdominal aortic aneurysms in infancy and early childhood. J Vasc Surg. 2016;64(5):1252–61.
27. Pellier I, et al. Occurrence of aortic aneurysms in 5 cases of Wiskott-Aldrich syndrome. Pediatrics. 2011;127(2):e498–504.
28. Barral X, et al. Surgery of the abdominal aorta and its branches in children: late follow-up. J Vasc Surg. 2006;43(6):1138–44.

29. Kaye AJ, et al. Complex vascular reconstruction of abdominal aorta and its branches in the pediatric population. J Pediatr Surg. 2008;43(6):1082–8.
30. Hasjim BJ, et al. National trends of thoracic endovascular aortic repair versus open thoracic aortic repair in pediatric blunt thoracic aortic injury. Ann Vasc Surg. 2019;59:150–7
31. Davis FM, et al. Pediatric nonaortic arterial aneurysms. J Vasc Surg. 2016;63(2):466–76 e1.
32. Gangopadhyay N, et al. Brachial artery aneurysm in a 7-month-old infant: case report and literature review. Plast Reconstr Surg Glob Open. 2016;4(2):e625.
33. Amjad I, Murphy T, Zahn E. Diagnosis and excision of an ulnar artery aneurysm in a two-year-old boy. Can J Plast Surg. 2010;18(1):e15–6.
34. Matsubara M, et al. Congenital-idiopathic superficial femoral artery aneurysm in a 7-year-old child. J Vasc Surg. 2011;53(6):1699–701.
35. De Luccia N, et al. Congenital external carotid artery aneurysm. Ann Vasc Surg. 2010;24(3):418.e7–10.
36. Benrashid E, et al. Mycotic saccular abdominal aortic aneurysm in an infant after cardiac catheterization: a case report. Ann Vasc Surg. 2015;29(7):1447.e5–1447.e11.
37. Mendeloff J, et al. Aortic aneurysm resulting from umbilical artery catheterization: case report, literature review, and management algorithm. J Vasc Surg. 2001;33(2):419–24.
38. Piercy KT, et al. Renovascular disease in children and adolescents. J Vasc Surg. 2005;41(6):973–82.
39. Stanley JC, et al. Pediatric renovascular hypertension: 132 primary and 30 secondary operations in 97 children. J Vasc Surg. 2006;44(6):1219–28; discussion 1228–9.
40. Kayssi A, et al. Management of acute limb ischemia in the pediatric population. J Vasc Surg. 2014;60(1):106–10.
41. Hogg RJ, et al. National Kidney Foundation's kidney disease outcomes quality initiative clinical practice guidelines for chronic kidney disease in children and adolescents: evaluation, classification, and stratification. Pediatrics. 2003;111(6 Pt 1):1416–21.
42. Selvin E, Burnett AL, Platz EA. Prevalence and risk factors for erectile dysfunction in the US. Am J Med. 2007;120(2):151–7.
43. Hoppe H, Diehm N. Percutaneous treatment of venous erectile dysfunction. Front Cardiovasc Med. 2020;7:626943.
44. Doppalapudi SK, et al. Endovascular therapy for vasculogenic erectile dysfunction: a systematic review and meta-analysis of arterial and venous therapies. J Vasc Interv Radiol. 2019;30(8):1251–1258 e2.
45. Benaragama KS, et al. Erectile dysfunction in peripheral vascular disease: endovascular revascularization as a potential therapeutic target. Vasc Endovascular Surg. 2020;54(8):707–11.

28 Biostatistics

Carlos Chavez de Paz and Allen Murga

Biostatistics and Epidemiology

Basic Statistical Concepts

- Statistics is a field of study concerned with the collection, organization, summarization, and analysis of data. When data analyzed is derived from biological science and medicine, we used the term biostatistics [1].
- Data may come from many sources: medical records, external sources, surveys, experiments.
- Descriptive Statistics: to describe and summarize the data.
- Inferential Statistics: to make inferences that can expand the data to a population.
- Variables: characteristics presented as values in different persons, places, or things.
  - Quantitative variable: can be measured or counted

C. C. de Paz
Department of Surgery, Cary Medical Center, Caribou, ME, USA
e-mail: cchavez@pineshealth.org

A. Murga (✉)
Department of Vascular Surgery, Loma Linda University, Loma Linda, CA, USA
e-mail: amurga@llu.edu

A. Murga et al. (eds.), *The Vascular Surgery In-Training Examination Review (VSITE)*,
https://doi.org/10.1007/978-3-031-24121-5_28

    Discrete variable: the possible values are either finite or countable numbers (e.g. number of patients, length of hospital stay)
    Continuous variable: the possible values can take any value in a particular limit (e.g. height, weight)
  - Qualitative variable (categorical): can be placed in different categories distinguished by some characteristic or attribute (e.g. race, gender)
- Measurement scales: the first step in any statistical analysis is to determine the level of measurement [2], which influences the type of statistical analysis that can be performed on it.
  - Nominal scale: names or categories (e.g. sex, race, ethnicity)
  - Ordinal scale: ranked categories, classifications (e.g. CEAP (CVD [3]), Rutherford (PAD) [4])
  - Interval scale: ordinal scale, the differences between units of data can be defined, and there is no meaningful zero (e.g. temperature, years)
  - Ratio scale: interval scale, and there is a meaningful zero (e.g. age, weight)

Inferential Statistics

- Uses random samples of data and makes inferences (predictions) about the population.
- Uses sample data from the population to answer research questions (test hypothesis)
- Population: complete collection of all elements/subjects to be studied
- Sample: a subset of elements drawn from the population
- Methods of sampling: convenience, simple random, systematic, stratified random, and cluster.

Descriptive Statistics

- Results that summarize a given data set, usually a sample of a population
- Data may be distributed in different ways: skewed to the left, skewed to the right, or sometimes is disarranged without any particular shape (See Fig. 28.1)
- In some cases, the data tends to be around a central value (e.g. mean) with no bias left or right, resembling a "Normal Distribution" (See Fig. 28.1d)
- Descriptive statistics show their results as **measures of central tendency** (summary) and **measures of variability** (dispersion) [5]
- Measures of central tendency
  - Mean: the sum of scores in the data set divided by the total number of scores. Is strongly affected by extreme values

$$\mu = \frac{3+3+7+9+10+10}{6} = 7; \quad \mu = \frac{3+3+7+9+10+100}{6} = 22$$

  - Median: the midpoint of the arranged $\frac{n+1}{2}$th observation of the dataset. Is not affected by extreme values

    From the set: 2, 5, 7, 16, 84; the midpoint is the $\left(\frac{5+1}{2}\right)$3rd observation = 7
  - Mode: the value in the data set that occurs most frequently. Sometimes there are more than one mode

    From the set 21, 45, 30, 25, 45, 21, 45; the mode = 45
- Measures of Variability: show the amount of dispersion present in a dataset; if the values are close to each other (small dispersion) or if they are widely scattered (greater dispersion)
  - Range: largest value – smallest value
  - Variance: measures dispersion relative to the scatter of the values about the mean
  - Standard deviation (SD): square root of the variance. In a normal distribution shows us the percentage of data that

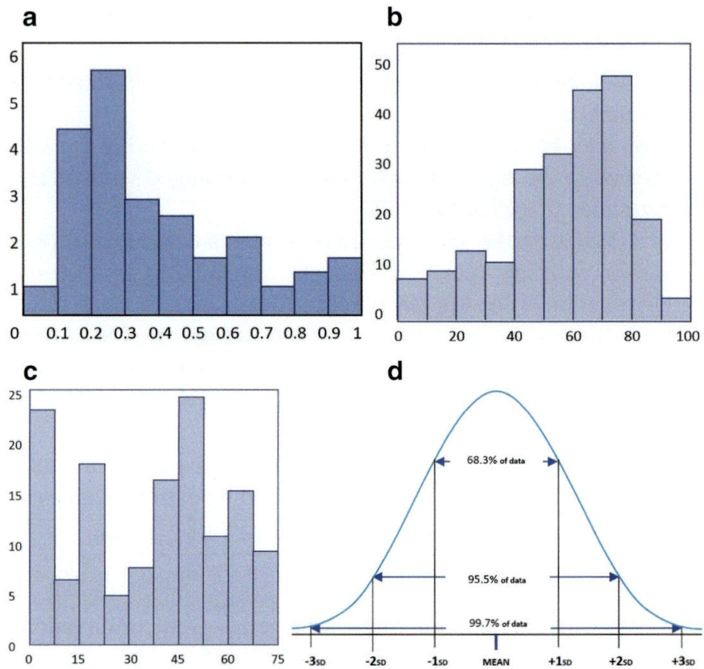

Fig. 28.1 (**a**) Distribution bar chart with frequencies skewed to the left. (**b**) Distribution bar chart with frequencies skewed to the right. (**c**) Distribution bar chart with frequencies disarranged. (**d**) Normal distribution of a dataset with the corresponding standard deviations from the mean

falls between 1, 2, or 3 SDs (68.3%, 95.5%, and 99.7%, respectively) (Fig. 28.1d).

– Coefficient of variation: standard deviation divided by the mean, used to compare dispersion between two or more groups.

Probability

- Probability is the likelihood (chance) of the occurrence of an event
- Observational probability will calculate probabilities from a sample using relative frequencies

- The **Law of large numbers**: summary results that are based upon a large number of independent observations (trials) which are less susceptible to the effects of variance (random error) when compared to results derived from fewer observations
- In probability, the **central limit theorem** (CLT) states that the means of a large number of independent random samples, each with a finite mean and variance, will approach a **normal distribution** (usually if the sample size is >30) (See Fig. 28.1d).
- The normal distribution can be used to model the distribution of many **variables** that are of interest. This allows us to answer probability questions about these random variables.

Estimating Population Parameters

- Estimate: process of using the data available from the sample to **estimate** the unknown value of the population parameter (statistic from the population)
- We can compute two types of estimates: a **point estimate** and an **interval estimate**.
- Point estimate: a single value used to estimate a population parameter.
- Interval estimate: a range of values that includes the parameter being estimated

Hypothesis Testing

- Null hypothesis ($\mathbf{H_ø}$): hypothesis to be tested, is a statement of status quo (no difference)
- Alternate hypothesis ($\mathbf{H_A}$): hypothesis that competes with the $\mathbf{H_ø}$, is a statement of what we believe is true if the sample data results in rejecting the null hypothesis
- Significance level (**α level**): is the probability of rejecting the $\mathbf{H_ø}$ when it is true. It is suggested that a probability of 1 in 20 (0.05), is a convenient cutoff level to reject the null hypothesis, but the significance level can change according to specific circumstances

- *p*-value: smallest value of $\boldsymbol{\alpha}$ for which the $\mathbf{H}_{\emptyset}$ can be rejected, or said in other words, the probability of obtaining a result more extreme than the result actually obtained when the null hypothesis is true [6]
- Confidence interval: shows an estimated range of values which is likely to include an unknown population parameter
  - The narrower the confidence interval is, the more precision it has
  - A wide interval may indicate that more data should be collected before making assumptions about the parameter
- Test statistic: is a value computed from the sample data that is used in making the decision about the rejection of the null hypothesis
  - Helps to evaluate whether the test statistic falls within the rejection region
  - Helps to decide if we reject or fail to reject the $\mathbf{H}_{\emptyset}$ at the pre-specified α level and make a conclusion
  - There are different hypothesis tests which use different test statistics based on the probability model assumed in the null hypothesis. The most common are:

    Z-test, to determine differences between two population means, used if the data has a known normal distribution

    t-test, similar to a *Z*-test but used if an unknown normal distribution, used for continuous or ordinal scales

    ANOVA, F statistic, similar to a *t*-test and can compare means of more than two groups

    Chi-square test, X^2 statistic, used for categorical variables (counts or frequency data)
- Type I error (α error): reject the $\mathbf{H}_{\emptyset}$ when it is true. The probability of committing a type I error is the same as α (the significance level)
- Type II error (β error): failing to reject the null hypothesis when it is false (See Table 28.1)
- Power: probability of rejecting the $\mathbf{H}_{\emptyset}$ when it is false [7]. This is defined by 1-β. Decreasing $\boldsymbol{\alpha}$ makes it harder to reject the null hypothesis and thus lowers the power (See Fig. 28.2)

Table 28.1 Hypothesis testing table

	Truth	
Decision	$\mathbf{H_\emptyset}$ is true	$\mathbf{H_\emptyset}$ is false
Reject $\mathbf{H_\emptyset}$	Type I error (α)	Correct
Fail to reject $\mathbf{H_\emptyset}$	Correct	Type II error (β)

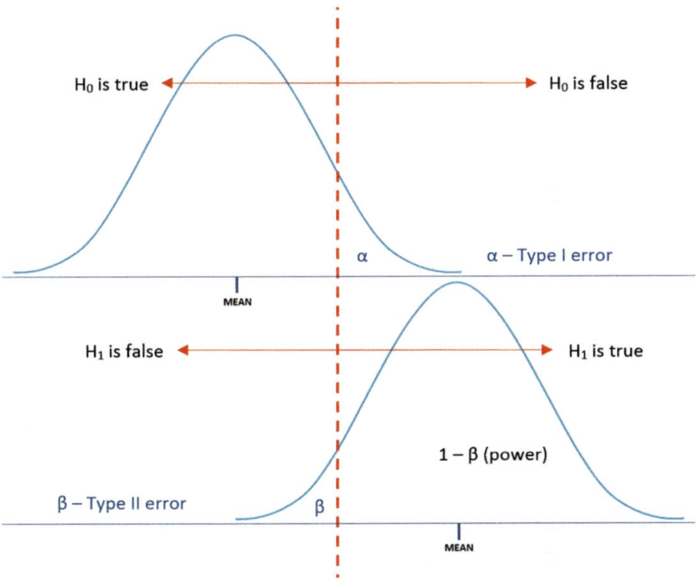

Fig. 28.2 Hypothesis testing graph: distributions of the null (H_0) and the alternate (H_A) hypothesis

Evaluating the Relationship Between Variables

- Correlation: measure of association between two continuous variables (strength). The direction and strength of the linear relationship are measured by the correlation coefficient (r).
  - If the variables X and Y have nonlinear relationship, it will not provide a valid measure of association
  - Correlation does not imply causation

- Simple linear regression: determines the linear relationship between two continuous variables and determines the equation of the best line that fits through the data
  - The regression equation is then used to predict the value of the dependent variable Y given the independent variable X. The dependent variable is continuous.
- Multiple linear regression: introduces two or more predictor variables into the prediction model
  - Multicollinearity: occurs when the predictor variables are so highly intercorrelated that they produce instability problems [8]
  - Overfitting: the inclusion of too many variables in the equation can lead to an equation that does not predict well the outcome [9]
  - Stepwise regression, forward selection, and backward elimination help with overfitting and multicollinearity problems
- Logistic Regression: method for predicting binary outcomes on the basis of one or more predictor variables. The dependent variable is binary (dichotomous). Measure of effect is the Odds ratio.
- Poisson Regression: uses a count dependent variable, is suitable for rate data. Measure of effect is Incidence Rate ratio.
- Proportional Hazards Regression: models the relationship between survival of a patient and a set of independent variables (e.g. age, comorbidity index, BMI). Measure of effect is Hazards ratio.

Epidemiology

- Definition: The study of the distribution and determinants of health-related states or events in specified populations and the application of this study to control of health problems [10]
- Descriptive Epidemiology: Study of the amount and distribution of disease within a population by person, place, and time.
  - Person variables: age, sex, race, social status

  - Place variables: natural boundaries, urban/rural differences, international comparisons
  - Time variables: secular trends, cyclic trends
- Types of studies
  - Observational: does not manipulate the exposure and does not randomize subjects

    Descriptive: useful to generate hypothesis, e.g. case reports, cross-sectional surveys, ecologic studies

    Analytic: generate and test hypothesis, suggest causality
    - Case-control: used for rare diseases. Less expensive. Start from the outcome and look for the exposures. High selection and information bias
    - Cohort: used for common diseases (outcomes). Start from the exposure and follow the development of an outcome. Can calculate incidence and risk ratio. Confounding and loss to follow-up may occur.
  - Interventional (clinical trial)

    Randomized controlled trials: experimental studies. The researcher manipulates the exposure and randomly assigns subjects to the exposed and unexposed. Eliminates selection bias. Strongest prove of cause and effect. Highest cost.
- Measures of effect: summarize the strength of the association between exposures and outcomes [11]
  - Rate: probability of occurrence of some particular event (outcome) in relation to a population and a measure of time.

    $$\frac{\text{number of events}^{*}}{\text{population at risk}} \text{ time specification}$$
  - Incidence:

    $$\frac{\text{number of new cases}}{\text{total population at risk}} (\text{at a given point in time})$$
  - Prevalence:

    $$\frac{\text{number of existing cases}}{\text{total population at risk}} (\text{at a given point in time})$$
  - Crude Mortality rate:

    $$\frac{\text{number of all deaths} (\text{at a defined period of time})}{\text{total population in the same period of time}}$$

  - Relative risk:
$$\frac{\text{Probability of the event in the exposed group}}{\text{Probability of the event in the unexposed group}}$$
  - Risk difference (excess risk, or attributable risk): $\text{Risk}_{\text{exposed}} - \text{Risk}_{\text{unexposed}}$
  - Number needed to treat (NNT): measurement of the impact of a therapy by estimating the number of patients that need to be treated in order to have an impact on one person

$$\text{NNT} = \frac{1}{\text{Risk}_{\text{unexposed}} - \text{Risk}_{\text{exposed}}}$$

- Screening Tests: widely used in medicine to assess the likelihood that members of a defined population have a particular disease (see Table 28.2).
  - Sensitivity: screening test's ability to correctly identify those individuals who truly have the disease.

$$\text{Sensitivity } \% = \frac{a}{a+c} \times 100 = \frac{\text{TP}}{\text{TP} + \text{FN}}$$

  - Specificity: screening test's ability to correctly identify those individuals who truly do not have the disease.

$$\text{Specificity } \% = \frac{d}{b+d} \times 100 = \frac{\text{TN}}{\text{TN} + \text{FP}}$$

  - Positive Predictive value (PPv): screening test's ability to identify correctly those individuals who truly have the disease (true positive) among all individuals whose screening tests are positive [12]. PPv increases with increasing disease preva-

Table 28.2 Screening test for a disease

	Disease		
Test result	Present	Absent	Total
Positive	TP (*a*)	FP (*b*)	$a + b$
Negative	FN (*c*)	TN (*d*)	$c + d$
Total	$a + c$	$b + d$	n

lence, therefore high-risk populations are the best targets for screening programs. It is a critical measure of the performance of a diagnostic method, as it reflects the probability that a positive test reflects the underlying condition being tested for.

$$\text{PPv }\% = \frac{a}{a+b} \times 100 = \frac{\text{TP}}{\text{TP}+\text{FP}}$$

- Negative Predictive value (NPv): screening test's ability to identify correctly those individuals who truly do not have the disease (true negative) among all individuals whose screening tests are negative [12]. NPV decreases with increasing disease prevalence.

$$\text{NPv }\% = \frac{d}{d+c} \times 100 = \frac{\text{TN}}{\text{TN}+\text{FN}}$$

Questions and Answers

1. A surgeon has designed a study in which he will compare the mean length of stay in days after the use of three different endovascular devices for the treatment of type A and type B aorto-iliac disease. The best statistic test is:
   (a) Correlation coefficient
   (b) Chi-square
   (c) ANOVA
   (d) Paired *T*-test
   (e) *Z*-test
2. Specificity is determined by:
   (a) False negatives/False negatives + True negatives
   (b) False positives/False positives + True positives
   (c) True negatives/True negatives + False negatives
   (d) False negatives/False negatives + True positives
   (e) True negatives/True negatives + False positives
3. The following type of study includes the outcome variable (e.g. severity of internal carotid occlusion) and tries to estimate the exposure variable:
   (a) Correlation
   (b) Case-control

   (c) Cohort
   (d) Randomized control trial
   (e) Logistic regression
4. A research group is studying the effect on survival after BKA for complicated type II diabetes. They obtained a couple of thousand patients from an established prospectively collected database. After stepwise elimination of variables, they would like to perform a multivariate analysis, the best statistical test would be:
   (a) Logistic regression
   (b) Cox proportional Hazards regression
   (c) Poisson regression
   (d) Simple linear regression
   (e) Meta-analysis
5. To analyze the data of a new screening tool for detecting skin perfusion of the lower limbs in patients with moderate to severe claudication, the following statistical test has a direct relationship with the incidence of the disease in a population:
   (a) Specificity
   (b) Sensitivity
   (c) Odds ratio
   (d) Positive predictive value
   (e) Number needed to treat

Answers: 1 (c), 2 (e), 3 (b), 4 (b), 5 (d)

References

1. Daniel WW, Cross CL. Biostatistics: a foundation for analysis in the health sciences. New York: Wiley; 2018.
2. Mertler CA, Reinhart RV. Advanced and multivariate statistical methods: practical application and interpretation. London: Routledge; 2016.
3. Eklöf B, Rutherford RB, Bergan JJ, Carpentier PH, Gloviczki P, Kistner RL, et al. Revision of the CEAP classification for chronic venous disorders: consensus statement. J Vasc Surg. 2004;40(6):1248–52.
4. Hardman RL, Jazaeri O, Yi J, Smith M, Gupta R. Overview of classification systems in peripheral artery disease. Semin Intervent Radiol. 2014;31:378–88.

5. Marshall G, Jonker L. An introduction to descriptive statistics: a review and practical guide. Radiography. 2010;16(4):e1–7.
6. Cohen HW. P values: use and misuse in medical literature. Am J Hypertens. 2011;24(1):18–23.
7. Krzywinski M, Altman N. Points of significance: power and sample size. London: Nature Publishing Group; 2013
8. Vatcheva KP, Lee M, McCormick JB, Rahbar MH. Multicollinearity in regression analyses conducted in epidemiologic studies. Epidemiology. 2016;6(2):227.
9. Ivanescu AE, Li P, George B, Brown AW, Keith SW, Raju D, et al. The importance of prediction model validation and assessment in obesity and nutrition research. Int J Obesity. 2016;40(6):887.
10. Porta M. A dictionary of epidemiology. Oxford: Oxford University Press; 2014.
11. Tripepi G, Jager K, Dekker F, Wanner C, Zoccali C. Measures of effect: relative risks, odds ratios, risk difference, and 'number needed to treat'. Kidney Int. 2007;72(7):789–91.
12. Trevethan R. Sensitivity, specificity, and predictive values: foundations, pliabilities, and pitfalls in research and practice. Front Public Health. 2017;5:307.

Index

A. Murga et al. (eds.), *The Vascular Surgery In-Training Examination Review (VSITE)*,
https://doi.org/10.1007/978-3-031-24121-5

N

O

P

S

T

FSC
www.fsc.org
MIX
Papier aus verantwortungsvollen Quellen
Paper from responsible sources
FSC® C105338

If you have any concerns about our products,
you can contact us on
ProductSafety@springernature.com

In case Publisher is established outside the EU,
the EU authorized representative is:
Springer Nature Customer Service Center GmbH
Europaplatz 3, 69115 Heidelberg, Germany

Printed by Libri Plureos GmbH
in Hamburg, Germany